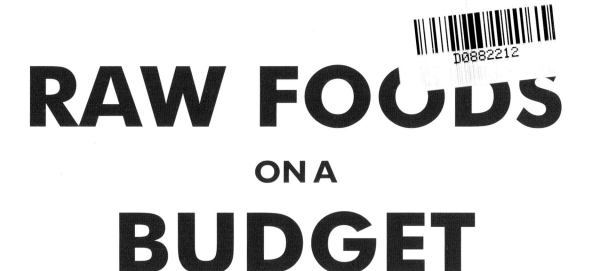

RAW FOODS
ON A
BUDGET

the ultimate program and workbook to
enjoying a budget-loving, plant-based lifestyle

BRANDI ROLLINS, M.S.

Editors

Rufiena Jones; GaBrilla Ballard; Alicia Ross-Beck, MSN, PNP

Beta Readers: Tamar Wallace, Cecelia Williams, Nancy Cullinan

The Special Color Edition

ISBN-10: 0982845847
ISBN-13: 978-0-9828458-4-4

When you get, Give.

When you learn, Teach.

-Maya Angelou

In every budget is the opportunity to experience

limitation or abundance.

The choice is ours...

-Brandi Rollins

Thank you Universe for this amazing gift.

It was an honor to serve as a vehicle for this book.

This book is truly a gift to us all.

Yay! Somebody realizes that we can't always afford the gourmet raw goodies and out-of-season produce! -Sue

You rock – I love your ideas and commitment to staying raw while saving money! -Marci

Love what you are doing! Can not use the standard excuse about expensive food/ingredients with you... -Jeanette

With a family of 6 to feed, two of those being pre-teen boys who NEVER stop eating, I need all the budget saving tips and meals I can get :-) -Donna

Raw food is changing my life - worth every penny - but I could use some ways to manage the budget. -Joyce

The information you are sharing, no one else seems to be talking about it, yet it's so necessary for success on raw. -Patricia

Just bought the book! Great resource... -Traci

TABLE OF CONTENTS

Preface   vii

Section 1: Introduction

Chapter 1: My Journey   1

Chapter 2: The Raw Foods on a Budget Program   9

Section 2: The Curriculum

Module 1 - Establish a Strong Foundation

Chapter 3: It's Not About the PRICE   15

Chapter 4: ENVISION the Life You Want!   17

Chapter 5: Choose YOUR TYPE of Raw Foods   27

Chapter 6: Create Your BUDGET!   29

Chapter 7: Improve HOW You Buy Food!   43

Module 2 - Redefine Your Local Food Environment

Chapter 8: Improve WHERE You Buy Food!   61

Chapter 9: GROW Your Own Food!   77

Module 3 - Take Care of Business at Home

Chapter 10: Improve How You STORE Food!   95

Chapter 11: Improve How You PREPARE Food!   101

Chapter 12: Improve How You EAT Food!   109

Section 3: Raw Start-Up Costs

Chapter 13: FOOD Start-Up Costs   131

Chapter 14: EQUIPMENT Start-Up Costs   145

Section 4: Recipes

My Un-Cooking Philosophy	154
Drinks	155
Breakfast	165
Light Salads and Soups	173
Salsas and Spreads	185
Main Dishes	195
Pies and Cakes	217
Cookies and Simple Pleasures	237
Ice Creams and Sorbets	247
Breads and Crackers	261
Dried and Frozen Foods	269

Afterword

	277

References

	284

Index

	285

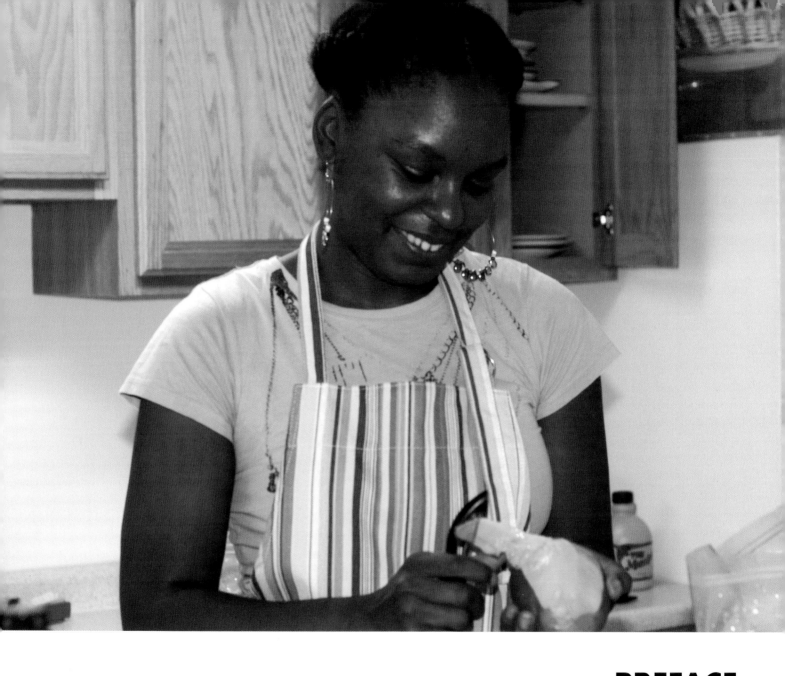

Why I Wrote This Book...

"How can I afford a healthy diet?"

I will admit, it's a hard question to answer, and for a while, we didn't have many good answers. The common solutions were to buy in bulk, take advantage of sales, shop at farmers markets, buy cheaper foods like beans and rice, and sprout your own greens. However, these answers were missing something and left many of us unsatisfied. Even as I write these tips, I feel that they are missing the bigger picture.

Raw Foods on a Budget was co-created with the Universe, a team of editors and readers, and myself to provide the world with real answers on how to enjoy an inexpensive, budget-loving, plant-based lifestyle. Designed as a program, this book goes beyond just listing the various ways of finding low-cost raw foods and, instead, takes a holistic, more thorough approach to food budgeting. This book was written with you in mind to teach you *how* to shop; *where* to buy inexpensive raw foods; how to *eat*, *prepare*, and *store* raw foods in ways that get you more bang for your buck; how to *grow* your own food for less; how to create and manage a *budget*; and how to improve your overall *relationship* with food and money.

A budget is more than about saving money or getting you out of debt, it's a tool for creating the life you want. And it doesn't have to limit or restrict your life. Ultimately, it's really what you make it. In this book, I advocate using a budget as a pathway to discovering real abundance. Abundance is not about having a kitchen stocked with produce, much of which goes to waste; it's about appreciating what you have and knowing that you will always have what you need. So, don't let this book sit on your bookshelf. Take advantage of these materials; this book is a gift to all of us.

Thank you to everyone who has helped this book evolve and manifest into a beautiful piece of work. I would first like to thank the Universe for seeing the potential in this book. When I first began writing *Raw Foods on a Budget*, I thought I would write a simple book that listed budget-friendly strategies. What the Universe had in mind was so much bigger and more comprehensive than anything I could have imagined. This book is a testament to the creative power of the Universe.

Thank you to my editors and dear friends, Rufiena Jones, GaBrilla Ballard, and Alicia Ross-Beck for your support, wonderful input, and continuous feedback. You continually pushed me to do my BEST. Thank you to my awesome Beta Readers: Tamar Wallace, Nancy Cullinan, and Cecelia Williams for your valuable feedback. For one whole year you volunteered as Beta Readers to give me feedback on every chapter and recipe, and I am honored to have your name on this book. Thank you to all of my readers who gave me feedback, let me know that I was on the right path, and continued to inspire me during this labor of love. And I would like to thank my book illustration team, Maurice Novembre and Alicia Ross-Beck, for making this book the best-looking book ever!

I would like to thank my mom for being the fantastic woman that you are. You are an amazing, inspiring woman and it is an honor to be your daughter. And I would love to thank my family and friends for their love and support.

About to get my Raw on a Budget on!
-Azmera

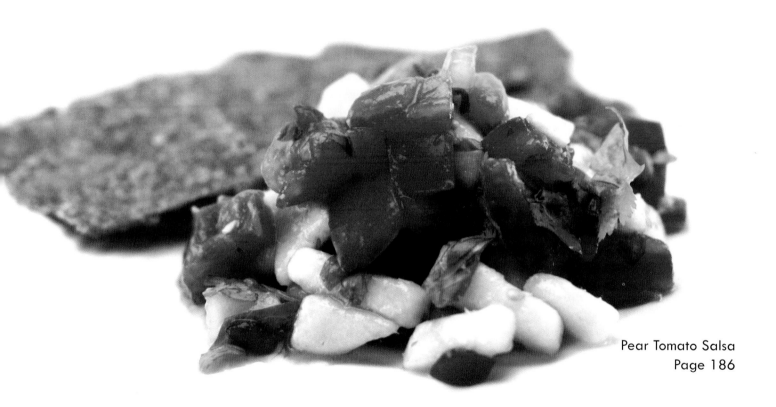

Pear Tomato Salsa
Page 186

SECTION 1

Introduction

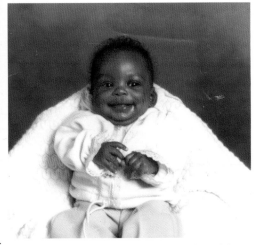

6 months old

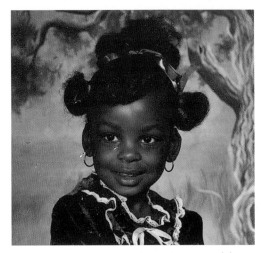

4 years old

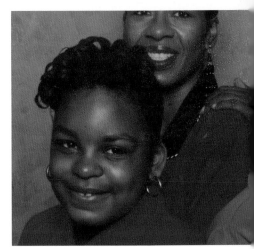

11 years old

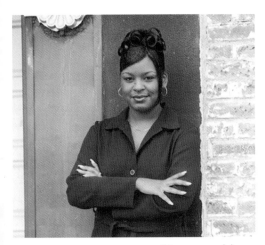

21 years old

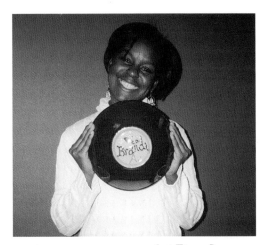

1st Time Raw
24 years old

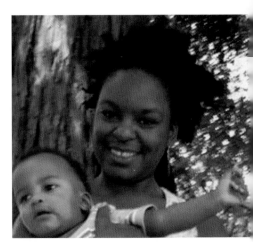

2nd Time Raw - Day 1
25 years old

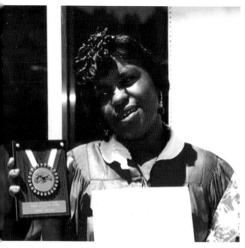

13 years old

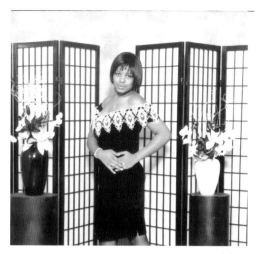

14 years old

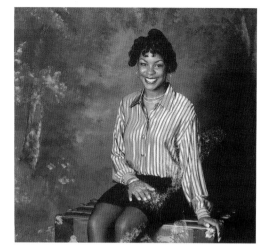

17 years old

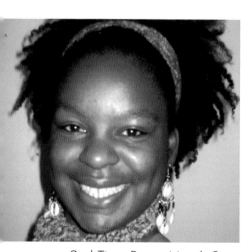

2nd Time Raw - Month 3
26 years old

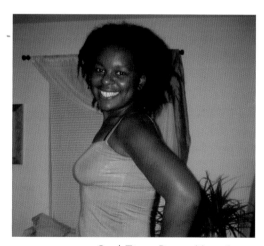

2nd Time Raw - Year 1
27 years old

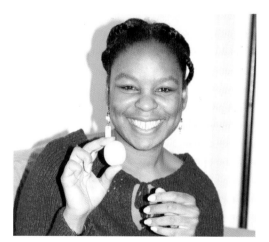

2nd Time Raw - Year 5
31 years old

CHAPTER 1

My Journey

As a child, my mom was my world. She was my favorite person and I aspired to be her "mini-me". My mother taught me everything from being a great person, to working hard, to following my dreams of becoming an artist and President of the United States. Yes, it's true...I did want to become President...well, until I learned that the work far exceeded the benefits. My mother also taught me about food. Like many women, my mother tried many diets including Weight Watchers™, Slim-Fast™, and the Cabbage Soup diet. Plus, she was the only person I knew who owned a Stairmaster (a piece of exercise equipmen which I still love to this day)! Being my mother's "mini-me", I thought that dieting was the coolest thing in the world, and I unconsciously aspired to become a dieter myself. I can even remember, one time, sneaking strawberry-flavored Slim-Fast™ powder to school to mix into my milk. Of course, it tasted disgusting and I had to throw it away.

By age 8, I was cooking. I could make Hamburger Helper, fried chicken, French fries, and killer pancakes. With the help of a 7th grade home economics class, I eventually added homemade cakes, cookies, and breads to the list. By high school, I was known as the Betty Crocker™ in my family and my diet was filled with fried-this and baked-that. Sadly, here's what a typical day looked like: for breakfast, an old-fashioned chocolate donut; for lunch, a bag of M&Ms™ and can of Mountain Dew™; for after school snack, 1-3 bowls of sugar-sweetened cereal; and for dinner, iceberg lettuce with fat-free ranch, and a baked potato and chicken breast (the only "healthy" meal of the day). In short, my diet was the opposite of good. Then I would work it off by spending 2-3 hours at the gym playing basketball, climbing stairs on the StairMaster™, and taking a 60-minute aerobics class. In a twisted way, it was balance.

My eating habits only worsened when I began college (who knew there was room for it to get worse!). I attended Centre College in Danville, Kentucky, a small liberal arts school, and for the first time, I could eat anything I wanted, anytime I wanted! I would stay up all night studying and eat a whole medium cheese pizza by myself, or eat chicken fingers, carrot cake, pasta, and French fries at the school cafeteria. Along with the stress of college, these eating habits eventually caught up with me, and I gained more than my freshman fifteen. And to make matters worse, I developed acne for the first time in my life. Augh!!!!!

Then it all changed when I was 22 years old. I had just devoured a plate of orange chicken and fried rice at a cheap Chinese food restaurant when I decided to call a close friend for some fun girl talk. As soon as she found out about the Chinese food I had just eaten, she gave me the talking-to of my life! She lectured me for close to three hours about my eating habits and I got the message: orange chicken...bad; fresh oranges...good! Well, maybe it wasn't fresh oranges... she was practicing the Atkins diet...so maybe it was orange-flavored bacon. Nevertheless, I got the message and this became my impetus to search for the perfect diet.

Over a period of two years, I experimented with several diets including the Atkins diet™, a plant-based indigenous diet, and an organic whole foods diet. These diets left me feeling better and with more energy, but I kept searching for a better way of eating. Then I found the raw foods diet and it rocked my world.

My raw foods journey began on September 21, 2004, after reading *Raw Power* by Stephen Arlin and David Wolfe. The book made so much sense that I converted from a whole foods diet to a 100% raw foods diet overnight! I was able to stay raw for three months and the only time I ate cooked food was on Thanksgiving and Christmas (I think I ate collard greens and turkey). Although I was a raw foodist for a brief amount of time, during this period, I learned who I really was. Many of the characteristics that I thought were me, weren't me at all; rather, they were a reflection of my poor diet. Eating raw foods taught me who I was and who I could be:

- I could be happy 24 hours a day. I couldn't get mad or stay upset. I would sing in traffic.

- I had tons of energy. I became a person who could jump out of bed and start their day; I no longer needed a 1-2 hour warm-up! I would wake up at 4am to make my food for the day, and work from 7am to 9pm at my two jobs.

- I did not have to have menstrual cramps. They completely went away during my first month as a raw vegan, which was pretty spectacular given that I had had menstrual cramps since I was 12 years old. As a raw vegan, I would have happy cycles. I couldn't believe it.

- I could live a life free of inflammation! Through raw foods, I learned that I was allergic to wheat and sugar. While I was eating a cooked diet, these foods were causing a lot of inflammation, which left me bloated and swollen. But, on the raw foods diet, I had become un-swollen for the first time in my life.

- I could see the world in a better way (literally). For the first time that I could remember I was seeing the world in 3-D. The world looked more defined and I could quickly see distances between far away objects.

- Overall, my first raw vegan experience taught me who I was. I was not a grouchy, tired person; rather, I was filled with unlimited happiness and joy every minute of every day.

So, why did I stop eating raw? Life and dating eventually caught up with me. I began eating Indian food, Chinese food, sushi, and other cuisine. Plus, I became tired of salads. At the time, I thought that being raw vegan meant eating tons of salads; so once I got tired of lettuce, I stopped eating salads and subsequently had difficulty staying raw vegan. I still ate mostly fruits and vegetables, but I slowly began cooking them, and I continued to eat cooked food for 2 years. During this period, I gained 40 pounds, my eyesight and hearing worsened, and I became fatigued. Keep in mind that I felt this way even though I was eating mostly vegetables, fruits, and seeds, and I consumed very little dairy, meat, non-organic food, and grains. I had returned to the cooked world, but I truly desired to become a raw vegan again. The raw food diet gave me the happiest time in my life and I wanted that joy again!

Becoming Raw Vegan...
The Second Time Around

In July 2006, I became a raw vegan again. Yay! My motivations were simple: 1) I wanted to be crazy happy; 2) I had just seen the movie "Breakthrough" (created by Storm and Jinjee Talifero--a documentary about a raw vegan family) and I decided that I wanted raw vegan babies; and 3) I didn't want a parasite like the one that had just come out of my friend. In addition, I was getting ready to start graduate school at Penn State University and I wanted the endurance to excel in my studies while pursuing all of my other interests like gardening, dancing, and sewing.

Although I was enthusiastic about re-entering the raw food world, I quickly learned that it would not be as easy as the first time. I can still remember sneaking a spoonful of brown rice off a friend's plate and dreaming of hamburgers (something I hadn't eaten in years). But I persevered, and after three weeks, I was fine. Then three weeks quickly turned into one year and I was still 100% raw! Yay!

Here are some of the changes I noticed after the first year:

- I lost weight. Around 30 pounds! It happened slower compared to the first time I was raw, possibly due to the stress of being in graduate school. I still have some weight to lose. One thing that I do love about being raw vegan is that my body gets this amazing shape. It's very feminine. I can move mountains with these hips!

- My eyes are clearer. They kinda sparkle. My vision is still the same; hopefully that will improve over time.

- My menstruation cycle is 1 day shorter and I feel less discomfort. Now I can feel it coming about 2 days prior, and a few minutes before it actually starts.

- My skin glows. It's pretty amazing. My face is also clearer and smoother.

- My BO is horrific. It means that I'm detoxing, but my sweat is like cologne.

- My temperament is pretty stable. However, the stress from graduate school keeps my mood slightly fluctuating, especially on the first day of my cycle. My body goes into hibernation, and if I don't have time to sleep it can be a dangerous situation (just kidding!). But overall, I am happy most of the time.

- In terms of sleeping, I still like to sleep 8 ½ hours. However, there was a period when 9-9 ½ hours was good. So maybe I need less sleep.

- My stool is very regular. I poop at least once a day and all floaters!

To date, I have been a raw vegan for 5 years. It has had its ups and downs, but overall, it has been an amazing experience. It has kept me happy despite the stress of being in graduate school, and I honestly don't think I would have accomplished as much without being raw vegan. With all this energy and focus, I have been able to work with several colleagues at Penn State University and other universities on multiple obesity-related research projects. Plus, I still have enough energy to work on my garden, spend time with family and friends, write books, and sleep 8 hours a night.

The Budget-Conscious Raw Vegan Emerges

Although I was excelling at being a raw vegan, I was not managing my money very well. I was completely convinced that because I was a raw vegan, I needed a lot of food. So, I would spend $500-600 a month of my "barely-above-the-poverty-line" student stipend to buy food from my local grocery and health food stores, and farmers markets. Despite my low income, I was buying too much and wasting too much. My wasted food would end up in my compost bin, but I might as well have been feeding my worms with cash because I was throwing money away. In the back of my mind, I knew something wasn't right, but I didn't want to change.

Then it happened! In the summer of 2007, the US economy crashed, setting forth a recession that forced me to change! It took two years for it to effect me, but when it did, it brought with it all of the consequences of my poor money management. All of a sudden the APR rates on my credit cards were astronomical! For the first time, I had to face the poor decisions I was making to afford my "abundant" raw lifestyle.

So, I began to downsize. There was very little room for unnecessary purchases, so I created a budget and for the first time, I had to stick to it. I cut back on unnecessary expenses like clothing and entertainment, and I made a plan to reduce my debt. In addition, I cut back on my food expenses: I downsized to one CSA farm share (i.e. a farm-based program where you receive a box of local produce every week; for more information see page 63), I stopped shopping at the more expensive "higher quality" grocery store and began frequenting the less expensive one, and I began taking my garden seriously and growing more of my own food. Although

I was making progress, I still felt uneasy. Believe it or not, I wasn't sure if I would have enough food. Plus, I liked being able to buy what I wanted when I wanted it.

As I stuck with my budget (it was tough), I began to experience small successes. I learned that I could eat just fine on one farm share, a lesson that saved me over $1100 in one year! Another success was the discovery of fruit picking. I grew up in a city, so the thought that you could go to a farm and pick your own fruit was foreign. At the time of this discovery, I was living in Buffalo, New York, for the summer, and the farm that provided my CSA was offering amazing prices for pick-your-own strawberries, raspberries, and blueberries. So, one afternoon after work, I took the plunge and picked a grocery bag of organic blueberries. I was shocked when I was only charged $8 for the bag. That's when I truly learned that high-quality produce didn't have to be expensive. This one event set forth a tidal wave of explorations into my local food environment for low-cost, high-quality raw foods, and I began to redefine this environment for myself. Instead of my food environment only consisting of my local health food store, the expensive, "higher quality" grocery store, and CSAs, it began to include stores like TJ Maxx™, a discount department store; the moderately-priced grocery store that sells some of the best greens in town; smaller family-owned farms that I had never visited before; and the produce shelf at Tait Farms that is often stocked with seconds (i.e. ripe fruits and vegetables that are sold at half-price). Through this process of discovery, I shifted from relying on my local grocery and health food stores to depending more on my local farms and garden. That was huge!

The downturn of the economy forced me out of my comfort zone of spending without thinking and gave me an opportunity to experience some amazing improvements in my life. My budget became my gateway to abundance, a healthy relationship with food and money (Amen!), and it gave me the freedom to do the things I wanted to do. I learned that abundance was not about having a refrigerator and counter space lined with produce; instead, it was knowing that I already had what I needed, that I would always be provided for and have what I need, and to appreciate and share what I have been given. Instead of being afraid that I would run out of food, now I share my creations with the world and give more of myself without fear. I honor the food that I have been given and the people I get to share it with. My budget had changed my life.

Today, I spend 50-75% less than what I used to spend on food. And because I am more connected with my local farmers, grow a lot of my own food, and eat-in-season, the food that I eat today is of better quality than the food I used to eat when I didn't have a budget! Who says that you need to sacrifice quality for low prices! Now that I have seen the opportunities a budget can provide, I want to help everyone enjoy a budget-loving raw food lifestyle, so that they too can experience the gifts that I have been given. This book is a gift to us all.

ARE YOU READY TO DISCOVER REAL ABUNDANCE?

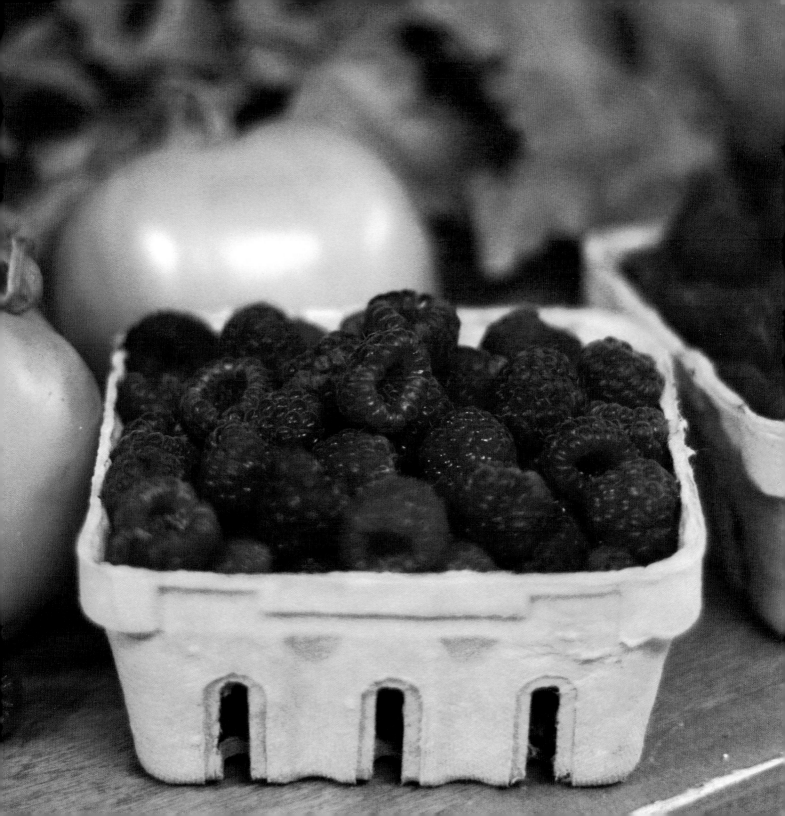

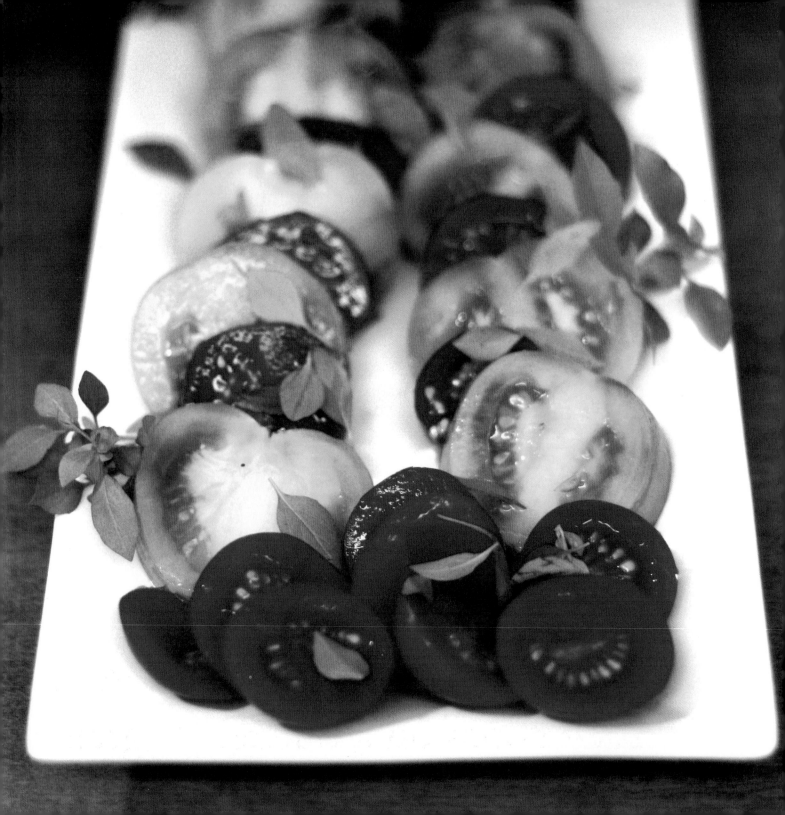

Where do I start?

-Danielle

Here! :)

-Brandi

CHAPTER 2

The Raw Foods on a Budget Program

Welcome to the first program devoted to teaching you how to live a budget-conscious, healthy lifestyle. It doesn't matter if you are 100% raw, high raw, raw friendly, vegan, vegetarian, or health conscious, the Raw Foods on a Budget program was created for people just like you who are trying to afford a plant-based diet. This program is unique in that it goes beyond the price of food and teaches you how to have a positive and abundant relationship with money and food. Wouldn't it be wonderful to feel confident that you will always have everything you need? That you would always be provided for? Well, that's living in a state of abundance and the purpose of this book is to guide you there.

Here's how it works! The curriculum is organized into three modules that will teach you how and where to buy food, and how to take care of your food once you bring it home.

MODULE 1
Establish a Strong Foundation

This first module focuses on YOU! Before we talk about locating inexpensive produce, you will have an opportunity to create and manage a budget, develop a positive and empowering relationship with your budget, choose the type of raw foods diet you want to create (e.g. simple or fancy recipes), and learn how to shop for food. These skills are a strong foundation that will support you as you begin your budget-conscious journey! Don't skip this module!

MODULE 2
Redefine Your Local Food Environment

It's common for people to have access to local sources for high-quality, inexpensive produce--they just don't know about them. Take this opportunity to step out of your comfort-zone of shopping at the local, expensive health food store and begin to explore your local food environment. In this module, you will acquire skills to connect with local farms, grocery stores, and even department stores in new cost-friendly ways. Plus, you will learn how to grow your own food the inexpensive way!

MODULE 3
Take Care of Business at Home

Now it's time to shift your focus back home and learn how to treat your produce in budget-friendly ways. In this module, you will learn how to store your fruits, vegetables, nuts, seeds, and oils in ways that keep them fresher longer; prepare raw foods in ways that stretch your dollar; and, unlearn unhealthy eating habits that cost you a pretty penny!

This book is a complete program that covers many dimensions to having a food budget, and often they are topics you haven't thought of and could most likely benefit from. Ideally, when working through this book, you will read it from beginning to end. However, it's also okay to jump to specific chapters, particularly ones that you can benefit from immediately. I just ask that you avoid sticking only to those chapters that you think you need. Each chapter is a wealth of knowledge and, when given the opportunity, can teach you so much.

Curriculum and Timeline

Here's the curriculum and suggested timeline for the Raw Foods on a Budget program. The length of the program, however, will ultimately depend on how much time you can devote to it. If you are short on time, don't be afraid to take it slow.

MODULE 1

Week 1   Envision the life you want, begin tracking your food expenses, and choose the type of raw foods you want to prepare on a regular basis. Read chapter 4 "ENVISION the Life You Want!" and complete all of the worksheets; read chapter 5 "Choose Your Type of Raw Foods" (very short); and read pages 30-31 of chapter 6 "Create Your BUDGET!"" and begin tracking your food expenses on the Food Expense Log (pages 36-38).

Week 2   Set your food spending goal(s) and create your monthly budget. It's good to set aside 3-5 hours to complete this task. Read pages 31-33 of chapter 6 "Create Your BUDGET!" and complete the worksheet on pages 39-41.

Week 3-6   Improve the way you buy food! Learn how to buy what you need and eat all you have by creating menu plans, shopping lists, and figuring out how much food you need. This will have the biggest impact on your budget. Read chapter 7 "Improve HOW You Buy Food!" and begin activity 1 on page 50. This activity can take 1-4 weeks to complete depending on how much food you currently have in your kitchen. When you have completed this activity, move on to Module 2.

MODULE 2

Weeks 7-9   Explore your local food environment for high-quality, low-cost produce by connecting with local farms, grocery and health stores, and more. Read chapter 8 "Improve WHERE You Buy Food!" and choose one activity from this chapter to do this weekend.

Week 10   Plan a garden! It doesn't matter how much land you have access to, you can always grow something! Read chapter 9 "GROW Your Own Food!"

MODULE 3

Week 11   Learn how to store your produce and create a produce monitoring system! Read chapter 10 "Improve How You STORE Food!" and complete activity 1 on page 100.

Week 12   Learn how to prepare raw food in ways that save you MONEY! Read chapter 11 "Improve How You PREPARE Food!" and complete activity 1 on page 108.

Week 13   Get more mileage out of your meals by improving the way you eat! Read chapter 12 "Improve How You EAT Food!" and complete all of the worksheets. And that's it! Your done!

Brandi has put together a very well organized (and tasty looking!) series of practical ways to...get the freshest nutrition possible, without the high cost...Give it a serious try. -Bob

Thanks again for the Book,
I'm loving it!!! :) !   -Kittora

So excited to learn this information.
-Melody

Brandi, this is amazing. You've invested a ton of work into this book! I am totally floored...   -Ann Marie

Brandi, I bought your book download today and I love it. Your writing style is so friendly and you seem to have thought of everything.   -Linda

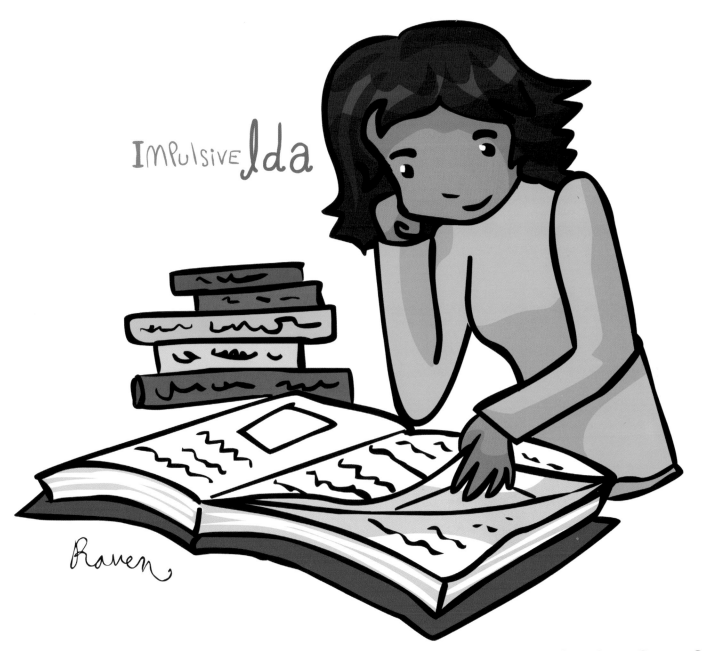

IMPULSIVE Ida

Raven

SECTION 2

The Curriculum

Module 1

Establish a Strong Foundation

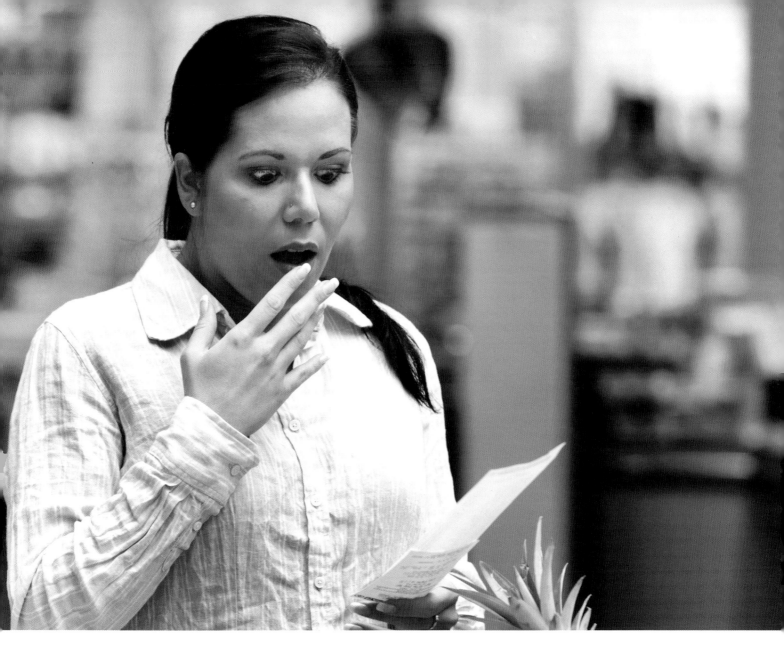

CHAPTER 3
It's Not About the PRICE

You may be thinking, "health foods are so expensive...so, what do you mean, it's not about the price?" The fact is that food prices play much less of a role in how much money we spend than we think, and this brief chapter will explain why!

STRATEGY 1
It's not about the price

Often when we think about having a food budget, we focus on the price of food. We become engrossed with clipping coupons, looking for sales, and buying in bulk, all in an effort to reduce the price of food. Although these are useful strategies, in most cases, it's the way that we shop, store, and eat food that weigh heavy on our budgets. Consider this:

- In the U.S., 60% of all grocery purchases are un-planned; in other words, they are impulsive buys.

- U.S. and U.K. households throw away 25% of their food, amounting to $48.3 and £12.2 billion, respectively, each year.

- In the U.S. and U.K., fruits and vegetables comprise 30-60% of all food that is thrown away.

- Households who value menu planning as a way to re-duce food waste tend to plan their meals around the foods that they want rather than what they already have.

- In the U.K., 2.7 metric tons of food is wasted because it spoils or is not used in time.

- In the U.S., Americans on average consumed 400 more calories per day in 2000 than they did in 1983.

As you can see, there are so many areas in our relationship with food and money that could be improved before we focus on the price of food. Think about it, how much food have you thrown away or overeaten in the last month? Now, estimate how much you paid for that food and ask yourself, what would have saved you more money: searching for lower prices or not wasting food?

So, why do we buy so much food? Many people are driven by the fear of running out or not having enough, the plea-sure of finding a great deal or being able to eat what they want, and/or buying food to cope with emotional states like stress. Plus, many of us were taught to want the American Dream when it comes to our kitchen. We want a refrigerator, cupboards, and counters filled with fresh fruits and vegeta-bles. Also, when we focus on the price of food, we focus on the problem being outside of ourselves. It's easier to blame the economy and the rising costs of foods, etc. While it's true that these factors do impact our budget, unconscious spending and overeating are such a HUGE problem, that even when there's a recession, we still continue to buy food to waste.

So, even if you don't believe it right now, tell yourself that it's not about the price. As you work through the program, you will come to understand that when you focus on your relationship with food and money, the possibility for growth is enormous. We can't control the price of food, but we can control how and where we buy food, and how we store, pre-pare, and eat our food.

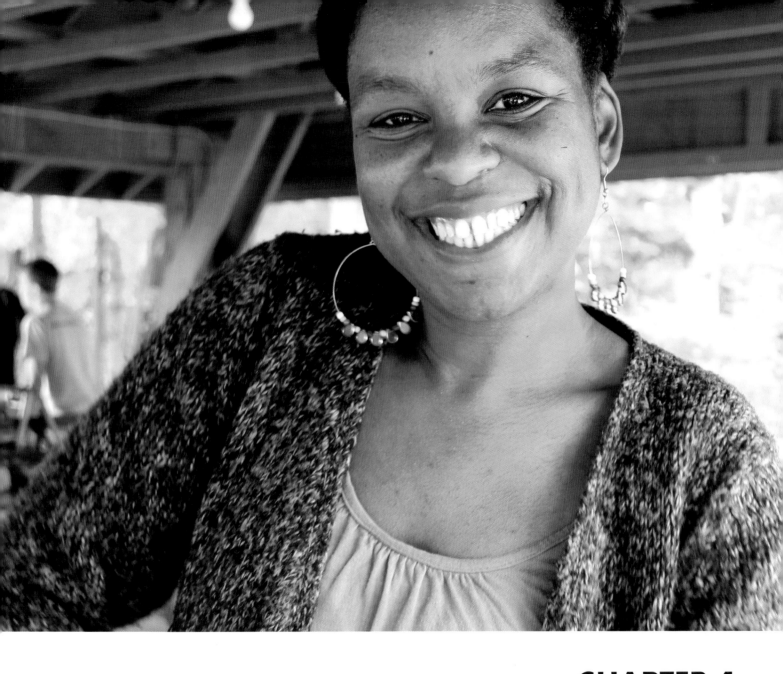

CHAPTER 4

ENVISION the Life You Want!

All too often, budgeting is viewed as a negative entity that limits or keeps us from enjoying the life we want. However, when we approach a budget from this standpoint, we are less likely to create or maintain one. For example, take my crazy friend, Impulse Ida, a resident of Shopville City. Like many of us, Ida is interested in having a budget, but she is having trouble sticking to one:

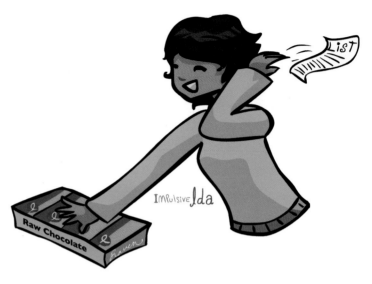

IMPULSIVE *Ida*

Ida's food expenses were getting out of control. Not knowing what to do, she consulted with her friend Frugal Francis. After a long conversation, Ida decided to create a budget. Even though she didn't want to limit her spending, she decided to do it anyway.

The first few days were great! She was able to buy only what she needed. Then one day, Ida had a huge craving for raw vegan chocolate, but she didn't have any in the house. As she considered going to the store to buy some, her willpower kicked in and she resisted her temptation…that is, until a few days later when it was time to go grocery shopping again. This trip was more difficult because Ida began to feel like her budget was limiting her. She couldn't have the foods she wanted. So, she broke down a little and splurged on one raw vegan treat. Well, that treat led to another treat the next day, then to a few more unplanned treats a few days later. The next thing she knew, Ida was back where she started with high grocery bills.

Ida could have helped herself stay on a budget by developing a positive attitude towards her budget. Instead of seeing it as a source of limitation, she could have viewed it as a vehicle to achieving the life she has always wanted. A budget can bring joy, abundance, and confidence to our lives if we set our intentions in that direction. Our thoughts become our actions, so if we focus on the limitations of a budget, then that will be our experience. However, if we focus on the beautiful experiences we want a budget to bring to our lives, these beautiful experiences will become a reality. In this chapter, I provide key strategies that will help you set your intentions towards a beautiful, budget-conscious raw food lifestyle.

STRATEGY 2
Know your reasons

It's important to know why you are making a commitment to eating raw foods on a budget. What are your reasons? Have you really thought about them? Knowing why you want to make these changes will help you stay on a budget. All too often, we commit to things without really clarifying to ourselves why we are doing them and what those reasons really mean to us. In my early attempts at creating a budget, I really didn't think about my reasons for doing it. I just wanted to spend less money on food and pay off debt. They were reasons, but they lacked a bigger vision. I wasn't clear as to how these reasons would change my experience in the world. So, when I was confronted with opportunities to spend a lot, I didn't have well-developed reasons to fight back. However, when I started my current budget, I envisioned what my experience in the world would be like without credit card debt and I saw myself as a happier and more generous person. This meant a lot to me. I also wanted to stop wasting so much food. Before my budget, I would let my taste-buds do the buying, rather than my brain, and I ended up wasting a lot of food. However, now my brain and taste-buds are good friends and they work together in buying my food. To help you identify your reasons for creating a raw foods budget, complete the worksheet on pages 22-23.

STRATEGY 3
Envision where you want to be

When starting a budget, it's useful to envision the person you would like to become and the life you would like to have. So many times, we enter a budget thinking I just want to pay off my bills, reduce my debt, and stop stressing about money; however, with this approach, we are always focusing on the negative things we want removed from our life. There is nothing wrong with this, but we can get a lot further by focusing on the positive things we want to invite into our life. For example, when I envision who I want to be as a raw food budgeter, it goes something like this.

> *I want to be a raw vegan who appreciates the food she has been given and shares it with others. I want to be organized and planful in making food purchases and monitoring my food so that none of it goes to waste. I want to use the money I am no longer throwing away (by wasting food) to pay bills and put into my savings account. I want to be the person who explores her backyard for food and focuses on eating a variety of local raw fruits and vegetables rather than the typical ones sold at the grocery store.*

Now, its your turn! Who would you like to be? Use the worksheet on pages 24-25 to guide you through this activity.

STRATEGY 4
Think abundantly

A budget provides an opportunity for us to remember that life is abundant. A budget encourages you to take advantage of the food you already have, rather than buying new food and wasting it. For example, often, we already have the ingredients for a wonderful salad or smoothie in our kitchen - we just don't know it because we are lacking the ingredients we *want* to use. You may have raw granola but no nut milk, or salad fixings but no olive oil. Rather than focus on what you lack, take this as an opportunity to create a new recipe that's just as or more delicious than the original. Abundance isn't about buying as much food as you want, it's about appreciating what you have and realizing that you already have everything you need.

STRATEGY 5
Enjoy the ride

A budget can be a fun experience if you let it! It's so easy for us to ruminate on our limited income; but, it doesn't have to be this way. A budget is a guide--that's all. We are the ones who make it into a negative entity lurking in the back of our minds, reminding us that we cannot have what we want. Rather than thinking this way, remind yourself of what you will be gaining by living on a budget.

Plus, having a budget can be fun! As I stuck to my budget, it surprisingly turned into a fun process where I rediscovered the things I already had and found out what I truly needed. It even brought me closer to my community and ignited a new level of creativity in my food preparation. So, as you read the chapters and create your budget, remind yourself that you have everything to gain during this process and that the biggest thing you will lose is your stress!

STRATEGY 6
Take pride in a half-empty fridge

When you buy the produce you need rather than the produce you want, you will find that your refrigerator and counters are not as full as they used to be. This can be a strange experience for some of us who are used to having a refrigerator filled with food and counters lined with bowls of produce. I will admit that it feels good to open my refrigerator and have so many wonderful options to choose from. Why wouldn't it? A full fridge looks better than an empty one, just like a furnished house looks better than a house with no furniture. However, all of this "fullness" has a price. It costs a lot to keep our kitchens filled with fresh produce. And just think about how much of this food goes to waste. When a refrigerator is full, we tend to forget about the foods we have, and it's easy for small food items to hide behind larger items and spoil.

The good news is that we can unlearn our preference for a full refrigerator. Just change your ideas about what a half-empty fridge means to you. For some of us, a half-empty fridge may mean a lack of abundance or even poverty; however, it can have a more positive meaning. For me, a half-empty fridge means that I am succeeding at living on a budget, and that I am appreciating and using all that I have while not wasting the abundance I have been given. So, take pride in your half-empty fridge! It's a sign of your success!

STRATEGY 7
Be kind to yourself

As you go through the process of transitioning to a budget-friendly raw foods lifestyle, you will undoubtably experience many successes and "failures". It's very easy to be hard on yourself when you make a large impulse buy or spend over budget; however, remember to be kind to yourself. This is a new pathway for many of you in that you are cultivating new budget-friendly behaviors and getting rid of poor, ineffective habits. So, it's important to be patient with the process and realize that the "failures" you may experience are not failures at all. In fact, as long as you learn something from the experience, every "failure" is a success. So, be kind to yourself, and if you allow it, every success and "failure" will become an opportunity to learn more and make improvements that lead to a better life.

FUN Activities

ACTIVITY 1:
What does a budget mean to you?

What are your reasons for creating a raw foods budget? What motivated you to buy this book? What did you hope to gain? What do you want to improve in your life? Now think about the fears you have about having a budget. What do you fear a raw foods budget will take away from your life? In my case, I feared that it would take away my raw junk food and impulse buys. Often when we don't deal with these fears, it becomes difficult for us to maintain our budget. Situations come up that ride on our fears and if we haven't identified solid reasons for having a budget, our fears may win and our budgets may fall apart. Use the worksheet on pages 22-23 to complete this activity.

ACTIVITY 2:
Envision who you want to be

Imagine that you are already reaping the rewards of your budget right now! Be vivid. Envision how a budget has changed the way you experience the world. What has a budget brought to your life? What everyday strategies do you use to maintain a budget-friendly raw vegan lifestyle? What qualities do you have and what does your life look like? What do you look like (physically and emotionally)? What does the variety in your diet look like? What type of raw foodist are you? What has your budget allowed you to accomplish in your life? What does it look and feel like to have your debts paid off? Answering these questions will help clarify to yourself exactly what you are working for. Use the worksheet on pages 24-25 to complete this activity.

WHAT DOES A BUDGET MEAN TO YOU?

In this activity, I want you to really think about why you want to live a budget-friendly lifestyle. All too often we rush into creating a budget without identifying first what it means to us. In the past, I have created a lot of budgets; however, almost none of them stuck because I didn't give myself the opportunity to truly invest in them. I never gave myself the time to think about what a budget was going to add to my life. So when situations came up where I felt limited by my budget, it was easy for me to ignore my budget. Almost all of these challenging situations brought my fears about having a budget to the forefront. Because I hadn't identified these fears, I never prepared myself to deal with them when they came up. Fortunately, we can use our reasons for having a budget to combat our fears. For example, when I am tempted to make an impulsive food purchase, it taps into my fear about not being able to buy the raw junk food I want. However, I am able to overcome this temptation by reminding myself what a budget will bring to my life, including being debt free and being able to freely share my food with others.

For this activity, list the benefits you want a raw foods budget to bring to your life and the fears you have about having a budget. To help you do this, I have provided my own responses to these questions in the table below. Use my responses as an example, and then complete the table on the next page for yourself.

Benefits	Fears
What benefits will a raw foods budget bring to your life?	*What do you fear a raw foods budget will take away from your life?*
1) It will reduce the amount of stress I experience everyday regarding my debt. I will be able to use the money I save on food to pay bills.	1) It will take away my ability to make impulse buys. I love being able to buy what I want or to see something yummy and just buy it.
2) To waste less food. I thought abundance meant having large amounts of fresh fruits and vegetables, but it doesn't feel right that I am wasting so much food. Something needs to change. I want a budget to help me discover what abundance really means.	2) I won't be able to buy the raw junk food that I sometimes crave.
3) To help me believe that I have enough food to share with others and will not run out.	3) I am nervous that I won't be able to eat out at restaurants when I want to. Although I don't eat out very often, sometimes I want to eat something decadent.

Benefits	Fears
What benefits will a raw foods budget bring to your life?	*What do you fear a raw foods budget will take away from your life?*
1)	1)
2)	2)
3)	3)
4)	4)

WORKSHEET
ENVISION YOUR SUCCESS

To begin this activity, grab a pen and this book, and find a quiet place to sit. Next, close your eyes and for 10 minutes imagine that you are experiencing the payoffs of your raw foods budget right now. What does your life look like? <u>Be vivid</u>. How do you feel? What do you look like? What are you eating? What are you wearing? How much are you spending? What have you accomplished? When you are ready, write down what you saw on the next page. Because this can be a strange activity for some of you, I have provided my own personal vision below.

<u>THIS IS WHO I WANT TO BE!</u>

I see myself living debt free. I see myself at the checkout of my local health food store using cash to pay for all of my food and feeling confident that there is enough money to cover my needs. I have identified my food needs and am shopping with a conscious state of mind. I don't give into my impulses to buy raw junk food and instead I choose to buy vibrant, fresh fruits and vegetables. I see myself returning home from a successful grocery shopping trip on a beautiful sunny day in my clean car. I pass my beautiful, prolific garden as I walk to my front door. Then I begin to put my food away into an almost empty, clean refrigerator. I have purchased the best local produce and all the vibrant colors glow in my white, sparkly refrigerator. Then I put the few dry foods I purchased into the freezer and/or mason jars. Next, I venture out into the garden to collect heirloom tomatoes, strawberries, black raspberries, cucumbers, peppers, basil, oregano, lettuce, and a variety of other fresh fruits and vegetables. It feels good to know that most of my food is coming from my home garden and that I am only buying what is necessary from my local health food store.

I see myself inviting friends over to my home to share our abundance over a meal. The sun is out and the sky is blue and I am wearing simple clothes that are light and breezy, yet reflect my individual style. In preparation for the meal, I have made several simple raw food dishes and am willing to share all of it with them. I am committed to giving them a beautiful experience. I have taken the time to pour love into preparing the food, rather than thinking about how much money it is costing me. And I feel confident that even if my friends don't bring food that I can eat, that I will be okay. I have enough. I am provided for, even if I can't see how it is going to happen. It will just happen.

As I sit with my friends and eat, I savor my food. I take my time to enjoy the life I have been blessed with. And I can taste the beauty in my life through the recipes I have created. I am not thinking about money even though I am on a budget. The money is just a means to an end and my focus is on the life I want to create.

NOW, IT'S YOUR TURN! WHO DO YOU WANT TO BE?

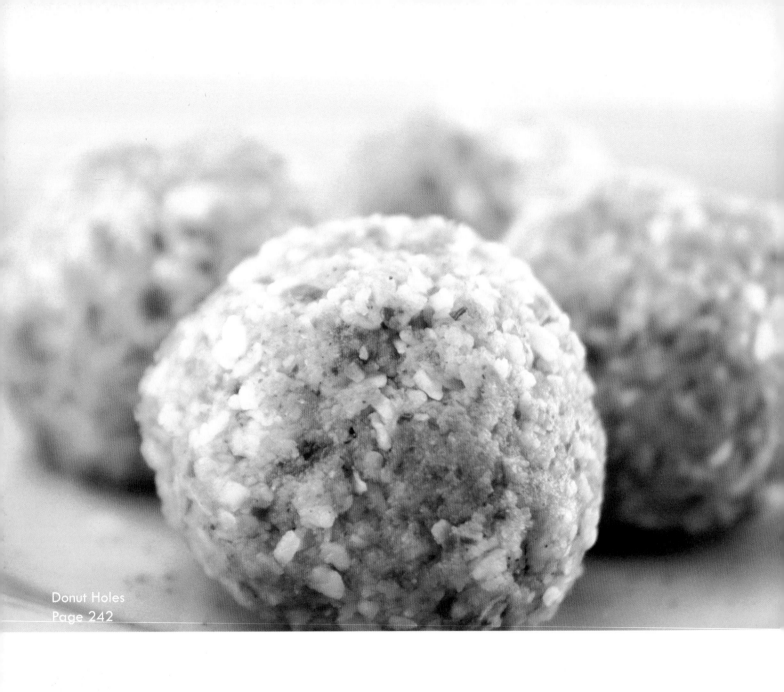

Donut Holes
Page 242

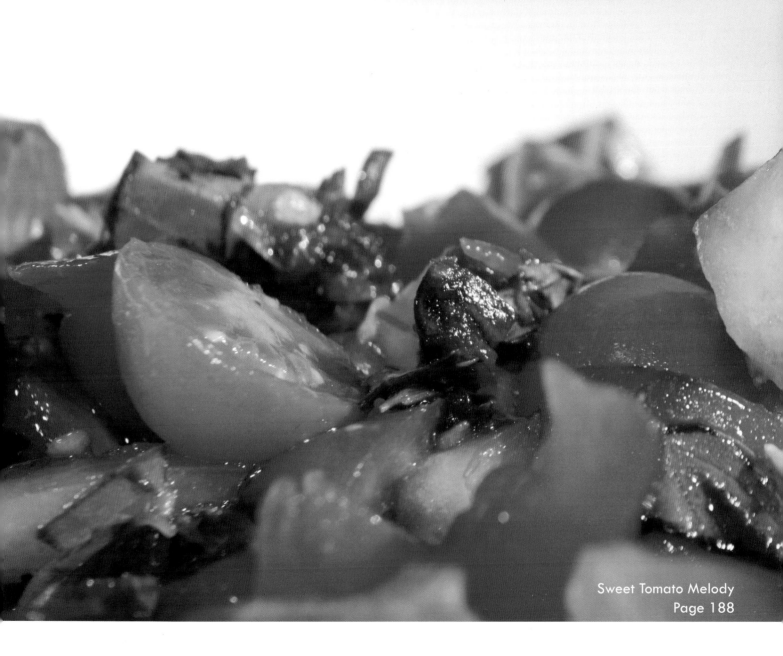

Sweet Tomato Melody
Page 188

CHAPTER 5

Choose **YOUR TYPE** of Raw Foods

Do You Want to create fancy raw food meals or do you want to keep them simple? Answering this question is important when creating a budget because it will determine how much you will spend to stock your kitchen with raw food and equipment.

So, what does a simple or fancy raw foods diet look like? Below are some quick definitions! I have also included a moderate category, which borrows a little bit from both worlds.

SIMPLE raw food meals require very little preparation and equipment. The recipes are simple, and fruits and vegetables are eaten in their whole food forms as much as possible. For example, a person may eat two whole apples for breakfast and chopped vegetables for lunch. Examples of simple recipes include my Corn Salad (on page 174) and Sun-Baked Gazpacho (on page 208).

MODERATE raw food recipes merge simplicity and advanced food preparation. These recipes include basic ingredients; however, some equipment is used like a blender, food processor, and/or dehydrator. Most of the recipes in this book are moderate raw food recipes like Donut Holes (on page 242) and The Best Pate Ever (on page 192).

FANCY raw food preparation stretches the imagination of what we think about raw foods. It consists of elaborate recipe preparation that utilizes ingredients from around the world and expensive equipment like high-speed blenders or juicers. This type of raw foods also requires the most planning as it can take 1-2 days to complete a recipe. I can't think of one recipe from this book that would fit the fancy category; however, my recipe for Candy Ice Cream Bars (on page 258) does come close.

When choosing the type of raw foods you want to create, consider the amount of time and money you can devote to preparing raw foods. Creating the perfect raw food kitchen is a balance between your taste preferences, finances, and time. If you prefer the flavors of fancy raw food cuisine, then you will need to devote more money and time to creating these meals. If you are on a very small budget and/or have very little time available to prepare meals, then a simple raw foods diet may better fit your lifestyle. However, choosing a simple raw foods diet doesn't mean that you can't create a moderate or fancy meal once in a while! Plus, it's okay to start with one type of raw foods diet and later graduate into another. It's completely up to you! My only recommendation is that you start small because it's more cost-effective to graduate from simple recipes to advanced food preparation than the other way around. Plus, keeping it simple or moderate from the start will translate to lower food and equipment start-up costs. In making your decision, you may find it helpful to review the costs associated with common raw food ingredients and equipment in chapters 13 and 14.

So tell me, what type of raw foods diet do you want to create?

Write Below

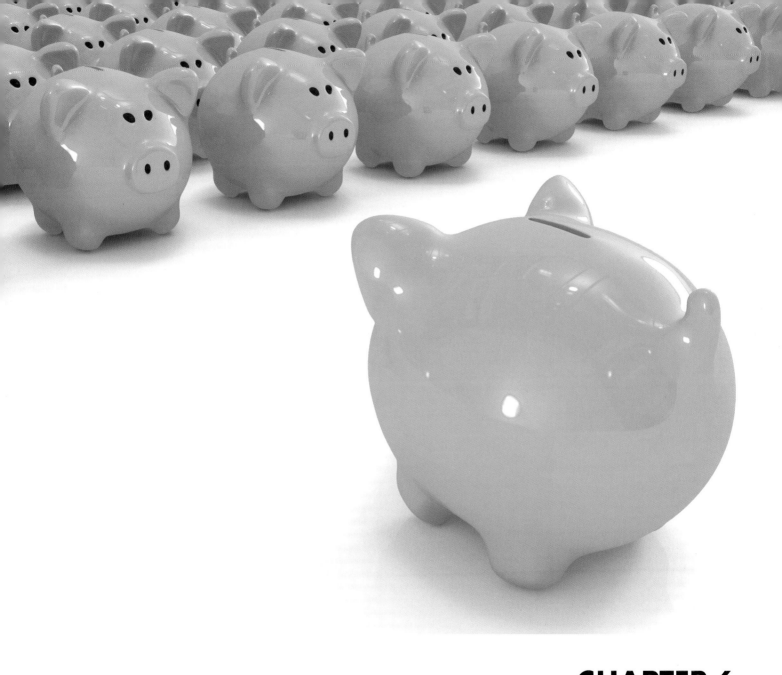

CHAPTER 6
Create Your **BUDGET!**

Take a moment and think about where you are in terms of having a budget. In our society, it's "normal" to be in the dark about how much money we spend on food. But now it's time to get out of the dark! Yay! In this chapter, I will help you to create a monthly budget, choose a budget managing system, and figure out how much you are currently spending on food and how much you can afford to spend!

Before we dive into this chapter, let's check in on our friend Impulsive Ida. Like many of us, Ida is interested in a raw foods lifestyle, but she is having trouble affording it.

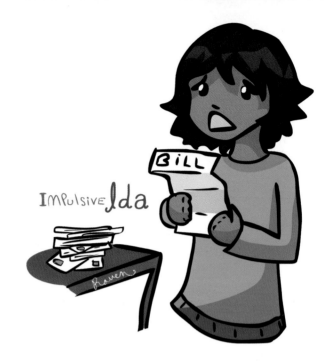

IMPulsive *Ida*

Ida has read many books on raw foods and she knows the diet back and forth, but when it comes to managing her food expenses, she is not doing so well. In fact, her food bills are making it difficult for her to stay raw because she keeps running out of food money before her next paycheck. As a result, she is faced with 2 options: eat "cheaper" cooked foods or use her credit cards. Because Ida is on a mission to improve her health, she uses her credit cards to cover her food expenses. However, with the recent downturn of the economy, her credit card interest rates are higher than ever and, subsequently, she has found it difficult to afford her accruing debt. Ida has tried to budget in the past, but she just can't seem to get her food expenses below what she can afford.

Ida's situation is not unique. In fact, I think that we all can see a little bit of ourselves in Ida. Like most people, Ida was not taught how to shop for inexpensive fruits and vegetables or how to live on a budget. Instead, she learned how to shop at grocery stores and how to buy A LOT OF FOOD (I mean you gotta keep that refrigerator full, right?). Given that most grocery stores charge high prices for fruits and vegetables, it's no wonder why Ida and many of us are struggling to afford the raw food diet. And it's no surprise that many people like Ida have used their credit cards to cover a portion of their food expenses. But, NOW A CHANGE HAS COME! By completing this chapter, you will have taken a HUGE step towards living a budget-loving, raw foods lifestyle!

This chapter is organized into 4 steps:

- Step 1: Figure out how much you currently spend
- Step 2: Figure out how much you can afford to spend
- Step 3: Set your first food spending goal
- Step 4: Create your monthly budgeting system

Give yourself some time when working through these steps. They are not meant to be done all in one day. Rather, begin Step 1 now and set aside 3-4 hours over the weekend to do Steps 2 and 3. And when you are comfortable with the first three steps, proceed to Step 4.

Think of this chapter as your budget starting point. Creating and managing a household budget is a HUGE topic that includes making and managing investments, and managing saving funds for education, etc. It's impossible to discuss all of this in one chapter. For recommendations on great budget books, refer to page 35.

Step 1
Figure Out How Much You Currently Spend

Before you can make progress towards living a budget-conscious, raw food lifestyle, it's important to see where you are. How much do you spend every week on food (both raw and other foods)? It's no longer okay to just have an idea or to simply not know. You are now on the raw foods on a budget path, where exact numbers are the rule, not the exception. So, make it your #1 goal this week to keep all of your food receipts and add them up at the end of the week. This will give you a starting point to work from. Because tracking

your expenses is essential to cultivating budget-loving habits, I strongly recommend that you continue to track your weekly food expenses on the Food Expense Log (on pages 36-38) for the length of this program. It's easy to overspend when you have no idea how much you are spending.

Tracking your food expenses is pretty straightforward. In short, you save all of your receipts and add them up at the end of every week. This includes receipts from grocery stores, restaurants, and wherever else you purchase food. If you are purchasing both raw and non-raw foods, then you will want to keep these expenses separate. It's a good idea to do this at the beginning because the strategies in this book may first affect your raw food expenses before they affect other food expenses. If you have a spouse, then ask them to give you their receipts (you can start a receipts' jar!). In addition, with so much technology today, your spouse can even take pictures of their receipts with their cell phone and send them to you, or you both can maintain an online spreadsheet using websites like Google™ Docs. Or, to avoid lost food receipts, you can take pictures of your own receipts!

Step 2
Figure Out How Much You Can Afford to Spend

To calculate how much you can afford to spend on food every month, you will first need to create a quick monthly budget for all of your expenses. If we don't know how much we can spend, it's easy to spend more than we have and accumulate debt. In this exercise, you will create a *monthly* budget. The budget is monthly because that's how frequent most people pay their major bills like housing, electricity, car insurance, etc. If you receive your paycheck every week or two weeks, just add up your total income for the whole month. Use the worksheet "The Launch-Pad Budget" on pages 40-39 to create your budget.

STRATEGY 8
Say YES! to the fun stuff

One of the great things about having a budget is that you can plan for the fun stuff and actually watch it happen! How many times have we set lofty vacation goals, only to watch time pass and nothing come to fruition. Having a budget helps you plan and make small contributions toward achieving your fun goals! And the fun stuff doesn't have to be expensive or extravagant. Fun stuff could mean saving up for a bus fare or rental car to visit a museum or go to the beach. Or, it could mean purchasing that raw food appliance you have been lusting after like a Vitamix™ blender or Samson™ juicer. Plus, including some fun stuff into your budget will help you stay on track. When we omit all the fun stuff from our budgets, our budgets are more likely to fail because we are depriving ourselves. A budget only takes away from your life if you let it. Remember, having a budget means saying NO to the things that don't matter like the impulse buys, so that you can say YES to the stuff that does matter, like vacations, time with your family, and great raw food equipment.

STRATEGY 9
Set aside money for infrequent bills

We all have those infrequent bills like our quarterly water bill or yearly car registration. To avoid surprises, plan for these bills. This may mean that you set aside a few dollars every month for your water bill, which may arrive every 3 months. Or, if you know an annual bill like your car registration will be arriving soon, begin setting aside some money 3-4 months ahead of time. It just takes a little planning!

STRATEGY 10
Give, give, give!

Participate in the circle of giving! It doesn't matter how much or little we have, we can always contribute something to the world. If you are very low on funds, give your time to a charity every month. Or, give someone an unexpected hug or share a beautiful meal with someone. Give in any way that you can, and don't feel bad if you can only give a little. The more you stick to a budget, the more you will save, and the more you can give. Living on a budget allows us to share with the world. The more we give, the more that is given to us in the forms of joy, beautiful friendships and experiences, amazing produce and meals, and financial security.

Step 3
Set Your First Food Spending Goal!

Now you are ready to set your first spending goal! Yay! Your first goal is simple: spend less on food than you budgeted in Step 2. If you're already doing that, then aim to spend 10-25% less than what you are currently spending. Avoid setting a very low amount for your goal unless you absolutely have to for income reasons. Really think about what your goal should be so that it's not unrealistic or unattainable. Although many of you will be able to cut your spending in half, it will be a gradual process with your savings increasing as you work through the program. So give yourself room to grow!

If you are purchasing foods for raw *and* cooked meals, then I recommend that you set two separate goals: one for your raw food bills and the other for your cooked food bills. You can record your goals on the Food Expense Log on page 36.

STRATEGY 11
Get your spouse and children on board

Talk with your spouse and children about having a budget. A sure-fire way to fail on a budget is to have a spouse and/or child who isn't on board, but if you do it right, they may become your biggest budget advocates!

The first step you can take with your spouse is to figure out where your money goes. It's often that when one person manages the finances the other spouse doesn't understand how much is paid towards the bills, especially the food bills. Communication is key to having a successful household budget. If your spouse is hesitant towards starting a budget, there are some techniques you can use to get them on board! Try including some fun money into your household budget, with which you and your spouse can do whatever you want. This way your spouse doesn't feel so constrained by the new budget. In addition, consider having meetings at the beginning of each month to discuss your successes from the past month and set goals for the upcoming month. Also, share your budget success as a family. When you save money as a family, celebrate as a family! Jump around the house! Make it an event! And lastly, find a budget book like *Get Financially Naked: How to Talk Money with your Honey* by Manisha Thakor and Sharon Kedar, and read the book together. This way you are both investing time into your budget and making it a part of your regular conversations.

When talking to children about budgeting, always keep it positive. Emphasize the rewards of living on a budget. Children don't always understand limitations or delaying gratification, but they understand rewards. Talk about the amazing activities you will be able to do as a family and what a budget will bring to the family as a whole. And make them a part of your budget success! You can even teach them about managing their own money with a piggy bank or their very own checking account. Read them children's books like *Do I Need It? or Do I Want It?: Making Budget Choices* by Jennifer Larson and *The Berenstain Bears' Trouble with Money* by Stan and Jan Berenstain. And lastly, always talk about your budget in a positive way. For example, if your child asks for an expensive item, say, "Well, that's not in our budget, but let's find some recipes (or toys) that are in our budget". Give them a positive alternative so that they won't focus on what they can't have.

Step 4
Create Your Monthly Budgeting System

Now that you have your budget and monthly spending goal, it's time to create a budget management system to support you in meeting this goal every month. A budget management system is simply a way to manage your budget every month. Often people create a budget only to stop using it after a few months. Having a budget management system ensures that you stick with your budget and, subsequently, reap the rewards. Budget management systems can range from the very simple envelope method (described below) to financial software like Quicken™. Whatever system you choose, you want it to be quick and to fit your lifestyle.

An easy budgeting system is the Envelope Method. This method is like creating multiple bank accounts for each of your budget categories (e.g. food, entertainment). To do this method, take a few envelopes and write the expense categories from your budget (e.g. food) on each envelope. Then insert the amount of money you have budgeted for that category into the appropriate envelope. What makes this system great is that once you've spent all of the money that's in one of your envelopes, that's it. Keep in mind that you do not need to create envelopes for fixed or one-time expenses like rent, electricity, or car insurance. Arrange for these expenses to be automatically withdrawn from your bank account. This way they are always paid on time and fewer expenses need to be managed. You can also create virtual envelopes using a spreadsheet software like Microsoft Excel™; however, the easiest and most reliable way to use the envelope method is to do it manually.

Other budgeting management systems include software like Quicken™ and Mint. Quicken™ is a very powerful computer software package that manages all of your expenses, retirement funds, business income and expenses, and more. In fact, if you have a business, it may be easier to use software like Quicken™ to manage both your business and personal expenses. Plus, as a time saver, Quicken™ can download transactions from your bank account(s) and investment funds. It's pretty amazing! Quicken™ costs from $30-80, depending on your needs. If you are not ready for Quicken™, you can start off by using Mint (www.mint.com), a free online budget management system that is owned by the makers of Quicken™.

STRATEGY 12
Find a budget system that works & stick to it

It may take several months to reap the benefits of a new budget system, so hang in there. For example, in the past it has taken me 3 or so months of budgeting to observe trends in how I spend money. When you have this data over time, you can see where the problems are and make informed changes to your monthly budget.

There may be times when you want to make small adjustments to your budgeting system to help it fit your lifestyle and that's okay. Just don't overhaul the whole system too early; otherwise, you will never know if it saved you money!

STRATEGY 13
DO NOT carry a balance on your credit cards

Most Americans are used to having some debt, to where it has become normal to carry a balance on their credit cards. However, when you are living on a budget, one of your goals is to STOP unnecessary spending and to pay off any debt you may have accumulated. So set firm boundaries with yourself and stay away from the plastic!

STRATEGY 14
Wait for those large expenses

Sometimes you may need to make large food expenses like buying 5 or 10 pounds of hemp seeds, or a bushel (about 35lb) of tomatoes from your local farm. When making large purchases, be as planful as possible. If you know ahead of time that you will purchase a large item, put some money aside after every paycheck so these expenses do not come as a surprise. For example, one winter I stashed cash away every month in preparation for refilling my home's oil tank (used for heating). It was great to have $400 saved to pay for a $600 oil bill!

There also may be times when a large expense just pops up! In this situation, the best thing you can do is to sleep on it. Wait 24 hours because you may find that you don't even need the large purchase. Or, you may find cheaper sources to get what you need, or even discover a less expensive substitute.

STRATEGY 15
Know your triggers!

Learn what triggers you to buy more than you need. Often stress is a huge trigger and encourages impulsive spending as a form of therapy. I know when I am stressed, I immediately want some chocolate. Or maybe taking your children with you to the grocery store sets off your impulsive shopping. Whatever it is, try to avoid these triggers when you shop. If you are stressed, avoid shopping until you're calm. If you can, leave your children at home and shop alone. A good way to identify your triggers is to ask yourself before you purchase something: "Do I need this?", "Why do I want this?", and "Is this in my budget?" It's usually the items that we don't need that can help us understand our triggers and overcome them.

MY FAVORITE LOW-COST BUDGET BOOKS

- *You're Broke Because You Want to Be: How to Stop Getting By and Start Getting Ahead* (2007), by Larry Winget

- *Get Financially Naked: How to Talk Money with Your Honey* (2009), by Manisha Thakor and Sharon Kedar

- *The Budget Kit: The Common Cents Money Management Workbook* (2008), by Judy Lawrence

- *The Pocket Idiot's Guide to Living on a Budget* (2005), by Peter Sander and Jennifer Sander

WORKSHEET
WEEKLY FOOD EXPENSE LOG!

It's so easy to ignore how much we spend on food...I mean everybody does it, right? However, this book is all about empowering you as a budget-conscious shopper and this worksheet is a HUGE step in that direction. Plus, by tracking your food expenses you can watch your food bills shrink as you implement the strategies in this book!

This worksheet has two parts. The first part consists of tracking your food expenses, and in the second part, you will set your food spending goals. Note that when doing part 2, you will first complete your budget on pages 39-41 to determine how much you can spend on food.

Part 1: Track your weekly food expenses in the table provided on the next page. Keep all of your food receipts and calculate the total amount you spent at the end of the week. If you purchase foods for raw and cooked meals, then keep these weekly food expenses separate.

Part 2: Write down your first set of spending goals! This goal is the maximum amount you want to spend on food each month. If you are spending more than you have budgeted for food, then your first goal is to spend less than this amount. However, if you are already spending less than you have budgeted for food, make your spending goal 10-25% less than what you are currently spending. If you purchase foods for raw and cooked meals, then I would recommend that you set two separate goals: one for your raw food bills and the other for your cooked food bills. I recommend keeping them separate at first because the strategies presented in this book may initially impact your raw food expenses before they influence your cooked food expenses. When you have consistently spent less than your first goal for several weeks in a row, set a new spending goal! This way you are always making progress!

RAW Goal	Other Food Goal

JANUARY

Week	Raw Food	Other Food	Total
1	_____	_____	_____
2	_____	_____	_____
3	_____	_____	_____
4	_____	_____	_____
5	_____	_____	_____
Total	_____	_____	_____

FEBRUARY

Week	Raw Food	Other Food	Total
1	_____	_____	_____
2	_____	_____	_____
3	_____	_____	_____
4	_____	_____	_____
5	_____	_____	_____
Total	_____	_____	_____

MARCH

Week	Raw Food	Other Food	Total
1	_____	_____	_____
2	_____	_____	_____
3	_____	_____	_____
4	_____	_____	_____
5	_____	_____	_____
Total	_____	_____	_____

APRIL

Week	Raw Food	Other Food	Total
1	_____	_____	_____
2	_____	_____	_____
3	_____	_____	_____
4	_____	_____	_____
5	_____	_____	_____
Total	_____	_____	_____

MAY

Week	Raw Food	Other Food	Total
1	_____	_____	_____
2	_____	_____	_____
3	_____	_____	_____
4	_____	_____	_____
5	_____	_____	_____
Total	_____	_____	_____

JUNE

Week	Raw Food	Other Food	Total
1	_____	_____	_____
2	_____	_____	_____
3	_____	_____	_____
4	_____	_____	_____
5	_____	_____	_____
Total	_____	_____	_____

JULY

Week	Raw Food	Other Food	Total
1			
2			
3			
4			
5			
Total			

AUGUST

Week	Raw Food	Other Food	Total
1			
2			
3			
4			
5			
Total			

SEPTEMBER

Week	Raw Food	Other Food	Total
1			
2			
3			
4			
5			
Total			

OCTOBER

Week	Raw Food	Other Food	Total
1			
2			
3			
4			
5			
Total			

NOVEMBER

Week	Raw Food	Other Food	Total
1			
2			
3			
4			
5			
Total			

DECEMBER

Week	Raw Food	Other Food	Total
1			
2			
3			
4			
5			
Total			

LAUNCH-PAD BUDGET

It's time to create your budget! How exciting! This worksheet will help you determine how much money you can afford to spend on food, after taking into account your other household expenses. As you continue on your budget path and begin saving money, you will undoubtably make adjustments to this budget.

When completing the worksheet, consider these tips:

- Food should always be one of your top priorities. People are quick to underfund their food category when, in fact, more money should be devoted to supporting their health.

- Be as accurate as possible when listing your expenses.

- If you are spending more than you have, you will need to adjust your numbers until your spending (and savings) matches your income.

- Every single dollar of your income should be allocated to the categories on this form. When you're done, your total income minus your total expenses should equal zero; in other words, your disposable income should be zero.

Income

Include all sources of your monthly income (i.e., salary/wages, social security, retirement, account interest, alimony/child support, real estate income, investment dividends, unemployment, food stamps, etc.).

Salary/Wages _____

Salary/Wages (Your Partner) _____

Other _____ _____

Other _____ _____

Other _____ _____

Total Income _____

Expenses - Housing & Utilities

Mortgage/Rent _____

Real Estate Taxes _____

Homeowner's/Renters Insurance _____

Repairs or Maintenance _____

Household Supplies/Furniture _____

Phone - Home _____

Phone - Cell _____

Cable _____

Gas _____

Water _____

Trash _____

Electricity _____

Internet _____

Other _____ _____

Other _____ _____

Total Housing/Utilities Expenses _____

Expenses - Health

Medical _____

Dental _____

Vision _____

Life Insurance _____

Medications/Prescriptions _____

Other _____ _____

Total Health Expenses _____

Expenses - Transportation

Car 1 Payment _____

Car 2 Payment _____

Gas & Oil _____

Car Maintenance _____

Public Transportation _____

Other _____ _____

Other _____ _____

Total Transportation Expenses _____

Expenses - Personal

Alimony/Child Support _____

Charity Contributions _____

Child/Day Care _____

Baby Sitter _____

Children's Activities _____

Clothing Maintenance (laundry) _____

Clothing Purchases _____

Memberships (gym, other) _____

Personal Care (grooming) _____

Tuition and School Supplies _____

Expenses - Food

Grocery - Raw Food Only _____

Grocery - Other Food _____

Restaurant - Raw Food Only _____

Restaurant - Other Food _____

Other _____ _____

Other _____ _____

Other _____ _____

Total Food Expenses _____

Expenses - Entertainment

Entertainment _____

Vacation _____

Events _____

Hobbies _____

FUN MONEY (entertainment) _____

Other _____ _____

Other _____ _____

Total Entertainment Expenses _____

Savings

Emergency Fund _____

Retirement _____

College _____

Other _____ _____

Other _____ _____

Other _____ _____

Other _____ _____

Total Savings _____

Gifts _____

FUN MONEY (personal) _____

Miscellaneous _____

Other _____ _____

Total Personal Expenses _____

Expenses - Debt

Credit Card 1 _____

Credit Card 2 _____

Credit Card 3 _____

Credit Card 4 _____

Credit Card 5 _____

Credit Line _____

Student Loan 1 _____

Student Loan 2 _____

Personal Loans _____

Other _____ _____

Total Debt Expenses _____

Summary

Insert your total income, expenses (housing & utilities, food, health, etc.), and savings here. Subtract total expenses and savings from your total income to arrive at your disposable income. You want your disposable income to equal zero. All of your money should be allocated to the categories on this form. This way you will have a plan for all of your money.

Total Income _____

Total Expenses (-) _____

Total Savings (-) _____

Disposable Income _____

I love the guide on meal planning and shopping, what a life saver that has been. I am no longer wasting food and money.

-Sherrie

I need this book!
-Nina

OMG, I have been looking for something like this for so long...

-HP

One of the most valuable tips I have learned is how to shop and eat everything before going to buy more food! Not only has it saved me a LOT of money, it has helped me to be creative with my foods.

-Shawnette

THANKS AGAIN FOR THE book. I'M LOViNG iT!!!

-Kittora

L-O-V-E the vision, the passion, and sincere desire to share your knowledge with so many people...

-Theresa

this is a great book! i followed one of your suggestions on how to shop more effectively, and it is saving me money. it was so simple and for some reason i never thought of it!

-Ashley

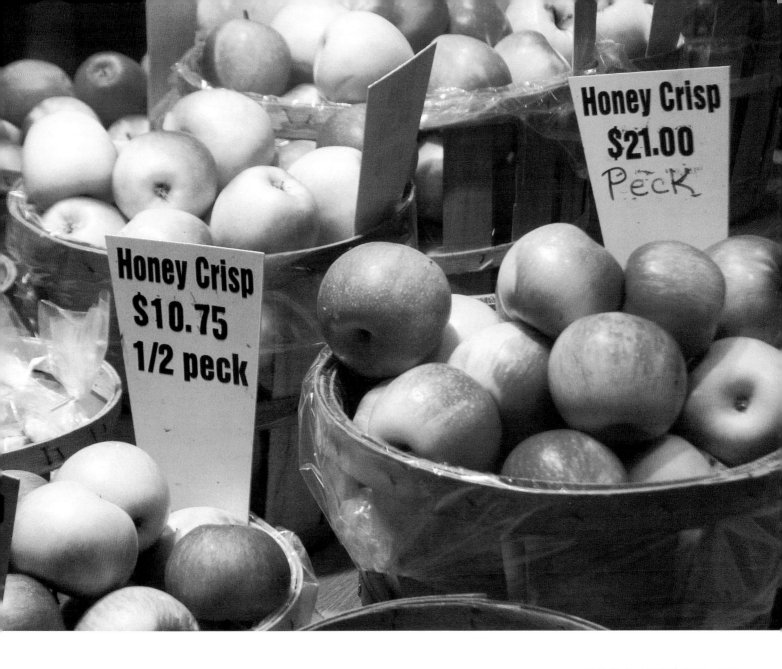

Honey Crisp
$10.75
1/2 peck

Honey Crisp
$21.00
PECK

CHAPTER 7

Improve **HOW** You Buy Food!

Before we dive into the many ways for finding low-cost, high-quality produce, it's important to first consider how you buy food. In fact, how you buy food is more important than where you buy food. For example, let's take our friend Impulsive Ida:

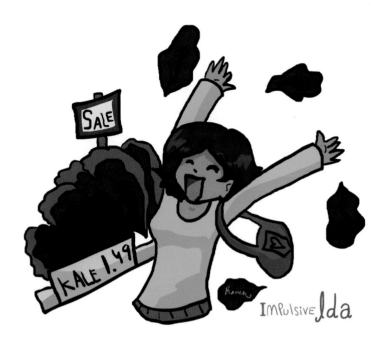

One Sunday morning before lunch, Ida goes to her local grocery store. To her surprise, she sees that her favorite kale is on sale! Typically, a bunch of kale costs $2.49, but now it's on sale for $1.49. Ida is super excited and buys three bunches (costing a total of $4.47), rather than the one bunch she normally purchases. One kale-filled week later, Ida managed to only eat two bunches of her kale and sadly the third bunch remained in the back of the refrigerator for weeks and Ida eventually threw it out. In the end, Ida wasted food and spent more money than she needed, even though she paid a cheaper price.

What did Ida do wrong? Ida needed a better sense of what she needed. At the grocery store, Ida 'wanted' three bunches of kale, but she only 'needed' two bunches. Plus, Ida went to the grocery store while she was hungry. She hadn't eaten lunch yet and experienced the "eyes are bigger than your stomach" effect. When we are hungry, we tend to buy more food than we can realistically eat. Lastly, Ida didn't have a plan for the kale she purchased. A sale can only save you money if you eat all of the food.

You may be asking yourself: Is this really a big deal? She only wasted one bunch of kale. The problem is that many of us impulsively shop on a regular basis so that we routinely buy way more than we need and waste a lot of food and money as a result. In the United States, an average of 60 to 70% of grocery purchases at supermarkets are unplanned (Underhill, 2008). This means that we are shopping like Impulsive Ida more than half of the time! So, it doesn't matter if the food is on sale or not, if we throw food away, we throw our money away. In order to take advantage of low-cost, high-quality produce and successfully stay on budget, we need to first learn HOW to shop for food.

STRATEGY 16
Buy what you need, eat all you have

This is one of the MOST IMPORTANT strategies in the whole book! If you always buy the food you 'want' rather than what you 'need', you will always spend more than you budget. I know it can be difficult to resist those immediate 'wants' like raw vegan chocolate, ice cream, cheesecake, and fruit and nut bars at the grocery store, but buying these 'wants' can wreck your budget. Plus, you can make these goodies at home for a much lower price. Just take a look at the dessert recipes in this book!

The first step to buying only what you 'need' is to figure out how much food you actually need. The easiest way to see how much food you need is to see how long it takes you to eat a specific amount of food. You can do this by eating all the perishable food in your kitchen before buying any new food. You might cringe at this idea. I know I did when it first came to me because it meant that I couldn't make any impulsive trips to the grocery store to buy a food I was craving. Nope, I had to eat all of my food until it ran out. Aughhh!

Although eating all you have may seem daunting, this exercise provides a great learning opportunity. First, it will teach you that you need a lot less food than you currently think you do! Second, this exercise will force you to be creative in new ways during your food preparation. For example, one week, I was down to a few carrots, celery stalks, and lemons. I had just returned home from the gym and was looking for something to eat. I am not a big carrot fan, so the thought of making a recipe primarily composed of carrots was not happening. I decided to try juicing the carrots with a few stalks of celery and a whole lemon. I also picked some parsley from my garden and juiced that, too. The juice came out so good that I included it in this book (see "Carrots Rejoice" recipe on page 160). What a nice surprise! Third, this exercise provides an opportunity for you to connect with your food. It's difficult to appreciate the food you have when you have a ton of it in your kitchen, simply because it's easy to forget about it. However, when you are buying what you need, all of the food you purchase has a place in your life.

You know that you only need three oranges instead of a 5lb bag and you know exactly when you are going to eat them. And lastly, after you do this exercise, you will find that you spend A LOT LESS the next time you buy food. You will shop more consciously because for the first time, you will know how long it takes you to eat a bunch of celery. You will feel empowered and in control of your spending, instead of feeling out of control and impulsive.

To help you determine how much food you need, complete Activity 1 "Learn how much you need by eating all you have" on page 50. This is the most important activity in the whole book and it can immediately save you a lot of money, so consider starting this activity today!

For guidance in buying the amount of food you need, consider implementing the next four strategies for planning your meals, using shopping lists, not shopping when you are hungry, and buying 3-4 days worth of food at a time.

STRATEGY 17
Plan your meals

Planning your meals will tell you how much food you need to buy as well as help you avoid food wastage. Meal planning may seem like a daunting task, but it really isn't. Most of us already plan some of our meals in advance. For example, many people prepare for the work week by buying their breakfast and lunch foods in advance (e.g. coffee, English muffins, deli meat, cheese, mayo, etc.). This is meal planning. Often parents buy their children's lunch foods (juice boxes, sandwich ingredients, cookies, chips) for the school week ahead of time. This is meal planning. Sometimes people buy ice cream and pies in advance for their after dinner dessert. This is meal planning. I think you get the point. The fact is that we do meal planning all the time; the only difference is that now the meals will be raw vegan.

Meal planning can be time consuming the first time you do it, but the more you do it, the more automatic and natural it will become. For example, when I go grocery shopping I have specific meals in mind for the next few days and I shop specifically for these meals. First, I think about the recipes I want for lunch and dinner for the next few days (I tend to hold a lot of recipes in my head) and then I shop specifically for those recipes. And then I will make these recipes 2-3 times until the ingredients run out. However, my thoughts would not be as organized if I hadn't gone through the process of planning my meals on paper. Plus, I also keep my meals simple. For instance, breakfast tends to be fruit rather than an elaborate raw vegan meal. I save the more fancy stuff or combination recipes for lunch and dinner. Snacks are whole fruits or cut-up veggies, or something I dehydrated over the weekend. Integrating simple meals throughout the day speeds up the meal planning process. To guide you in creating your first raw meal plan, a worksheet has been provided on pages 57-58.

STRATEGY 18
Use a shopping list

The logic is simple: if you have a shopping list, it's easier to resist impulse buys. Like I mentioned before, 60-70% of our grocery purchases at supermarkets are unplanned (Underhill, 2008). Just think about how much money we could save if we reduced our impulse buys!

In creating a shopping list, begin by creating a meal plan, as described in strategy 17. Then take your meal plan and write down all the ingredients required for each recipe. This will keep your shopping list focused; however, you may find that a few non-meal plan items will creep onto the list. To determine if these items are justified purchases, first ask yourself "is this a need or a want? If the item is a need then keep it on the list, but if it's a want then drop it like a bad habit. Once you have your shopping list, look around your kitchen to see if you already have some of the items you need. To guide you in creating your first shopping list, a worksheet has been provided on page 59.

STRATEGY 19
Don't shop when you are hungry

An easy way to prevent impulsive buying is to avoid shopping when you are hungry. When some people are hungry, they tend to buy more food than they normally would (Mela, Aaron, & Gatenby, 1996; Nisbett & Kanouse, 1969) *and* they are more likely to buy unhealthy snack foods for immediate consumption (Read & Leeuwen, 1998). For raw vegans, this may mean that we splurge on expensive raw snack foods like cookies, chocolate, and crackers to satisfy our immediate hunger rather than waiting to eat a delicious, more affordable meal at home. If you know that you tend to buy more food when you are hungry, satisfy your hunger first and then go shopping. But, if you find yourself hungry while shopping, buy a quick snack like an apple or bag of nuts first before you begin shopping. You will have to checkout twice, but it will save you money in the long-run.

STRATEGY 20
Buy 3-4 days worth of food

I am often asked this question: "For how many days should I buy food?" While my answer varies slightly for each individual, it involves a balance between not buying too much food, not having to go grocery shopping too often, and not wasting food. I find that 3-4 days worth of food helps me to balance this equation. You may want to follow a similar strategy because it's so easy for food to be forgotten. Plus, you may find that the food you buy for 3-4 days actually lasts 5-6 days. That's 2 extra days! This can occur because you might miss a planned meal or snack (e.g. someone treats you to lunch, you are not hungry, or you eat a meal not on your menu plan), or you have leftovers from the last meal. Plus, eating raw foods is about eating fresh foods, so you wouldn't want old produce sitting in your fridge anyway.

When you buy 3-4 days worth of food, you will probably visit your local grocery store or farms 1-3 times a week. This may be more frequent than you wish to shop; however, it comes with the raw food territory. In order to have fresh fruits and vegetables, they must be purchased often. But, you can reduce the amount of time you spend shopping by having a shopping list, visiting stores that are located close to each other, or only going to the grocery store when necessary. For example, I typically visit my local health food store once a week, so I schedule it when I know I will be in the area. However, when I don't need to go, I don't go. I also schedule blocks of time to do big grocery shopping trips. On Tuesday afternoons, I pick up my CSA farm share from a nearby community center, visit a produce shop at a local farm, and then visit my local health food store. If I need to, on Saturday mornings, I visit an international market and 1-2 grocery stores. These excursions only take me 1-1½ hours per trip. This is a small price to pay for good health.

STRATEGY 21
Buy what's in season

There are so many reasons to buy what's in season. For one, fruits and vegetables are cheaper when they are in season. For example, I can buy one quart (i.e. 4 cups) of blueberries for $3 when they are in season; however, when they are not in season, ½ pint (i.e. 2 cups) will cost me $3.99 at the grocery store. Tomatoes are another good example. I can buy 17 pounds (1/2 a bushel) of organic tomatoes through my CSA program for $7.50; however, when tomatoes are not in season, I can only purchase one pound for $3.99 at the grocery store. As you can see, it's cheaper to buy produce when it's in season. Plus, produce tastes much better when it's in season. For example, in Pennsylvania, strawberries in June taste much better than the strawberries sold at grocery stores in December. Just because you can buy a strawberry in the winter doesn't mean that its edible or tastes good. Moreover, out-of-season produce tends to be shipped long-distances from other states and countries. Large chain grocery stores are able to stock out-of-season produce like strawberries, apples, and melon in the winter because they are grown in countries like Mexico and New Zealand. So much pollution is created by shipping produce such a long distance. Also, in order to ship fruits and vegetables long distances, they are picked when they are unripe. Unfortunately, this impacts the nutrient content of the produce. The longer fruits and vegetables are allowed to ripen on the vine, the greater their nutrient content. Because local, in-season fruits and vegetables are picked when they are ripe, they typically have a higher nutrient content than produce that's shipped long distances. And lastly, when you buy what's in season, you support your local economy. So, support your local farmers by buying in-season produce from farmers market, farm stands, and CSA programs.

Eating by season can be a little daunting, especially when you see strawberries, blackberries, and other juicy fruits all year round in your grocery store. However, there are ways to help you adjust to eating by season. One way is to join a CSA program. Farms only grow what's in season, so it's very unlikely that you will receive out of season produce. Another useful strategy is to taste a food like blueberries while it's in season, so that you can appreciate its full flavor, and then taste it again when it's out of season. I did this when I was desperate for blueberries one winter. After tasting the out-of-season blueberries, I immediately tossed them out because they had no flavor whatsoever (creepy!). Another strategy is to gorge on a fruit or vegetable while it's in season. For example, when strawberries are in season, I eat pounds and pounds of them. Then at some point, I am done with them and don't really miss them until they return the following season.

To help you determine when specific fruits and vegetables are in season, pages 52-55 display seasonal harvest charts for the northeastern, midwestern, southern, and western regions of the United States. You should be able to find these foods (and more) when they are in season at your local farms, farmers market, and grocery stores. Note that farms frequently store vegetables and grow leafy greens in greenhouses during the winter, so many foods like beets, carrots, onions, potatoes, leeks, apples, and lettuce mixes will be available all winter long. If you are located outside of the United States or wish to have a seasonal chart that is more specific to your state or locale, you can create your own seasonal harvest chart on page 56. Seasonal harvest charts for countries outside of the United States can often be found on websites like www.pickyourown.org and your government's Department of Agricultural website.

When reviewing the seasonal harvest charts, keep in mind that they are estimated timetables. Weather and soil conditions can delay or speed up the maturity of crops. In addition, the charts may not display all of the produce you have access to locally, so talk to your local farmers about the produce grown in your area.

STRATEGY 22
Think variety!

Let's enhance how you think about raw foods. In fact, this is probably one of the most important topics in the whole book because it impacts your budget as well as your ability to maintain a raw vegan diet. Many of the raw food recipes out there involve the same few expensive ingredients like coconut, cacao, cashews, agave, dates, avocados, kale, etc. For many raw vegans, this translates to a diet composed of a limited variety of foods. This is problematic for two reasons: number one, these ingredients are expensive and, number two, eating a limited array of foods may become boring and result in you returning back to a cooked foods diet. But it doesn't have to be this way! There are plenty of vegetables and fruits that you can purchase from local farms and grow in your own garden, in addition to the selection found at your local grocery store.

Another benefit to eating a wide variety of plants is that it helps our bodies receive a wide variety of nutrients. Our prehistoric ancestors had access to hundreds of different kinds of edible plants compared to the 30 or so sold in most grocery stores (Bond, 2000). Just think about what this means for our bodies when we focus on a few foods. If we eat oatmeal for breakfast everyday or apples all the time, we are only giving our bodies a limited spectrum of nutrients. Thus, for optimum health, it's necessary that we eat a variety of plants and fruits.

There are several ways to increase the variety of fruits and vegetables in your diet! One strategy is to eat by season. This ensures that a variety of different foods will be entering and leaving our food environment all the time. Another strategy is to grow plants that you normally don't have access to like purslane, magenta magic (a type of mustard green), lambs quarters, etc. in your garden. A third strategy is to be open to new foods. You may find that when you visit your local farms, they are growing vegetables and fruits that you have never seen before. This may seem intimidating, but farmers are happy to tell you what they grow and how to prepare it. And if you end up not liking the taste of a new food, just tell yourself "I am learning to like it" and try preparing it in a different way. Preferences are learned, so give yourself time to learn to like a new food.

STRATEGY 23
Forage for your foods

In a society where almost all of our food is purchased from grocery stores, it's easy to forget to look for food in our own backyards. For example, every year during the early summer, my roommate and I would pick black raspberries that grow next to the wooded area around our house. Foraging can really be that easy. I have some friends who pick dandelion greens or miners lettuce growing in their yards for salads. And usually the wild fruits and vegetables you pick will have more nutrition and flavor than the ones sold at grocery stores.

Although I encourage people to forage, I don't support going outside and just eating anything that looks familiar. Foraging can be dangerous if you don't know what you are doing. Sometimes it's difficult to discriminate a poisonous plant from a safe one, so it's important to learn how to forage. Think about it: we all have been taught from a very young age about how to shop at a grocery store, but we have never learned about the wild edibles that naturally grow around us. Luckily, in many cities (big and small), there are "how-to" forage classes that teach you how to forage for local edible plants. The best way to find a foraging class is to talk to your local health food stores and/or search online using the keywords, "forage, wild, edibles" and your city name. Another option is to find a friend who routinely forages for fruits and vegetables, and tag along with them the next time they go foraging.

FUN Activities

ACTIVITY 1:
Learn how much you need by eating all you have

For the next few weeks, commit to eating all of your perishable foods (e.g. fruits, vegetables, food that has been hanging out in your kitchen for a while) before you buy any additional food. Through this activity you will learn how much food you actually need.

First, write down all of the food you have in your house on a piece of paper and place it on the refrigerator. This way you will know exactly what you have right now. Second, begin eating all the food on that list until every item has been crossed off. Keep in mind that you don't have to finish foods like spices or that 25lb bag of cashews you have in your cupboard. While it's good to include them on your list so that you know what you have and continue to eat them, don't feel pressured to eat them all while you are doing this activity. And lastly, pledge that you will not buy any additional food until you have eaten all of the foods on your list. Also, avoid going to the store while at work or when on the go; just tell yourself that you are committed to eating what you already have.

You may encounter difficulties while completing this activity. When I first did it, it was hard to resist buying cherries and grapes from the grocery store. I wanted things I didn't have. However, once I began to get low on produce, I started to feel this sense of accomplishment. And I became more creative. I started making juices and dishes that I wouldn't have thought of if I had been purchasing what I wanted. In addition, some of you may encounter difficulties if you have children. In general, children are more impulsive than adults and they want what they want, when they want it. The solution is to get them involved. Children are easier to please if you make it fun! You may run out of their favorite food, but you can involve them in creating a fun new recipe! Or you may run out of their typical lunch foods. Don't fret because this is an opportunity to create new lunch foods. Instead of their usual lunch, send your child to school with a yummy smoothie (using the frozen fruit that has been sitting in your freezer), some delicious crackers, and some cut up veggies with a delicious, new dip that you both created. Just make sure the smoothie is frozen when you pack it so that it has time to defrost by lunchtime. This may be more work than packing their usual lunch, but you are teaching your child about being resourceful, creative, and budget-conscious!

ACTIVITY 2:
Plan your meals and create a shopping list

Plan your meals for the next 3-4 days! It takes practice to get into the habit of doing this, so start today. Planning your meals not only helps you buy what you need, but it eases your transition to raw foods. It's easier to stay raw when you have a plan. To create a menu plan, browse through the recipes section of this book, and then use the guide and worksheet on pages 57-58.

Once you have created your menu plan, consider creating a shopping list (use the worksheet on page 59).

ACTIVITY 3:

Buy 3-4 days worth of food and see how long it lasts

This is a great activity to see how long the food you purchase actually lasts you. In my experience, 3-4 days worth of food actually lasts me 5-6 days. That's 2 whole days longer than I had planned! Typically, the food lasts longer because I will miss a planned meal or I will eat an unplanned meal (e.g. someone treats me to lunch).

To do this activity, simply buy 3-4 days worth of food and eat it until it runs out. It's helpful to make a list of the foods you purchased and tape it on your refrigerator. Be sure to write down the date you purchased this food. As you eat the foods on the list, cross them out. When you have crossed-out every food, then simply count how many days it took you to eat all of this food. Keep in mind that some foods don't need to be included on the list like spices because they last a long time. In addition, you may have bulk foods like a 5 pound bag of cashews and it's unrealistic that you would eat that many cashews in 3-4 days. Although it should still go on the list, don't expect to eat bulk foods like these in 3-4 days.

ACTIVITY 4:

Go foraging

This week, look online for a foraging class in your area. Using a search engine like Google™, type in the keywords "forage, wild, edibles" and your city name, and see what comes up. Also, contact your local health food stores to ask them about local classes and don't forget to look on their bulletin board(s). A simple, cheap strategy for learning how to forage is to find a friend who safely forages and to go with them on their next outing.

Sources for Seasonal Charts

NORTHEAST

Pennsylvania Department of Agriculture. Pennsylvania produce: Simply delicious. Retrieved from http://www.pafarmnews.com/Articles/2007/070207_PDA_seasonalchart.htm. Connecticut Department of Agriculture. Connecticut grown crop availability calendar. Retrieved from http://www.ct.gov/doag/lib/doag/images/season.jpg. New York State Department of Agriculture. New York state fruit and vegetable harvest calendar. Retrieved from http://www.agmkt.state.ny.us/HarvestCalendar.html.

MIDWEST

Illinois Department of Agriculture. Illinois...what's in season. Retrieved from http://www.agr.state.il.us/agrihappenings/farmers.php. Iowa Department of Agriculture and Land Stewardship. Produce availability calendar. Retrieved from http://www.agriculture.state.ia.us/Horticulture_and_FarmersMarkets/harvestCalendar.asp. University of Missouri Extension and University of Illinois Extension. (2009). To market...to market: A guide to locally grown food in the east central Missouri area. Retrieved from http://extension.missouri.edu/ecregion/market/MarkettoMarket2011.pdf.

SOUTH

Louisiana Department of Agriculture and Forestry. Louisiana harvest calendar. Retrieved from http://www.ldaf.louisiana.gov/portal/Portals/0/MKT/Farmers%20Market/LOUISIANA%20HARVEST%20CALENDAR.pdf. Georgia Fruit & Vegetable Grower's Association. Availability chart of GA grown produce. Retrieved from http://gfvga.org/georgia-grown/availability-chart-of-ga-grown-produce/. Kentucky Department of Agriculture. Kentucky proud produce: Produce availability guide. Retrieved from http://www.kyagr.com/marketing/farmmarket/documents/PRODUCEAVAILABILITYGUIDE.pdf.

WEST COAST

The Center for Urban Education about Sustainable Agriculture. Fruit and nut calendar. Retrieved from http://www.cuesa.org/seasonality/charts/fruit.php. The Center for Urban Education about Sustainable Agriculture. Vegetable calendar. Retrieved from http://www.cuesa.org/seasonality/charts/vegetable.php. Oregon Department of Agriculture. Oregon grown fresh produce: Seasonal availability. Retrieved from http://www.oregon.gov/ODA/docs/pdf/pubs/produce_calendar.pdf?ga=t. Tri-county Farm Fresh Produce. Season guide. Retrieved from http://www.tricountyfarm.org/season-guide.

NORTHEASTERN REGION OF THE UNITED STATES

BASED ON PRODUCE AVAILABILITY CHARTS FOR PENNSYLVANIA, NEW YORK, AND CONNECTICUT

	JAN	FEB	MAR	APR	MAY	JUN	JUL	AUG	SEP	OCT	NOV	DEC
Apples							■	■	■	■	■	■
Blueberries							▨	▨				
Cherries							░					
Grapes								▨	▨			
Melon							■	■	■	■		
Nectarines								▨	▨			
Peaches							■	■	■			
Pears								■	■	■	■	■
Plums, prunes							▨	▨	▨			
Raspberries						░	■		░	░		
Strawberries						▨						
Asparagus				■	■	■						
Beets							▨	▨	▨	▨	▨	▨
Broccoli						■	■		■	■		
Cabbage							■	■	■	■	■	■
Carrots							▨	▨	▨	▨	▨	▨
Cauliflower						░	░	░	░	░		
Celery	▨	▨										
Corn							■	■	■	■		
Cucumber							▨	▨	▨			
Lettuce					■	■	■	■	■	■		
Onions							■	■	■	■	■	
Peas					▨	▨						
Peppers								░	░	░		
Spinach					▨	▨			▨	▨		
Squash, summer						■	■		■	■		
Squash, winter									▨	▨		▨
Tomatoes							■	■	■			
Turnips	■	■							■	■	■	■

SEASONAL HARVEST CHART
MIDWESTERN REGION OF THE UNITED STATES
BASED ON PRODUCE AVAILABILITY CHARTS FOR ILLINOIS, IOWA, AND MISSOURI

	JAN	FEB	MAR	APR	MAY	JUN	JUL	AUG	SEP	OCT	NOV	DEC
Apples						X	X	X	X	X	X	
Blueberries						X	X	X	X			
Cherries												
Grapes							X	X	X	X		
Melon							X	X	X	X		
Nectarines						X	X	X	X			
Peaches							X	X	X			
Pears							X	X	X	X		
Plums, prunes							X	X	X			
Raspberries						X	X					
Strawberries					X	X						
Asparagus				X	X	X						
Beets						X	X	X	X			
Broccoli					X	X	X	X		X	X	X
Cabbage					X	X	X	X	X	X	X	
Carrots						X	X	X	X			
Cauliflower					X	X						
Collard Greens					X	X						
Corn							X	X	X	X		
Cucumber					X	X	X	X	X			
Kale					X	X				X	X	
Lettuce				X	X	X				X	X	
Peas					X	X	X	X	X			
Peppers							X	X	X			
Spinach				X	X	X			X	X	X	
Squash, summer					X	X	X	X	X	X		
Squash, winter							X	X	X	X		
Tomatoes							X	X	X	X		
Turnips					X	X	X				X	

SEASONAL HARVEST CHART
SOUTHERN REGION OF THE UNITED STATES
BASED ON PRODUCE AVAILABILITY CHARTS FOR LOUISIANA (LA), GEORGIA (GA), AND KENTUCKY (KY)
ABBREVIATIONS IN THE CHART INDICATE WHEN A FOOD IS ONLY AVAILABLE FOR THAT STATE.

	JAN	FEB	MAR	APR	MAY	JUN	JUL	AUG	SEP	OCT	NOV	DEC
Apples							■	■	■	■	■	
Blueberries						■	■					
Citrus	LA	LA	LA									LA
Grapes						■	■	■	■			
Melon						■	■	■	■	■	LA	
Nectarines					LA	LA						
Peaches						■	■	■	■			
Pears								■	■	■		
Plums, prunes						■	■	■				
Pomegranates									LA	LA	LA	
Raspberries						KY	KY	KY	KY			
Strawberries				■	■	■						
Pecans									GA	GA	GA	GA
Asparagus			■	■	■	■						
Beets	LA	LA	LA	LA	LA	KY,GA	KY.GA	KY,GA	KY,GA	■	LA	LA
Broccoli	LA	LA	LA	LA	LA					LA	LA	LA
Carrots	GA,LA	GA,LA	GA,LA	GA,LA	GA,LA							LA
Cauliflower	LA	LA	LA	LA	LA							LA
Collard Greens	GA,LA	GA,LA	GA,LA	■	■	■	■	■	■	■	■	GA,LA
Corn						■	■	■	■	■		
Cucumber						■	■	■	■	■		
Kale	LA	LA	LA								LA	LA
Lettuce	LA	LA	LA	LA								LA
Peas							GA	GA	GA	GA		
Peppers						LA			LA	LA		
Spinach	LA	LA	LA									LA
Squash						■	■	■	■	■		
Tomatoes						GA					LA	
Turnips	GA,LA	GA,LA	GA,LA	LA	LA							LA

WESTERN REGION OF THE UNITED STATES

BASED ON PRODUCE AVAILABILITY CHARTS FOR CALIFORNIA (CA) AND OREGON (OR)

ABBREVIATIONS IN THE CHART INDICATE WHEN A FOOD IS ONLY AVAILABLE FOR THAT STATE.

	JAN	FEB	MAR	APR	MAY	JUN	JUL	AUG	SEP	OCT	NOV	DEC
Apples	OR	OR	OR	OR	OR	OR	■	■	■	■	■	OR
Avocado	CA	CA	CA	CA	CA	CA	CA	CA	CA	CA	CA	CA
Blueberries					CA			OR	OR			
Cherries				CA	CA		OR					
Citrus	CA	CA	CA	CA	CA	CA	CA	CA	CA	CA	CA	CA
Grapes							CA	CA			CA	CA
Melon					CA	CA					CA	
Peaches, Nectarines							■	■	■	■		
Pears	CA	CA									CA	CA
Plums, prunes					CA	CA	CA					
Raspberries						■	■	■	■	CA	CA	
Strawberries			CA	CA	CA	■	■	CA	CA	CA		
Almonds								CA	CA	CA	CA	
Hazelnuts										OR	OR	OR
Walnuts	CA	CA	CA	CA	CA	CA				■	■	■
Beets	CA	CA	CA	CA	CA	CA					CA	CA
Broccoli	CA	CA	CA	CA	CA	CA					CA	CA
Carrots	CA	CA	CA	CA	CA	CA						
Cauliflower	CA	CA	CA	CA			OR	OR				
Collard Greens	■	■	■	■		■	■	■	■	■	■	■
Corn							CA	CA			CA	
Cucumbers						CA					CA	
Kale	■	■	■	■	■	■	■	■	■	■	■	■
Lettuce	CA	CA	CA	CA								CA
Peas				CA	CA						CA	
Peppers							CA	■	■	■	CA	CA
Spinach	■	■	■	■	■	■	■	■	■	■	■	■
Squash						■	■	■	■	■	■	■
Tomatoes						CA					CA	

MAKE YOUR OWN LOCAL SEASONAL HARVEST CHART

YOUR LOCATION: _____

Local Foods	JAN	FEB	MAR	APR	MAY	JUN	JUL	AUG	SEP	OCT	NOV	DEC

WORKSHEET
PLAN YOUR MEALS FOR THE NEXT 3-4 DAYS!

This worksheet will help you create your very first raw food menu plan! Yay! To help you get started, I have created an example menu plan. When creating your own menu plan, keep the following tips in mind:

- Many of the meals and snacks can have the same recipe. This will reduce the amount of ingredients you need to purchase and the time it takes to prepare your meals.

- Most of the recipes have more than one serving, so depending on how many people you are feeding, you will likely have leftovers. Incorporate these leftovers into your menu plan.

- Many of the recipes listed in the example menu plan use similar ingredients. Using an ingredient once is very expensive, but reuse an ingredient in several recipes and you will get your money's worth.

- Notice that on Thursday, I have planned to eat leftover fruits and vegetables. I expect that there will be leftover fruits and veggies from the recipes I made earlier in the week because there are always leftovers!

	Breakfast	Lunch	Dinner	Snack 1	Snack 2
Monday	Beet Greens Smoothie	Lemon Green Yum Kale Salad	Spaghetti + Beet Dessert Soup	Sea Vegetable Crackers	1 Banana
Tuesday	1 Banana + 1 Apple	Miso soup	Italian Salad + Peach Ice Cream	Sea Vegetable Crackers	3 Freezer Fig Cookies
Wednesday	Kale Green Smoothie	Lemon Green Yum Kale Salad	Spaghetti + Peach Ice Cream	Sea Vegetable Crackers	1 Apple
Thursday	1 Banana + 1 Apple	Italian Salad	Lemon Green Yum Kale Salad + Sweet Plum Sorbet	Sea Vegetable Crackers	3 Freezer Fig Cookies
Friday	Leftover fruit	Make recipe from leftover greens and veggies	Miso Soup + Sweet Plum Sorbet	Sea Vegetable Crackers	Leftover fruit and veggies

NOW, IT'S YOUR TURN!

	Breakfast	Lunch	Dinner	Snack 1	Snack 2
Monday					
Tuesday					
Wednesday					
Thursday					
Friday					
Saturday					
Sunday					

CREATE YOUR SHOPPING LIST!

Now that you have planned your meals for the next 3-4 days, it's time to create your shopping list. First, find all of the recipes listed on your meal plan and begin listing the ingredients and amounts you need for each recipe. You may find that several recipes call for the same ingredient. Rather than listing that one ingredient multiple times on your list, create a running tally of the amounts required for that ingredient (as shown in the example below).

Ingredients	Individual Amounts Needed for Each Recipe				Total Amount Needed
Olive oil	1 tbsp	+ ¼ cup	+ 3 tbsp	=	½ cup
1 _____	_____	+ _____	+ _____	=	_____
2 _____	_____	+ _____	+ _____	=	_____
3 _____	_____	+ _____	+ _____	=	_____
4 _____	_____	+ _____	+ _____	=	_____
5 _____	_____	+ _____	+ _____	=	_____
6 _____	_____	+ _____	+ _____	=	_____
7 _____	_____	+ _____	+ _____	=	_____
8 _____	_____	+ _____	+ _____	=	_____
9 _____	_____	+ _____	+ _____	=	_____
10 _____	_____	+ _____	+ _____	=	_____
11 _____	_____	+ _____	+ _____	=	_____
12 _____	_____	+ _____	+ _____	=	_____
13 _____	_____	+ _____	+ _____	=	_____

Conversion tips:
1 tablespoons = 3 teaspoons
1 cup = 16 tablespoons
1 pint = 2 cups
1 quart = 2 pints or 4 cups

Module 2

Redefine Your Local Food Environment

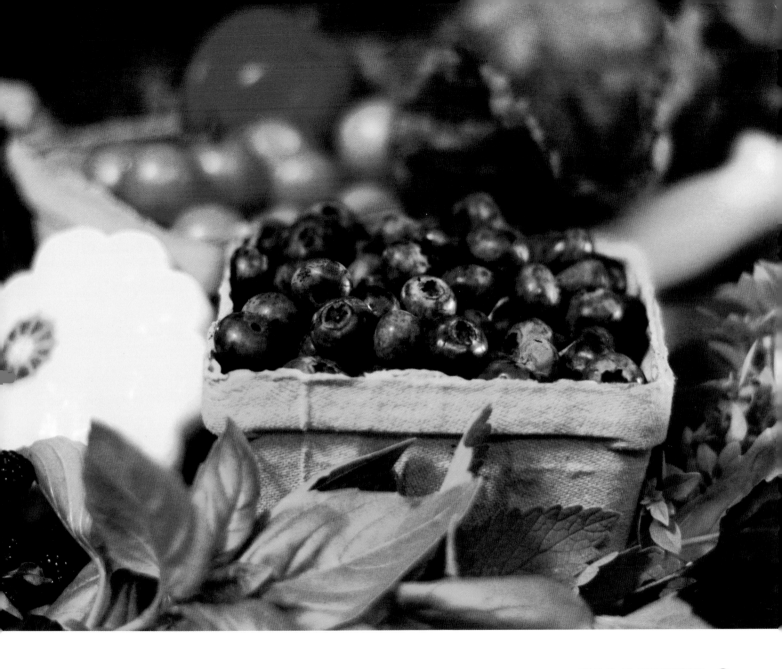

CHAPTER 8

Improve **WHERE** You Buy Food!

Now, it's time to learn how to find inexpensive, high-quality fruits, vegetables, nuts, seeds, and oils. Yay! In this chapter you will find a ton of strategies for locating high-quality produce through local farmers, grocery and health food stores, online websites, and even discount department stores. Because this chapter has so much content, I have organized these strategies by food source:

- Local farms
- Health food and grocery stores
- Internet and other sources

But before we go through the strategies, first let's revisit our friend Impulsive Ida. She could use a little help in finding low-cost fruits and vegetables.

Every Sunday morning, Ida buys her groceries for the week. Although she lives in a city with multiple health food stores, she likes to frequent a major health food store to buy all of her food. Ida likes where she shops, but she wishes her grocery bills were lower and that she had better access to a variety of fruits and vegetables. What is Ida doing wrong?

There are several simple strategies that Ida could use to increase her access to high-quality, inexpensive produce. For example, rather than purchasing all of her groceries from one store, Ida could visit multiple health food stores, grocery chains, and farmers markets. She could also visit local farms directly to purchase fruits and vegetables, join their

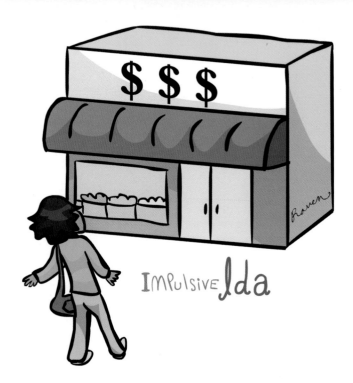

IMPULSIVE Ida

Community Supported Agriculture (CSA) program, and/or go fruit picking. By using the simple strategy of shopping around, Ida would be able to find the best produce at the lowest price. But this is not the only strategy she could have used! This chapter contains 17 strategies that both Ida and you could utilize to find inexpensive, high-quality produce. Enjoy!

Buying Food from Local Farms

The best way to eat raw foods on a budget is to buy the majority of your produce from one or more local farms. This may seem intimidating if you have never visited a farm, but it's my goal that this chapter will give you all the tools you need to connect with your local farmers. There are so many ways we can obtain fresh produce from our local farm(s) including CSA programs, local farmers markets, fruit picking opportunities, and produce stands or markets located on the farms themselves.

STRATEGY 24
Join a CSA program

CSA stands for Community Supported Agriculture and it's a way for individuals like you and me to buy produce straight from our local farms. Typically in a CSA program, an individual will sign up for a 'share', entitling them to a box of fresh fruits and vegetables every 1-2 weeks. It's that easy, and the benefits are huge! First, the produce is fresher and cheaper than the fruits and vegetables available at most grocery stores, and often it's cheaper than the produce sold at farmers markets. Second, CSAs help to support your local farms and community. CSAs are a type of cooperative business structure that allow individuals to purchase a share of the harvest from a farm for a specific season (e.g., summer, winter). This model benefits the farm because it provides them with cash up front to purchase seeds, compost, irrigation supplies, labor, and to plant and grow the produce. In other words, you invest in your local farms and in return they help you to invest in your health by providing you with fresh fruits and vegetables.

The price of a share can range from $200 to $700, depending on the farm, geographical region, season, length of the share, and whether the produce is certified organic. The best way to think about the cost of a farm share is to figure out how much it will cost you per box. For example, one summer, I paid $650 for a share that lasted 6 months, so it only cost me $24 per week. And because I shared the produce with a roommate, I only paid $12 per week!

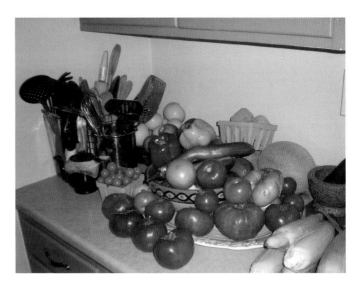

1 week of produce from my CSA farm share!

As you can see from the picture above, CSA programs provide you with a bounty of in-season produce. Often this produce is grown organically and/or using sustainable methods. Shares mostly contain vegetables and fruit, but they can also come with herbs, flowers, and other farm products. For example, in the past, I have received organic heirloom tomatoes, kale, collards, bok choy, parsley, lettuce, peppers, onions, cucumbers, garlic, yams, basil, oregano, raspberries, watermelon, cantaloupe, blueberries, strawberries, and the list goes on. However, keep in mind that the variety and quality of produce you receive will depend on weather and soil conditions. So, if the summer is very rainy, this will impact the quantity and flavor of the produce you receive. Actually, that is another reason to get to know your farmer. They can give you details on how well the fruits and vegetables are growing, and what you can expect to receive in your box. Lastly, farms often sell additional produce and products like olive oil and honey at the CSA distribution location. Sometimes, they even sell produce grown by other farmers. For example, my CSA program sells peaches from another local farm during the summer, and they even sell organic oranges, tangerines, tangelos, and grapefruit from an organic farm located in Florida during the winter.

The structure of CSA programs differ from farm to farm. Some farms only offer shares during the summer, while others offer shares during the summer and winter, or all year-round. I have seen farms that offer a separate vegetable share and fruit share. Though less common, fruit shares often contain fresh local fruits like cherries, peaches, nectarines, blueberries, strawberries, apples, and whatever else is grown on the farm. In addition, the shares can come in different sizes such as small, medium, and large. And, some farms distribute produce in a pre-arranged box while others permit you to choose the foods you want in limited or unlimited quantities.

There are several things to consider when looking for a CSA program. First, think about when during the week you can pick up your share. If you can only pick up your share on specific days of the week or on the weekends, this will limit which farms you can sign up with. Typically, farms have 1-2 pick-up dates/times during the week. In addition, many farms distribute shares off-site at community centers or health food stores while others only distribute shares at the farm, so be sure to factor in the location when selecting a CSA. Next, consider the types of produce the farm provides in the share. Fortunately, many farms have websites so you can easily find out what they grow. If the farm doesn't have a website, call the farm to obtain a produce list. Once you narrow down the farms to the ones that fit your criteria, decide whether it's important to have a share with a certified organic farm. If you are considering non-organic farms, ask the farm what type of pest control methods they use. Some farms follow organic or sustainable methods but are not certified organic due to the high costs of becoming certified. The last factor is price. You will obviously want the farm that will give you the best price. To do a price comparison between farms, figure out how much each share or box of produce will cost you per week by dividing the total price of the CSA program by the number of weeks you will receive your share. For example, I paid $650 to join a CSA program that lasted 27 weeks; when you divide 27 weeks into $650, you get 24, which meant that I only paid $24 per week.

Lastly, there are ways to reduce the cost of joining a CSA program. In some states like New York, farms accept food stamps as payment. Some farms even offer discounted shares or scholarships to low-income families, and/or work-share opportunities for CSA members to work on the farm or at distribution locations in exchange for a reduction in share costs. For example, my farm offered a $24 credit for every work shift (about 2.5 hours every 3 weeks) a customer completed on share distribution days and all the customer had to do was distribute boxes from the truck. That's $216 in savings for the whole season!

A great website to find your nearest CSA is www.localharvest.org/csa/. Or do a Google™ search for CSA programs offered in your city.

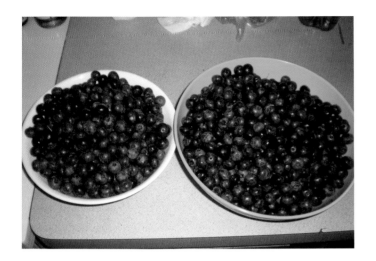

like to pick, locate farms that offer fruit picking or "pick your own". A great website to find "pick your own" farms is through www.pickyourown.org. This website will tell you what your local "pick your own" farms are growing, what produce they allow you to pick, whether they are certified organic, and if there is a produce stand or market located on the farm. Once you identify one or more farms, search for them online and see if they have websites. If they don't have a website, call for fruit picking dates, a list of produce that is available to pick (now and later in the season), and prices. Use this information to choose the best farm(s) that fits your needs. Now, the only thing left to do is to pick!

STRATEGY 25
Go fruit picking!

Fruit picking or "pick your own" is when you go to a farm and pick the fruit yourself. I experienced my first fruit picking experience a couple of years ago in Buffalo, New York, and I couldn't believe how inexpensive the produce was. After my day job, I would spend an hour picking strawberries and easily come up with a whole flat (12 pints) of organic, splendid strawberries for only $15. What a great way to celebrate the end of the day! Blueberries were my favorite to pick. I would pick pounds and pounds of them, and pay very little. One summer, I picked enough organically-grown blueberries to fill a grocery bag (shown above) and I only paid $8! This would have cost me almost $100 at the grocery store.

If you would like to go fruit-picking, first identify what's in season. Take a look at the seasonal harvest charts on pages 52-55 to get started. Once you know what you would

STRATEGY 26
Visit your local farmers market

Farmers markets are a great way to access locally-grown, inexpensive, high-quality fruits, vegetables, oils, nuts, and seeds. Plus, they support your local economy, help you connect with local farmers, and are a lot of fun. Farmers markets often sell prepared dishes and drinks, have free music and children's activities, and host community events. It's not surprising that farmers markets are more popular than ever! Did you know that the number of farmers markets in the United States has increased from 2,863 to 6,132 since 2000 (United States Department of Agriculture-Agricultural Marketing Services Division, 2010)? That's an increase of 114%! So, it's likely that you already have one or more farmers markets near you!

Where do you start? First, you need to find your local farmers market(s). A great place to start is to visit: www.localharvest.org/farmers-markets. Once you find one or more farmers markets, try looking for their website(s) online. Farmers markets that have websites typically list the variety of produce and products that are sold at the market, times and dates of operation, and the type of payments accepted (e.g. cash only, debit and credit cards, WIC vouchers, food stamps, etc.). Once you have this information, it's time to visit the market(s) you found; however, don't just start buying all kinds of produce when you get there. Carefully observe the prices, quality, and type of produce offered at the market. If they don't offer the type or quality of produce you want, then leave. Now you know that this market is not for you, at least during that time of year.

In general, when you shop at farmers markets, it's best to have some kind of strategy. Not all farmers markets are created equal in the type and quality of produce sold, amount of organic produce available, and prices. For example, when I lived in Oakland, California, I would visit three farmers markets on Saturdays. At the time, these markets differed widely in prices so I would first stop at the least expensive market and buy all the organic produce I could find that was on my shopping list. Next, I would stop at the moderately priced market and buy what the last market didn't have. Lastly, I would visit the most expensive market to buy the produce that neither one of the other markets didn't have like my favorite lettuce. As you can see, I had a strategy. By visiting multiple markets, I maximized my access to a variety of produce and was able to shop around for the lowest prices.

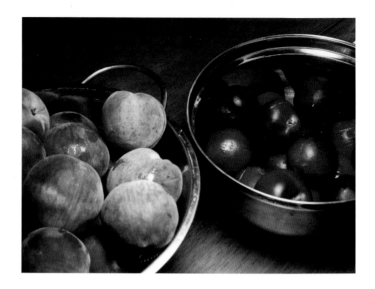

STRATEGY 27
Wait for cheaper prices

If you have ever visited a farmers market 10-20 minutes before it closed, you may have noticed that some farmers began selling their produce at cheaper prices. They do this because it's more profitable to make some money off of the remaining produce than to bring it back to the farm where it will spoil. This is where you step in. One day, visit your local farmers market 15 minutes before it closes and check whether the prices have been reduced. Keep in mind that by using this strategy, you run the risk of missing out on the produce you wanted because it sold out. Typically, I don't use this strategy because I don't want to risk not getting the produce I want. However, this strategy may be useful to people who are very low on cash. And it may naturally occur when you are running late anyway!

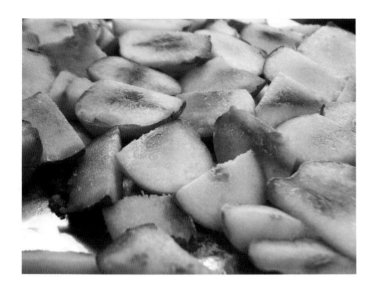

Seconds are great because they are ripe and ready to use when you buy them. This means that you don't have to wait several days for the peaches to ripen to make Peach Ice Cream (recipe on page 251)! Yippee! During the summer, I make a habit of buying seconds and using them to make quick sorbets like sweet plum sorbet (recipe on page 252).

Consider buying seconds to freeze. If you like smoothies, you can freeze seconds and then use them for future smoothies. Because the fruit is ripe when you freeze it, it will taste better than the frozen fruit you buy at the grocery store and it will be cheaper. For example, the peaches I bought as seconds cost me less than one dollar a pound. However, if I would have purchased frozen peaches from the grocery store, they would have cost me $2.50 for 3/4 lb and they wouldn't have tasted as good. Plus, don't my frozen peaches look fabulous (shown on top left)!

STRATEGY 28
Buy "seconds"

"Seconds" is a termed applied to ripe produce that needs to be sold immediately. To encourage people to buy seconds, farms typically discount them 50% or more. For example, both of my local farms offer seconds on a variety of fruits like peaches, nectarines, strawberries, and plums all at half-price! One time, I purchased 4 quarts of juicy, ripe peaches and 2 quarts of luscious nectarines for only $10 (shown above)!

STRATEGY 29
Buy in bulk; freeze or dry the rest

This is one of my favorite strategies. I just love the deals I get when I buy produce in bulk from my local farms. Every year, I pick or purchase extra boxes or flats of strawberries, rasp-

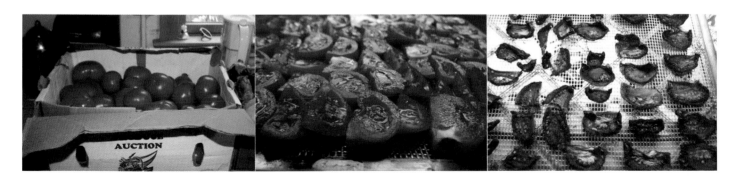

berries, blueberries, and tomatoes while they are in season and then I freeze them in preparation for the winter. I also dehydrate a ton of tomatoes and use them in crackers and sauces. For example, one summer, I purchased half a bushel of canning tomatoes (~17 lbs; picture shown on page 67) through my CSA program for only $7.50. I dried the whole box over one week and came out with 3-4 quarts of dried tomatoes that tasted like candy (see recipe on page 270). I like using these homemade 'sun-dried' tomatoes in a variety of recipes like my Fresh Italian Salad (page 179), Fresh Herb Spaghetti (page 197), Sweet Italian Crackers (page 262), and 'It Can Take It' Kale Salad (page 209).

The produce I freeze also provides me with some relief during the winter months when the variety of produce available is limited. For example, during the summer, I purchase organic raspberries by the flat for $30 (or $2.50 per half pint) and then I freeze them to use for smoothies in the winter. I also freeze tomatoes whole and use them for flatbread recipes (see recipes in "Breads and Crackers" section) and tomato sauces (e.g. Fresh Herb Spaghetti on page 197). One of my favorite things to freeze are herbs and leafy greens like basil, parsley, chard, kale, collards, etc., and to use them in pates, flatbreads, and sauces. Frozen leafy greens like kale can be used in green smoothies. During parts of the year, you can buy these greens at basement prices from farms and sometimes you can even get them for free! For more information about preparing for the winter, read my first book, *Confessions of an East Coast Raw Vegan: A Guide to Eating Raw Foods on the East Coast.*

STRATEGY 30
Shop around

If you have more than one farm in your area, then visit all of them. All farms are different, so don't just settle for one. Some farms offer a variety of produce, while others are cheaper, may be certified organic, or provide a CSA program. For example, I used to belong to two CSA programs in my area. One farm distributed their shares in prepackaged boxes while the other farm allowed us to pick the produce we wanted, though mostly in limited quantities. Even though both farms practically grew the same produce, one farm offered more fruit like blueberries, raspberries, and melons. The other farm was awesome because they allowed me to take unlimited quantities of heirloom tomatoes, parsley, kale, and basil during certain parts of the summer, and they sold local fruits and vegetables in their produce shop. So, as you can see, I benefited from both farms in different ways.

Buying Food from
Health Food/Grocery Stores

STRATEGY 31
Buy from co-ops and smaller health food stores

There are so many benefits to shopping at cooperative (co-op) grocery stores and smaller health food stores. I find that smaller stores offer local produce that is often more flavorful and less expensive than what is found at major grocery chains. For example, I can buy some of the best local cantaloupe for $1.50 and watermelon for $3.00 at my local health food store, whereas my local grocery stores can't match this quality or price.

Not all health food stores are the same, so be sure to shop around. Some offer a variety of produce while others focus more on dry goods and supplements. Plus, some stores offer cheaper produce than others. For instance, my favorite health food stores have been Fresh-Rite in Buffalo, NY, where I could always count on finding amazing lettuce and dark leafy greens; Stanley's in Chicago, IL, a produce store that offers some of the best deals on produce that I have ever seen; Clark's Nutrition and Natural Food Market in Riverside, CA, a store that has some of the cheapest produce I have seen in California; Rainbow Grocery in San Francisco, CA, which in my opinion is the best co-op grocery store in the world; Berkeley Bowl in Berkeley, CA, which sells the widest variety of produce I have ever seen in a store; Nature's Food Patch in Clearwater, Florida, which has one of the best raw pizzas I have ever tasted (and it's affordable); and Nature's Pantry in State College, PA, a store that has supported my raw vegan lifestyle for the past 5 years by selling high-quality nuts, seeds, dried fruits, spices, and local produce.

STRATEGY 32
Buy from Asian and International markets

Shopping at Asian and international markets is a great way to obtain a lot of inexpensive produce. In fact, most people don't realize how much money they could save if they shopped at these markets. Often, Asian and International markets sell a wide range of produce like mangos, coconuts, peaches, durian, tomatoes, watermelon, ginger, garlic, daikon, bok choy, lettuce, basil, cilantro, and the list goes on. The downside is that these markets don't tend to carry organic produce. However, even non-organic produce is healthier than a hamburger. And at the very least, consider buying your coconuts from these markets. They are cheaper and fresher than the coconuts sold at other markets and grocery stores. Keep in mind that not all Asian and International markets are the same. Some markets sell more produce than others. So, shop around.

STRATEGY 33
Form or join a buying club

A buying club is an organized group of individuals or families who pool their resources and time to purchase high-quality, healthy foods in bulk from a warehouse distributor. Buying clubs allow individuals like you to save money on retail prices because the products are purchased directly from distributors. The easiest way to become a member of a buying club is to join an existing one. A buying club requires quite a bit of work to create and maintain it, including finding members to join, locating a distributor, placing orders, bookkeeping, finding/renting a location (e.g. community center) to have the products delivered, and sorting and distributing the products once they have arrived. You can find a buying club near you at http://www.unitedbuyingclubs.com/index.htm or do a Google search to find buying clubs in your state.

Another quick alternative to forming a buying club is to order items in bulk with several other people. In this case, you and your friends would order several items in bulk from a local health food store or online.

STRATEGY 34
Buy from bulk bins

Try to buy everything from bulk bins. It's increasingly popular for health food stores to sell nuts and seeds, dried fruits, spices and teas, oils, vinegars, sweeteners (e.g. agave and honey), and nut butters in bulk. Some stores even sell soap, hair shampoo and conditioner, seaweed, and fermented foods in bulk. Buying in bulk saves you money in two ways: first, you are not paying for the cost to package the food, and second, you can choose how much you need. For example, a 2.5 ounce bottle of organic cinnamon ($4.50) costs twice as much as that same amount in bulk ($2.15). Plus, with a 2.5 ounce bottle of cinnamon I have to buy 2.5 ounces, but what if I only need 1-2 teaspoons for a recipe? If I bought this small amount of cinnamon in bulk, it would cost me less than 10 cents, however, if I bought the bottle, it would cost me almost $5!

If your local health food store doesn't offer a item you want in bulk, you may be able to ask them to order it from one of their distributors. For example, every Fall I ask my health food store to order a 25lb bag of sunflower seeds from their distributor, and I store the seeds in my deep freezer. Not only do I save $15, but I am able to buy sunflowers seeds while they are in season, which means fat, juicy sunflower seeds all year long.

Lastly, consider buying sale items in bulk. If you see one of your favorite foods on sale, it may be worth buying extra and then freezing or drying them to eat later. For example, during the month of May, a local grocery store had amazing manila mangos for a great price, so I bought 8 of them and froze them (shown on the right in a gallon-sized bag). So,

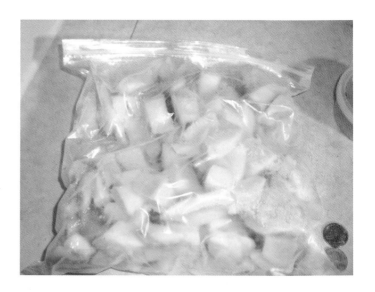

instead of buying frozen mangos for green smoothies from the store, I froze my own and saved $5.

When buying in bulk, it's important to have a plan for the food you buy. If you buy it and it goes to waste, then you haven't saved any money (in fact, you wasted money). Buying in bulk is only a savings if you eat all of the food.

STRATEGY 35
Keep an eye out for sales

This is really a given, but even I sometimes forget to use this strategy. I am so used to the foods I buy not being on sale, but the truth is that often fresh produce and raw food products do go on sale. If you know that a certain product or food will be on sale soon, plan to buy a lot of it so that you can stock up at a lower price. But be careful not to buy too much. It's not a good idea to buy tons of food simply because it's on sale. If it's nuts, seeds, or oils, I like to buy no more than 1-2 months worth when they are on sale because I know that my food preferences change over time. It's reasonable to expect that your tastes will change as the seasons change; so, it may take you longer than you think to eat all of the foods you bought on sale.

STRATEGY 36
Buy "seconds"

Yes, I mentioned this strategy in the previous section on buying produce from local farms, but it applies to grocery stores as well! Many grocery stores sell "seconds" (i.e., fruits that are ripe and need to be sold immediately). In my experience, I find that most major grocery chains do not offer seconds, but many smaller co-ops and health food stores do. And usually the food is 50% off the regular price. That's a huge discount! For example, I purchased 5 lbs of "second", organic, fair trade bananas at 49 cents a pound from a co-op in Pittsburgh. They were regularly priced at 99 cents, so I saved $2.50. Plus, I like my bananas to be very ripe before I eat them, so it was nice that they were already ripe and ready to go when I purchased them!

STRATEGY 37
Shop on produce delivery days

Often, it's cheaper to shop on days that produce is delivered to health food and grocery stores. On delivery days, the produce is fresher and less bruised, which means that it will last longer at home and save you money. Plus, grocery stores will often have sales on the days that produce is delivered in an effort to sell as much as possible before the produce loses its aesthetic appeal. So, talk to the produce staff at your local grocery and health food stores and ask them on which days their produce is delivered and if they plan to put any of it on sale.

STRATEGY 38
Don't buy convenience produce

In a busy world, convenience produce is a nice idea. The produce is already washed, cut up, and packaged nicely so you can eat it immediately; however, this convenience comes at a heavy cost. Convenience produce is much more expensive than regular produce and often isn't as tasty. For example, a one pound container of prewashed, ready-to-eat organic spring lettuce costs me $6 at my local grocery store. However, if I buy the lettuce by the head, I can get one pound of organic lettuce for $2.49 at the same store. So, for the same price as the convenience spring lettuce, I can buy almost three pounds of organic lettuce heads. What a huge difference! And there really is no difference in preparation time. I still have to wash the lettuce (it's always a good idea to wash pre-washed foods) and put it in a salad spinner. Another type of convenience food that people like to buy is pre-cut fruit, but I just don't understand it. I can buy a whole pineapple for the same or lower price as one small container of pre-cut pineapple. And at least with a whole pineapple, I can make sure I select one that is ripe and sweet. You don't have any idea how your pre-cut fruit will taste until after you buy it.

There is another reason to bypass convenience produce. Often convenience produce isn't as fresh as regular produce. There have been so many times when I have opened 1lb containers of salad mix and the lettuce had wilted in the middle. I have also bought prepackaged guacamole only to find out when I opened it that it had begun to ferment. So, bypass the convenience produce and head straight for the less expensive, fresher regular produce. It may take you a bit longer to cut and wash your own fruit and vegetables, but your wallet will thank you! Plus, you can always create your own convenience produce at home!

Buying Food Online and from Other Sources

STRATEGY 39
Buy foods from low-cost websites

There will be times when you need to buy specific items online. For example, I regularly buy hemp seeds and seaweed in bulk online because they are cheaper online and I don't have access to these items in bulk at my local grocery stores. The key to ordering foods online is to find the lowest price for the food(s) you want from sites that offer free or low-cost shipping. Some online stores are more expensive than others, so you may have to order your items from multiple websites. For example, I order my hemp seeds through www.amazon.com and even though they sell nori seaweed, I only order seaweed through www.pangaia.cc because they are cheaper. Ordering foods from multiple websites can be a little tricky because you have to factor in the multiple shipping costs, but it can be done.

When ordering online, consider partnering with a few friends to buy the items in bulk. You may not be able to afford 1 gallon of agave by yourself, but when you split it between 2 or 3 people, the cost becomes more reasonable. And if you and your friends spend enough, your order may qualify for free shipping.

If you are looking for low-cost websites, check out the budget-friendly, Raw Foods on a Budget online store (www.rawfoodsonabudget.com), which will be launched in October 2011. In the meatime, visit these great sites: www.pangaia.cc, www.rawfoodworld.com, and www.seaveg.com.

STRATEGY 40
Shop at discount stores

This is probably one of my favorite strategies and the one people expect the least. Many discount department stores like T.J. Maxx™, Tuesday Morning™, and Ross™ stock gourmet foods like high-quality olive oils (organic and non-organic), agave, and raw honey in their housewares sections. At my local T.J. Maxx™, I can usually find a 24 oz bottle of olive oil for only $9.99, whereas this bottle would have cost me at least $15 at any of my local grocery stores. And not only is it the same product, but it also tastes the same! I am very picky about oils and honey, and I will pay extra for great taste, but now I don't have to!

FUN Activities

Buying Food from Local Farms

ACTIVITY 1:

Join a CSA program!

Here are the steps for joining a CSA program. First, search for local CSA programs at www.localharvest.org/csa/ and make a list of available programs. Because some programs have their own website, check to see if you can find each program online. If they are not online, you will have to call the farm to ask about their CSA program schedule, the type of produce offered, the pick-up location, and program costs. Also make sure to ask if you get to select the produce or if it comes in a prepackaged box. Ask them about the sizes of the farm share (e.g. family size, individual size, large, medium, etc.), the average number of pounds that come in a share, whether separate fruit and vegetable shares are available, and whether the produce is organic or sprayed with pesticides. Make a list of all this information so that you can compare the advantages and disadvantages of each CSA program. In addition, you might find it useful to estimate how much each program will cost you per week. For example, if the CSA program will provide you with 13 weeks of food, divide the total cost of the share by the number of weeks. Use the cost per week amounts to do a price comparison between CSA programs.

ACTIVITY 2:

Visit your local farmers market(s)!

Make a commitment to visit your local farmers market this coming weekend! If you are lucky and have several farmers markets, go to a different one each weekend until you figure out which ones you like best. Every farmers market is different, and they can differ in the type of produce offered, number of farms that sell organic produce, and prices. I have even seen the same farm at two different farmers markets offering two different prices on the same produce. So shop around and have fun.

ACTIVITY 3:

Find and visit a local farm!

You may be surprised to find out that your nearest farm is a lot closer than you think. One time, I found a strawberry farm right around the corner from my mother's house! You can find local farms at www.localharvest.org or www. eatwellguide.org. If the farm has a website, look it up to see what kinds of produce are available, and whether the farm sells produce on site, has a CSA program, and/or offers fruit picking. Also, make sure the farm is open to the public and call ahead before you visit the farm just in case the information on the farm's website is inaccurate. Now all you have to do is go! Why not go this coming weekend?

Buying Food from Health Food/Grocery Stores

ACTIVITY 4:
Check out your local Asian or international market

Find and visit a local Asian or international market. If you are lucky, you will have access to more than one. Sometimes these markets can be intimidating because the food labels are often in a different language. However, with raw foods this should not be problem. You don't need a label to identify a mango or coconut. Consider making a plan to visit one or two of these markets this weekend. Take your time to browse and get comfortable. If you have any questions, talk to the staff. In my experience, I have found the staff at these markets to be extremely nice and helpful. Also, ask them if they have any discounts for buying foods like coconuts in bulk.

ACTIVITY 5:
Find and visit your local cooperative (co-op) grocery store!

I just love a good co-op. They have the best produce, and shopping at these stores is a great way to support your local economy. Consider visiting one this coming weekend! Also inquire about joining the co-op. Co-ops are member-owned and by becoming a member you receive a discount on your purchases.

ACTIVITY 6:
Do your own produce price comparison!

In this activity, you will compare the prices found at your local large grocery store to the prices found at your local co-op or health food store. This activity will help you decide where you should buy your produce and other food items. Using the worksheet on page 75, first make a list of the items you want to compare at both stores. Next, visit the large grocery chain, locate each item on your list, and then write in the worksheet the prices for each item. Also remember to rate the quality of each item (1=low, 4=high). Next, visit the co-op and do the same thing. Once you have all the prices and quality ratings, compare them.

ACTIVITY 7:
Practice buying in bulk

Make a list of the foods you eat on a regular basis and try to purchase these items in bulk. For example, I eat sunflower seeds, seaweed, and hemp seeds almost everyday. Because I eat these foods very often, buying them in bulk helps me to stay on budget. For example, I can buy a package of 10 nori sheets for $5, but I can get 50 sheets for $14 if I buy them online. That is a savings of $11! And given that I eat at least 100 sheets of nori per month, buying in them bulk saves me $22 a month.

Buying Food Online and from Other Sources

ACTIVITY 8:
Forage for goodies at local discount department stores!

Often discount department stores like T.J. Maxx™, Ross™, and Tuesday Morning™ sell gourmet foods like olive oils, honey, agave, and balsamic vinegar. And usually these foods are cheaper at these stores than they are at grocery and health food stores. So, visit a local discount department store and see what you can find!

DO YOUR OWN PRICE COMPARISON!

In this activity, you get to do your own price comparison! How exciting! Using this worksheet, first list up to 13 foods that you typically buy or would like to purchase from your local grocery store. Next, visit your local, major grocery store and write down the prices and quality of your listed foods. For example, if you have oranges on your list and the oranges you find are of poor quality then give it a rating of 1. However, if the quality is superb then rate it a 4. Lastly, visit your local co-op or health food store, locate all 13 foods, and write down the price and quality of each food. Once you have completed the worksheet, compare the quality and cost of each item. This activity will help you determine the type of items you should buy from each store on a regular basis.

Food Items	Price at Major Grocery Chain	Quality Rating	Price at Co-op/ Health Food Store	Quality Rating
1		1 2 3 4		1 2 3 4
2		1 2 3 4		1 2 3 4
3		1 2 3 4		1 2 3 4
4		1 2 3 4		1 2 3 4
5		1 2 3 4		1 2 3 4
6		1 2 3 4		1 2 3 4
7		1 2 3 4		1 2 3 4
8		1 2 3 4		1 2 3 4
9		1 2 3 4		1 2 3 4
10		1 2 3 4		1 2 3 4
11		1 2 3 4		1 2 3 4
12		1 2 3 4		1 2 3 4
13		1 2 3 4		1 2 3 4

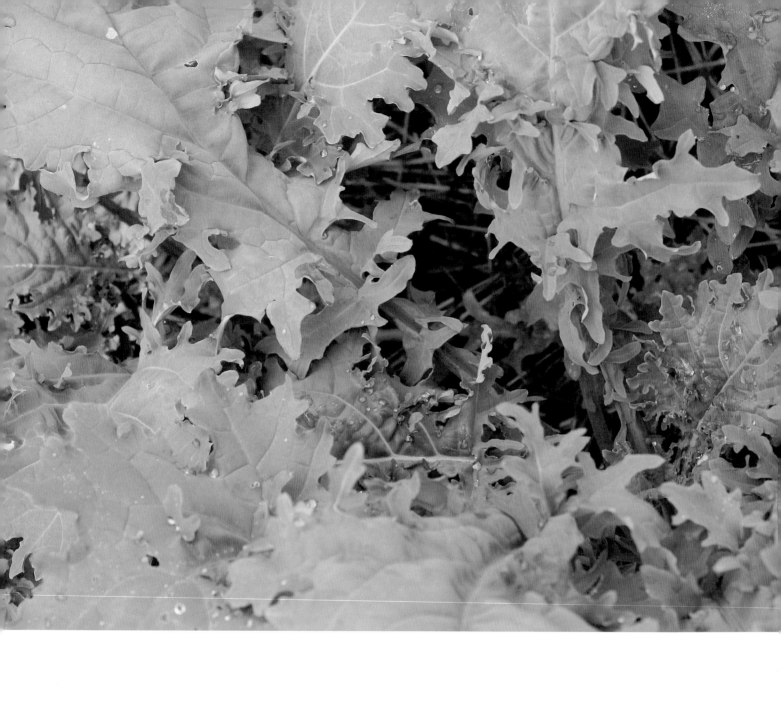

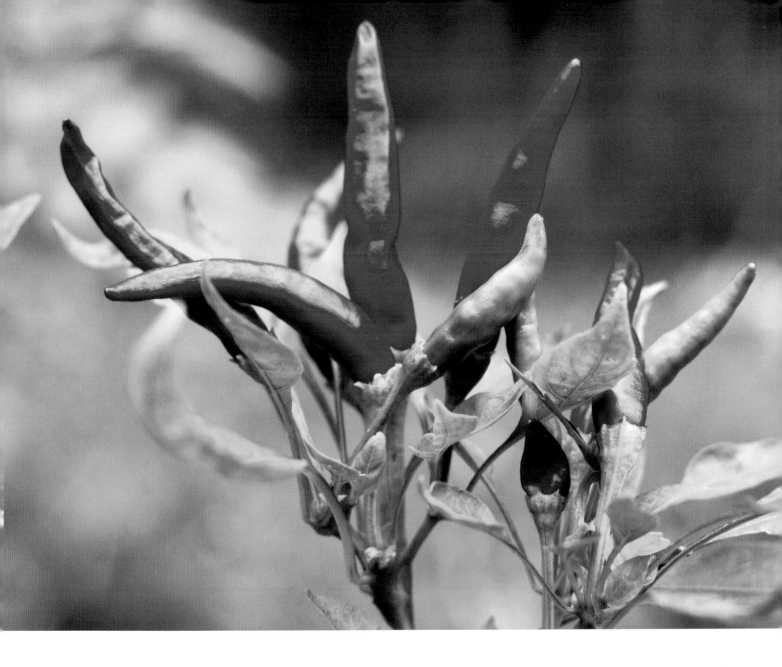

CHAPTER 9
GROW Your Own Food!

Get Ready, Get Set, let's garden! You

don't need a green thumb, a ton of tools, a lot of money, or even land to have a garden. A garden can be as simple as you make it, such as a pot of herbs in your kitchen or a small 2x5 foot garden in your backyard (shown on page 79). Plus, the benefits of gardening are endless! Growing your own fruits and vegetables is the best way to obtain high-quality fruits and vegetables at the lowest cost.

There are many benefits to gardening! Gardening is an opportunity to connect with Mother Nature and the food you eat. So much of our food is purchased at grocery stores, making it easy to forget that our food comes from a large, diverse ecosystem of plants, microorganisms, and wildlife. Another benefit to having a garden is that you get to determine how your food is grown. If you want an organic garden, then you can have one. In many cases, this is much easier (and cheaper) than finding and purchasing produce from a certified organic farm. Having a garden also reduces the amount of time from when a food is harvested to when it's eaten. Typically, the fruits and vegetables that are sold at grocery stores have travelled long distances and have been stored for one to three weeks before they reach your kitchen. This can result in significant nutrition loss as the nutrients in fruits and vegetables begin to degrade quickly after harvest. But, when you have your own garden, you can pick fruits and vegetables right before you eat them, thus minimizing nutrient degradation. Plus, when you have a garden, you can pick what you will use. So, rather than buying a head of lettuce from the store, you can pick exactly what you need.

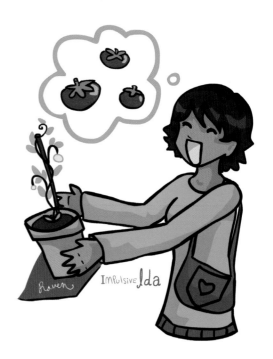

So, where do you start? There are many ways to start a garden and some are better than others. The goal of this chapter is to present the most cost-effective methods to starting the garden you have always wanted. But, before you learn what to do, first, I will show you what not to do. Here's our friend Impulsive Ida:

It's spring…the sun is out…and all signs of the winter have passed! It's a marvelous day and Ida can't help but smile as she walks up to the grocery store. But before she enters, Ida spots a beautiful display of ready-to-transplant tomato plants (shipped in this week from God knows where). She stops to view the plants and immediately begins to fantasize about tasting amazing tomatoes grown with her very own hands. So, she decides to buy 2 tomato plants (at $3.99 a piece) to plant in her small backyard. Al-

though she doesn't have a garden, she figures that she could easily prepare a small area in her backyard for the two plants. Well, the thought was easier than the action. It took Ida 3 weeks to make time to prepare the backyard. Eventually she got it done and put the tomato plants in the ground. Sadly, over the next 2 months, the tomatoes didn't grow like they did in her fantasy. The plants were producing fruit, but many of the leaves were discolored and chewed up by some unknown pest, and the fruits were weighing the stems down, which caused the fruits to quickly rot as they stayed in contact with the soil. She quickly did some research online and learned that the tomatoes she purchased needed some kind of physical support. She rushed to her local nursery to purchase tomato cages, but they were sold out for the season. She ended up using stakes and twine, but the plants were still having problems standing up. In addition, Ida learned that her plants were suffering from late blight and hornworms, two major pests of tomato plants. Sadly, by the end of the growing season, Ida had only enjoyed 2 small tomatoes from her garden.

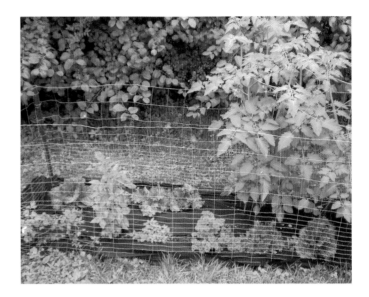

As you can see from Ida's experience, gardening is a process. No one becomes a master gardener overnight; however, there are several steps that Ida could have taken to get the most from her garden. The most important step that Ida overlooked was planning her garden. Like many of us, Ida was drawn in by the romantic ideas of tasting juicy fruits and vegetables that were grown with her own hands. She really didn't know what she was doing because she had not prepared herself to create a successful garden. Ida could have benefited from doing some initial research on how to grow her specific variety of tomatoes. By doing this, she would have learned about her plants' soil, water, and sunlight requirements, as well as how to prepare her backyard to meet these requirements.

To prevent you from taking the same path as Impulsive Ida, in this chapter, I will show you how to create a successful garden in a budget-friendly way! The chapter is organized into two sections: the first section presents seven strategies to guide you in planing your garden, and the second section provides seven strategies to help you find low-cost/free gardening materials.

Strategies for Planning Your Garden

STRATEGY 41
Start small

The idea of growing your own food is exciting, but sometimes this enthusiasm can translate into long store receipts and a lot of unused gardening supplies. So, start small, particularly if this is your first garden. Plus, there are benefits to starting small. It's often the case that we don't know what we are signing up for when we create our first garden. Gardens need attention and it's not enough to plant some seeds and come back a few months later to pick the fruit. Just like babies, seeds need tender loving care and protection, as well as nurturing as they grow. They need to be well-fed and watered, and protected from pests like aphids, deer, chipmunks, rabbits, and, in some cases, bears. For example, I have two gardens at home that cover 400 square feet of land. The first garden is right outside of my front door and I use it to grow sun-loving plants like tomatoes, strawberries, cucumbers, and peppers. And I have to admit that because of its location, I give it the most attention. In the second garden, located on the side of the house, I grow leafy greens, raspberries, and some sun-loving plants. Unfortunately, this garden receives less attention and it shows. This garden isn't as pretty and the plants don't grow as well. If I could do it all over again, I would just have one large garden covering 300 square feet in the front of my house. And it would have been easier for me to learn this if I had started small instead of starting big. Plus, I would have saved a lot of time and money as well. It has been 2 years since I created the second garden and there are still seeds and gardening supplies I haven't used yet!

Another benefit to starting small is that it gives you the time to learn the characteristics of your growing environment (soil, sun exposure, and water conditions). For example, soils can range from being sandy to clay-like, to having an abundance of microorganisms to barely having any, to having a low pH to being more alkaline, etc. Because soils can vary so drastically, it's not the case that you can throw a seed into the ground and watch it grow into a masterpiece. There may be soil amendments (e.g. compost, sulfur, etc.) that need to be made to prepare the soil for your specific plants. For example, last season I learned that strawberries like an extra boost of phosphorous in the soil, so I purchased a bag of bone meal (the only source of phosphorous I could find at the time; rock phosphate is a great vegan source) and sprinkled it into the compost that I was adding to the soil. And it worked! The strawberries were twice as big as they were last year and the most flavorful I have ever tasted! Another characteristic of your growing environment is the amount of sunlight it receives. If you plan to grow fruits like strawberries, tomatoes, cucumbers, etc., they require at least 6-8 hours of sun. In contrast, plants like lettuce and dark leafy greens prefer cooler temperatures and less sun. Therefore, it's ideal that you choose a location for your garden that will allow you to grow the fruits and vegetables you want to eat. The final major characteristic of your growing environment are the water conditions. How much rain will your garden receive during the growing season? Ideally, your plants will receive 1-inch of rain water per week, but if they don't, you may have to water the plants yourself. Keep in mind that you don't want your plants to receive too much water as this may cause their roots to rot; therefore, it's important that your plants have proper drainage. A simple way to achieve this is to place your garden on a patch of land that's on a slight incline. Overall, soil and water conditions, and sun exposure are important factors when starting a garden, and it works to your benefit to start small so that you give yourself the time to learn about them.

STRATEGY 42
PLAN it out!!!

It can be so tempting to buy a few vegetable or fruit plants at the grocery store, return home, and plant them into the ground. However, often when we do this, our plants don't grow very well or they simply die. This happens because we haven't planned out how we should take care of these plants. Do we have the right soil, an adequate amount of nutrients in the soil, the right amount of sun exposure, and enough time to take care of the plants, etc.? The benefit of creating a garden plan is that it forces you to outline exactly what you want to grow, when you will grow it, what materials you need, whether amendments to the soil are needed, and how much sun and water your plants will need. Plus, when you have a plan, it's easier to find a gardening book that will fit your needs. There are so many books out there, and having a well-thought out garden plan will help you find the perfect book for you.

Step 1. Decide what you want to grow. This first step is simple and fun! Using the worksheet on pages 91-93, list all the plants that you would like to grow right now. Remember to keep it small. After you finish making the list,

SIMPLE PLANTS TO GROW

Name	When to Plant	Sun & Temperature	Soil	Water	Major Pests
Tomatoes	Early spring	Sun to full sun >45 degrees F	Any type pH: 5.5 to 7	Normal to moist	Aphids, cutworms, hornworms, flea beetles, nematodes
Romaine Lettuce	Spring, summer, fall	Full sun in spring/fall; Partial shade in summer	Rich, well-drained, loose loam pH: 6.2-6.8	Keep moist, frequent short watering	Slugs, aphids, leaf hoppers
Strawberries	Early spring	Full sun	Light, dry, well-drained pH: 5.8 to 6.5	Frequent, thorough watering; 1-2 inches of water per week	Slugs, spider mites, birds, deer

go back through it and indicate the time of year its needs to be planted, the amount of sun exposure required (i.e. how many hours), type of soil required (e.g. pH), and the amount of water required for each plant. Also consider the type of protection your plants will need. Because there are a lot of pests that can potentially harm your plants, just consider the major pests for now. Keep in mind that some of these pests will be animals like rabbits and groundhogs. An easy, though time-consuming, solution can be to put up a fence, and in the case of groundhogs, make sure that the fence goes 6-inches deep into the soil. Hanging aluminium pans is a great deterrent for ground hogs and birds as well. You can find more of this kind of information on the Internet, or by looking through your seed packets or gardening books. To help you get started, I have provided this information for several easy-to-grow fruits and vegetables in the table on page 81.

Step 2. Decide where you CAN grow your garden. Once you have your list, you will be in the perfect position to choose the location for your garden. The biggest factor in choosing your garden's location is the amount of sunlight it receives. Although the soil condition and rate of rainfall are important, you can easily fix these by amending the soil with compost or watering your garden more often. It's practically impossible to add more sunlight. If you have mostly sun loving plants on your list like tomatoes, peppers, cucumbers, and fruits, then you will need an area that receives at least 6 hours of sun exposure a day. However, if leafy greens like romaine, kale, and/or collards, dominate your list, then an area with less sun exposure would be best. To determine the amount of sun exposure that an area receives, simply count the number of hours of direct sunlight it receives on a sunny day. The same goes if you plan on growing a container garden (shown on next page). Be sure that the location you plan to place your containers meets your plants' sun requirements. If you would like to grow your garden indoors, such as an herb garden, then you will need a windowsill that receives a lot of sunlight. You can even add additional lighting such as an indoor grow light.

So far, I have talked about gardening as though you had a space for one. But what happens when you don't have space for a backyard garden or even a container garden. Two great options are to participate in a community garden or rent a small plot of land. Community gardens provide opportunities for local residents to grow their own fruits, vegetables, and flowers. Though the guidelines vary, in general, a community garden is a public space owned by local governments and not-for-profit associations that are maintained by the gardeners themselves. Some community gardens allow you to have individual plots for personal use, while others are collectively grown and shared. To find a community garden near you, visit the American Community Gardening Association at www.communitygarden.org. The second option for obtaining land to grow a garden is to rent a small plot of land from the Cooperative Extension office at your nearby university or college. For example, the Cooperative Extension office at Penn State offers 10' x 10' plots for only $10 for the whole growing season. They may also offer a Master Gardener program, where you can learn how to grow fruits, vegetables, and flowers. For example, the University of California (UC) Cooperative Extension office in Los Angeles county (http://celosangeles.ucdavis.edu/Common_Ground_Garden_Program) offers Master Gardener and Victory Gardener programs, provides opportunities to participate in community gardens, and helps to support several gardens at local schools and homeless shelters.

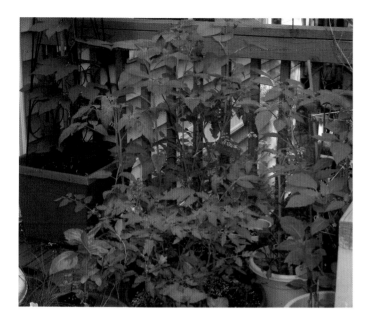

Step 3. Find the perfect fit. Now that you have your list and garden location, it's time to evaluate whether you can actually grow the specific plants on your list in your garden location. If your list contains sun-loving plants but the location of your garden doesn't receive at least 6 hours of sun, then remove these plants from your list or choose another garden location. If only one part of your garden receives a lot of sun, then plan to put your sun-loving plants there. You may also have plants that require specific soil conditions such as blueberries, which require a more acidic soil; however, if the necessary changes can't be made to fit your plants' requirements, remove these plants from your list. Also, consider whether the water conditions of your garden location fits the needs of your plants. It may be that because of where your garden is located (e.g., dry climate with a lot of sun exposure), your plants will require frequent watering. If you cannot provide enough water to meet their needs, consider removing the water-loving plants from your list and growing more drought-tolerant ones instead (or finding drought-tolerant varieties of your original plants). It's better to grow what will be successful than to waste space, money, and time on trying to grow a plant that will grow poorly and only produce one to two fruits (or leaves).

Step 4. Be practical. At this point, you have chosen the plants that you want to grow. Now, let's focus on what you need to grow. Is your list too long? If this is your first garden, keep the list short. Think of it this way: you can either learn from growing 2-3 plants really well or growing 6-8 plants poorly. Next, think of all the materials you will need to buy to grow those plants. Remember that buying a plant is the cheapest part, so leave room for the additional expenses that may come up. And, think about how much time you have. You may only have a few hours a week to devote to your garden, but this may not be enough for a large garden. Be realistic with how much time you have, otherwise, your plants will be neglected and grow poorly.

STRATEGY 43
Focus on cash crops

When planning your garden, you may be tempted to grow a whole variety of fruits and vegetables. I know I always am! However, you may get more miles out of your money and time if you focus on growing cash crops, that is, fruits and vegetables that are normally expensive for you to buy at the store. For example, heirloom tomatoes are very expensive to purchase at grocery stores, which is pretty crazy considering how easy they are to grow. In fact, an heirloom tomato plant can produce so many fruits that it becomes difficult to keep up with it. Another example is parsley. I have several bunches of parsley growing in my garden, however, because organic parsley is only $0.99 a bunch at my local grocery store, it really isn't worth my time to grow it. Rather, I could use this time to focus on growing raspberries, which are expensive to buy. So, consider growing the pricier fruits and vegetables when creating your gardening plan. However, if you really want to grow a specific plant, don't let this stop you. Just go for it!

STRATEGY 44
Don't do it alone

Creating and maintaining a garden can be a lot of work and very expensive. When I created my two 20 x 10 ft. gardens, I had three people (2 roommates and a friend) helping me turnover the soil, put in the water hoses, and set up the fence. And some of my friends even helped me weed, put in new plants, and take care of the garden. And since we shared the cost of the garden (i.e. time and materials), we also shared the profits. This saved me a whole lot of money and time! Plus, it was nice to share big gardening milestones with my friends.

STRATEGY 45
Educate yourself

The longer you garden, the more you will learn about the gardening process. You will learn from your trials and errors, as well as from observing your plants. However, you might want to speed up the learning process by attending free workshops, volunteering at a local nursery, and/or tak-

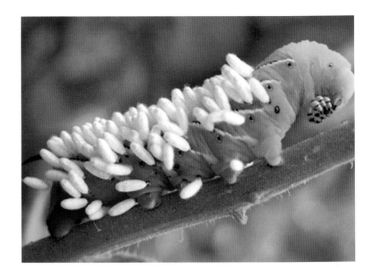

ing a Master Gardener's course. Check with your local farms and health food stores for information about free or low-cost gardening classes. Your county extension program office may also offer free workshops on gardening and composting. Also contact local nurseries to see if they have opportunities to volunteer. Be sure to mention that you are interested in learning more about gardening and plants so that they give you tasks that meet your interest. In addition, you may be able to find a local Master Gardener's program. The Master Gardener's program originated in 1972 to provide research-based gardening information to home gardeners. The program is available through local universities in 48 states in the United States and three Canadian provinces. Having gone through the program myself, I can honestly say that this course helped me gain a deep appreciation of gardening and the diverse ecosystem of microorganisms, insects, and animals that inhabit and surround my garden. The course is low-cost and scholarships may be available. For more information about Master Gardening programs, visit the American Horticultural Society website (http://www.ahs.org).

STRATEGY 46
Learn the life cycles in your garden

When you create a garden, you are creating a small city for insects, birds, microorganisms, and larger animals. Life goes where life is, and a key to gardening is learning how to interact with the life cycles of these organisms in ways that support the growth of your plants. For example, the tomato hornworm (also referred to as the tobacco hornworm; shown on the top left) is a major pest of tomato plants. The tomato hornworm is a type of moth that is in its larvae stage (i.e., the juvenile form that many insects undergo before metamorphosis into adult form) and feeds on the foliage of your tomato plants. Just a handful can massacre your tomato plants in a week or so! However, you can allow nature to take care of these pests for you. Because you have a garden, you may have also attracted the parasitic braconid wasp. Don't worry, these wasps are your friends. They are predators to several common garden pests including aphids, caterpillars, beetles, and stink bugs, and they consider the hornworm to be a delicious "meals-on-wheels" buffet! Basically, the female wasp lays her eggs into the bodies of a hornworm and, as the eggs hatch, the wasp larvae feed internally. You will see the wasp larvae emerge from the hornworm in their white cocoons (shown on left), and when you do, leave the hornworm alone. These wasps have taken care of the hornworm for you and will continue to do so all season long. Although, you may be thinking, "Wasps! Why would I want to keep wasps in my garden? Is it worth the trade off?" Yes! These wasps are rarely longer than 1/2-inch, so you barely notice them! Just allow nature to do the work for you!

Overall, as you continue to garden and connect with the soil, you will begin to learn the life cycles of the organisms that inhabit your garden, and, with time, interact with them in ways that encourage the healthy growth of your fruits and vegetables.

STRATEGY 47
Acceptance

Gardening is a process, so it's important to accept where you are. No one becomes a perfect gardener overnight. It may happen that your first crop of fruits and vegetables don't look like the perfect produce sold at farmers markets. That's okay because it takes time to learn how to garden. For example, consider my first garden: a container garden on the rooftop patio of my apartment in Oakland, California. The weather was great, but somehow I couldn't get anything to survive. When a plant did produce a fruit, the bugs got to it before I did. However, my next container garden was better. I did more research and it showed. My plants were healthier and produced some fruit. And every year since then, my garden has substantially improved and now I am able to produce enough food to reduce my food costs. But, it took 4 years of mistakes and lessons to figure things out…and I am still learning. So, remember to appreciate where you are in the gardening process and give yourself the opportunity to learn.

Strategies for Finding Low-Cost or FREE Gardening Materials

STRATEGY 48
Composting

Compost is the black gold of the gardening world. It's the best way to put nutrients back into the soil and is the least expensive as well. According to Compost.org, compost improves soil texture, structure, and aeration by loosening clay soils and improving the water-holding capacity of sandier soils. Plus, compost adds naturally-produced nitrogen, potassium, and phosphorus to your soil, which reduces the need for additional soil amendments like commercial fertilizers. In addition, according to the United States Environmental Protection Agency (www.epa.org), compost helps to:

- suppress plant diseases and pests

- produce higher yields of fruits and vegetables

- amend contaminated, compacted (e.g. clay soils), and marginal soils

- remove solids, oils, grease, and heavy metals from storm water runoff

The best way to get compost is to produce it at home. For example, many gardeners maintain a backyard compost pile consisting of leaves, lawn clippings, and other organic matter (see table below for acceptable materials). Compost piles are easy to create and maintain; all you have to do is start a pile of acceptable organic matter and mix it up (with a shovel) every time something new is added. The worms and fungi

WHAT CAN YOU COMPOST?

Yes	No
Clean paper	Black walnut tree leaves and twigs
Coffee grounds and filters	Coal and charcoal ash
Cotton rags	Dairy products (e.g. butter, milk, sour cream)
Eggshells	Diseased or insect ridden plants
Fruits and vegetables	Fats, grease, lard, or oils
Grass clippings	Meat or fish bones and scraps
Leaves	Pet wastes
Nut shells	Yard trimmings treated with chemical pesticides
Shredded newspaper	
Tea Bags	

Source: Environmental Protection Agency (http://www.epa.gov/epawaste/conserve/rrr/composting/basic.htm#todo)

will break up the materials and a year later, your compost will be ready.

A quicker way to generate compost is to do vermicomposting (i.e. worm composting). Basically, you add food scraps (e.g. non-meat items like vegetable tops, fruit peels, egg shells, coffee grounds) and other organic materials to a small or large bin containing red worms (you can buy these bins or create your own). The worms quickly turn your scraps into nutrient-rich "castings" that can be used in your garden. The process is more involved than managing a compost pile; however, it's a convenient way to recycle food waste and is ideal for people who do not have outdoor space for a compost pile. For more information on composting, visit http://www.epa.gov/epawaste/conserve/rrr/composting/index.htm.

When starting your own compost pile or bin it's often useful to first check with your county, city, or municipality because they may offer low-priced or free composting bins, composting workshops, and even FREE compost! Composting has become increasingly popular among these public entities because it reduces the amount of waste that ends up in their landfills. According to the EPA, yard and food waste togeth-

PLANTS SUITABLE TO GROW IN CONTAINERS

Herbs	Vegetables	Fruits
Anise	Beets	Blackberries
Basil	Carrots	Blueberries
Caraway	Cabbage	Raspberries
Chervil	Swiss Chard	Strawberries
Chives	Cucumbers	
Coriander (Cilantro)	Eggplant	
Dill	Kale	
Fennel	Lettuce	
Marjoram	Mustard Greens	
Mint	Onions, Green	
Parsley	Peppers, Bell	
Summer Savory	Squash, Summer	
Thyme	Tomatoes	

Source: West Virginia University Extension Service (http://anr.ext.wvu.edu/lawn_garden/herbs/container_gardening#fn1)

er make up 23% of the US waste stream, which makes composting a huge money saver for cities and counties. Many municipalities are starting composting programs, in which yard waste is collected from residents at curbside similar to the way trash is collected and then taken to a central location to be composted. The compost is used in public works projects like maintaining public parks and a significant portion is sold or given away. For example, twice a week during the spring and summer, my city drops off large piles of compost at local parks for residents to pick up for FREE. Or, if I prefer, I can go to the Solid Waste Authority and pick up 35lb bags of compost for $3 a piece. The downside to using public generated compost is that many residents may have used fertilizers, pesticides, and other chemicals in their yard, so you cannot control the chemicals that end up in this compost. Nevertheless, it's a nice way to get some initial compost.

STRATEGY 49
Find free or low-cost land

If you have a backyard, you already have access to "free" land, but what if you rent an apartment or live in California (where even if you own a home, you may only have access to 2 feet of usable soil). As mentioned in Strategy 42, one option is to start a container garden. A container garden is simply a garden of plants growing in containers. Although most plants prefer to be grown in the ground, you can surprisingly grow a large variety of fruits, vegetables, and herbs in containers (shown in the table on page 87). My first two gardens were container gardens. Although I have had more success with growing herbs and leafy greens in pots, I have also grown heirloom tomatoes that reached 6 feet tall. And now, it's popular to grow tomatoes in upside-down containers. For $10 or $15, you can buy a kit containing a pot, hanging tools, and tomato seeds. As long as the toma-

toes receive at least 6-8 hours of full sun per day, you can hang them and grow them anywhere. For help in making your own hanging tomato container, do a Google search for "hanging tomatoes". In addition, as mentioned in Strategy 44, if you absolutely have no space, you may be able to rent or obtain a free plot of land from a community garden and/or the Cooperative Extension office at your nearby university or college. Refer to Step 2 in Strategy 42 for more information on these programs.

What if you have the space for a garden, but the soil is unusable or there is no soil at all (i.e., gravel or cement)? One option is to create a lasagna garden. Lasagna gardening is a way to build a garden from the ground up. The garden is built by creating layers of different materials like newspaper and compost. For example, the first layer can be newspapers, the next straw, then compost and humus, followed by newspapers, straw, compost, and humus again. This is also a nice way to avoid digging up thick grass. You can just layer these organic materials on the grass, and the worms, fungi, and other microorganisms will breakdown the grass for you. For more information about lasagna gardening, check out the amazing book, *Lasagna Gardening: A New Layering System for Bountiful Gardens* by Patricia Lanza.

STRATEGY 50
Save your own seeds

Seeds are one of the most expensive materials in the gardening process. If you have the space and are ambitious like me, you will want to grow a large variety of plants; the problem is that seed costs can quickly add up, especially if the seeds are certified organic. A quick way to get "free" seeds is to save your own seeds from the produce you buy. This can be done with many fruit bearing plants and legumes like melons, loquats, and peas. For example, the next time you are eating a magnificent watermelon (with seeds), just save a handful of the seeds. Wash them and allow them to dry out on newspaper or a paper towel for several days. After they have dried, place them in a sealed, plastic bag and now they are ready to use. Some seeds require a little more work such as tomato seeds. To save tomato seeds, the seeds must be fermented to remove the gel coating, which inhibits seed germination. To do this, slice open a tomato and squeeze the pulp and seeds into a glass jar. Fill the jar with water until it's 3/4 full, and stir and set aside for a few days. After a few days you will notice a smelly mold residue collecting at the top of the water. Soon the water will clear and the good "alive" seeds will sink to the bottom. This process will take 4-5 days, and when it's done, just remove the water and mold, and pour the seeds onto a piece of newspaper or paper towel and allow them to dry. Once they are dry, you can store them in a sealed, plastic bag.

STRATEGY 51
Participate in seed exchange programs and events

This is a fun and easy way to obtain new seeds. Seed Exchange programs are grass-roots organizations that facilitate the sharing of seeds among communities of gardeners. For example, the Seeds Savers Exchange (www.seedsavers.org) is a 35 year-old non-profit aimed at saving the diverse garden heritage of North America by building a network of individuals committed to collecting, conserving, and sharing heirloom seeds and plants. Although a small fee is required for membership (to help support the organization), members exchange seeds by listing their available seeds in the annual Seed Savers Annual Yearbook, which is sent out every Fall.

If a member finds a particular seed they want, he or she will contact the member who has the seed, and that's it. There are other seed exchange programs all over the world, including the Appalachian Heirloom Seed Conservancy in the United States, the Heritage Seed Library in the United Kingdom, and the Seeds' Savers Network in Australia. There are also free online seed exchange programs such as the Backyard Gardener Seed Exchange (www.backyardgardener.com/seed-exchange/wwwboard.html), Seed Exchange - GardenWeb (www.forums2.gardenweb.com/forums/exseed/), and Seed Swaps (www.seedswaps.com).

There may even be annual seed-exchange events in your area that are hosted by local horticultural societies, gardening groups, Master Gardening programs, and environmental non-profits. The easiest way to find out about these events is to contact your local nursery or Master Gardener's program, or search online.

STRATEGY 52
Create a test garden in your kitchen

This is something I came up with when I started learning about gardening. Basically, you keep a few black plastic containers filled with seed-friendly soil on your kitchen windowsill and every time you find a seed in your fruits or vegetables, stick one of them into the soil. Sometimes the seed grows and sometimes it doesn't, but that's a part of the process. More often than not, the seed will grow into a plant that you can transplant into your garden. In the past, I have planted seeds from dates, loquats, watermelon, peas, and cantaloupe. Although the plant did not always survive (e.g. the date plant), it was a fun and cool process to be a part of.

STRATEGY 53
Borrow tools from a friend!

If you are starting your first garden, you may find it useful to borrow some of the more expensive gardening tools from a friend. For example, a spading fork, a tool used for aerating the soil and transplanting, can easily cost you $20 or more. This can be expensive when you already have other more basic gardening supplies (e.g. gloves, a trowel, twine, shears) to buy. So, save yourself some cash and ask a friend (or neighbor) if you can borrow a tool or two.

STRATEGY 54
Check online for free or low-cost gardening supplies

There is nothing like receiving expensive stuff for free! To keep the costs low for creating and maintaining your garden, consider using websites like Craigslist™ and The Freecycle Network™ to find free or low-cost gardening supplies in your area. Craigslist™ (www.craigslist.org) is an online network of communities that feature online classified advertisements for items for sale and free stuff, as well as jobs, housing, and personals. When I started my first container garden, I used Craigslist™ to find several free and low-cost, used plant containers. Another good resource for free and low-cost materials is the Freecycle Network™. The Freecycle Network™ is made up of 7.5 million people from around the world interested in reusing and keeping used "good stuff" out of landfills. Here's how it works: you sign up for a local Freecycle group (e.g. I am signed up for the Centre County Freecycle) at www.freecycle.org, and every time someone posts a free item or is looking for an item, you will receive an email. It's that simple.

Like any other website, it's important that you use caution when using Craigslist™ and the Freecycle Network™. Although most of the individuals who use these websites are trustworthy, a few individuals have used these websites for violent crime. More often than not, you will be asked to pick up the free or low-cost item from a person's home; however, avoid this if possible. Or, ask the seller to leave the free items on the curb in front of their house. Overall, just use the same precautions online that you use offline. Here are some safety tips taken from the Craigslist™ website (http://www.craigslist.org/about/safety):

When meeting someone for the first time, remember to:

- Insist on a public meeting place like a café

- Do not meet in a secluded place, or invite strangers into your home

- Be especially careful when buying/selling high value items

- Tell a friend or family member where you're going

- Take your cell phone along if you have one

- Consider having a friend accompany you

- Trust your instincts

CREATE YOUR OWN GARDENING PLAN!

This is the most important step you can take towards creating the garden of your dreams. Creating a garden plan will force you to make choices up front about what plants to grow, when and where to plant them, what soil amendments to make, how often to water them, and how to protect them. Overall, a gardening plan will help you get the most from your efforts, money, and time.

PART 1: WHAT MY PLANTS NEED!

List the plants you want to grow and their growing requirements in the worksheet provided on page 92. Write down the following information for each plant. You can usually find this information on the seed packet or by searching online.

- **Plant Name.** Provide the name of the fruit, vegetable, or herb that you would like to grow.
- **When to Plant.** List the time of year when your plants need to be planted into the soil.
- **Sun & Temperature.** Write down the sunlight and temperature requirements of your plant. Does it need to grow above a certain temperature like tomatoes? Does it need 6+ hours of full sun like watermelon?
- **Soil Conditions.** Does your plant have soil requirements? Does it require a certain pH or moist soil conditions?
- **Water Conditions.** List the water conditions for your plant. Does it need more or less than 1-inch of water per week?
- **Major Pests/Other Requirements.** What are your plant's major pests? Does your plant have any other requirements (e.g. needing physical support)?

PART 2: HOW I WILL KEEP MY PLANTS HAPPY!

Write down all the ways you plan to meet your plants' requirements in the worksheet provided on page 93.

- **Week/Month to Plant.** List the week and month that you will plant your plant.
- **Sun & Temperature.** Write down the planned location of your plant. Be sure to choose a spot where their sunlight needs will be met. Also, indicate how you will protect your plant from very cold and very hot weather.
- **Soil Amendments.** List the soil amendments you will make to nurture your plant (e.g. compost).
- **Watering Schedule.** Write down how often you will water your plant and by what means you will water your plant (e.g. by hand, using soaker hoses or ollas).
- **Protection from Pests/Other Needs.** Indicate how you will protect your plant from major pests and what you will do to meet any additional needs.

Because there is limited space on the worksheets, consider using extra sheets of paper if you have a lengthy plant list.

PART 1. WHAT MY PLANTS NEED!

Plant Name	When to Plant	Sun & Temperature	Soil Conditions	Water Conditions	Major Pests/Other Requirements
Soctia Tomatoes	Early spring (after the last frost)	> 45 degrees F Full Sun	Any type, but likes to have a rich soil	Very thirsty plants	Hornworm, aphids, late blight, early blight. Physical support like a tomato cage or bamboo stake.

PART 2. HOW I WILL KEEP MY PLANTS HAPPY!

Week/Month to Plant	Sun & Temperature	Soil Amendments	Watering Schedule	Protection from Pests/ Other Needs
Plant in last 2 weeks in April or early May (make sure the last frost date has passed).	Plant in a spot that receives 6+ hrs of sun and when it's > 45 degrees outside. If temps drop, cover plants.	Add compost when plants are transplanted. Put down straw for mulching.	1-inch of water every week. Install soaker hoses to conserve water and ensure that it reaches the roots.	Use compost to enhance plant's defenses. For early blight, mulch with straw to prevent soil from touching leaves. Pray for parasitic braconid wasps for hornworms. If I see a hornworm, pick it off. Buy tomato cages.

Module 3

Take Care of Business at Home

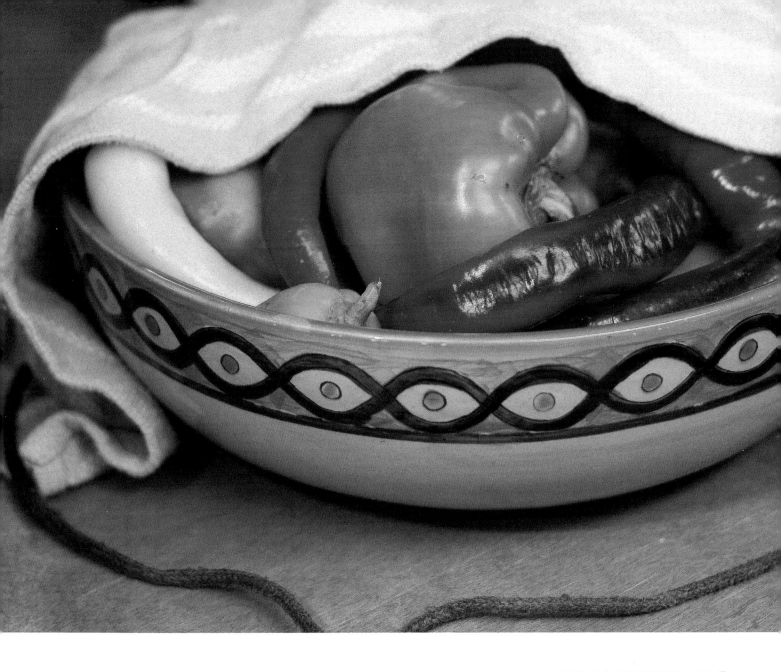

CHAPTER 10

Improve How You **STORE** Food!

Now that you know

how and where to shop for inexpensive fruits and vegetables, nuts, seeds, and oils, this chapter will show you how to store them in ways that prolong their freshness. Before we jump into the strategies, let's see what Impulsive Ida is up to!

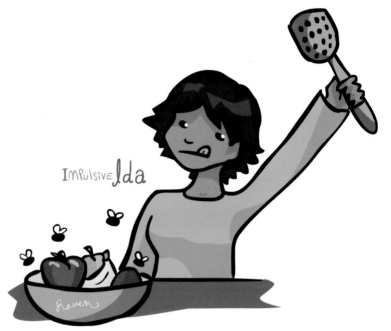

Ida returns home from a big grocery shopping trip. She spent a little more money than she needed to, but she is thoroughly satisfied with her purchases. Ida begins to put her food away and she does what most people do: the leafy veggies are placed in the refrigerator in the thin plastic bags she packed them in, fruit goes into a bowl on the counter, and oils and dry goods (i.e., nuts and seeds) are put into the cupboard.

Like most of us, Ida isn't doing anything wrong, she just could use a few tips to get the most out of her food.

STRATEGY 55
Protect unrefrigerated fruits and vegetables from fruit flies

If you leave your fruits and sweet vegetables (e.g. sweet peppers, tomatoes, onions) on the counter, cover them with a cloth to protect them from the common fruit fly. Fruit flies deposit mold spores under the skin of fruits and vegetables to increase the speed at which they spoil. In other words, they make your food go bad faster. An easy way to prevent fruit flies from having contact with your fruits and vegetables

is to put them into a bowl and cover them with a cloth. I like to take a shoestring and tighten the cloth around the bowl (shown on top right). Or, you can place your fruits and vegetables in a cloth bag. What you don't want to do is to put them in an airtight container, which will make your food spoil regardless.

STRATEGY 56
Protect your greens from moisture

The fastest way make your greens spoil is to keep them wet. Unfortunately, many people are not aware of this, and it's normal to store greens in plastic bags that have leftover "store water" sitting at the bottom. Then over time, additional moisture accumulates in the bags as yours greens sit in the refrigerator. This adds up to a lot of moisture!

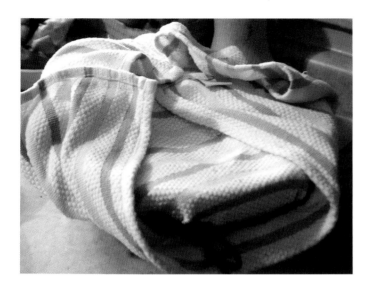

To protect your greens from excess moisture, first, pour out any store water from the bottom of your produce bag. Then place a paper towel at the bottom of the bag or along the sides to protect the greens from any new moisture that may accumulate. This small change will also help you get more mileage out of those flimsy, plastic produce bags you get at the grocery store.

STRATEGY 57
Use produce containers or bags

In the past few years, refrigerator produce containers and bags have increased in popularity. These containers and bags keep your fruits and vegetables fresher, longer by allowing them to breathe. This prevents ethylene gas buildup and excess moisture from accumulating. Some containers like Kinetic Go Green Premium Nano Silver™ are lined with silver nano technology to prevent mold, fungus, and other mi-

croorganisms from growing. I personally own this brand of container, and they keep my lettuce crisp twice as long. So, rather than my lettuce going bad after one week in a flimsy, plastic bag, my lettuce remains crisp for up to 2 weeks when I keep it in my Nano Silver container. These containers come in handy when you accidently buy too much food or when it takes you longer to eat the food you purchased. And they are very affordable! I purchased my container for $8.99 at T.J. Maxx and have been using it for over a year. You can also find these containers at the Raw Foods on a Budget Store (www.rawfoodsonabudget.com). Produce bags are also reasonably priced and come in an assortment of materials like organic materials, nylon, and plastic.

When looking for plastic containers, try to find one that is Bisphenol A (BPA) free. BPA is a chemical that has been used to manufacture hard plastics for over 40 years. The problem is that trace amounts of this chemical leach from the container into the foods, particularly when the food is heated (U.S. Department of Health and Human Services, 2008). BPA has been linked to poor reproductive outcomes, however, the jury is still out on proving the direct harmfulness to adults. In my opinion, people should avoid it all together. Thankfully, many manufacturers produce BPA free plastic, and you can find them in most grocery stores. You can identify these plastics by looking at the bottom on the container, and if the triangle has a 1-5 in it, then it's BPA free. If it has a 6 or 7, then the plastic contains BPA.

STRATEGY 58
Take care when storing your oils

Fatty acids in oils are sensitive to heat, light, and air, and when exposed to these elements, they begin to oxidize. What does that mean? Basically, the oils began to spoil. This is why many oils like olive, flaxseed, and hempseed come in dark bottles. If your oils come in a clear glass bottle, store them in a cool, dark place. To protect your oils from excess air, be sure to tightly close the bottle lids between each use. And if you live in a hot climate or you don't plan on using the oils right away, store them in the refrigerator.

Not all oils are the same. Oils that are saturated or have high concentrations of antioxidants like vitamin E are more stable and resistant to oxidation. Stable fats include butter, and coconut and palm oils. These fats can be stored for over one year. Other oils are less stable, like flaxseed and hempseed oils, and are best kept in the refrigerator. Olive oil contains a high amount of oleic acid, which protects the oil from spoiling; therefore, it can be kept out of the refrigerator. As a general rule, try to purchase small amounts of oils (i.e. 1-2 bottles) and use them within a month or two. This way you are only buying what you need and you are always eating fresh oils.

For more information about oils and fats, check out the book *Know Your Fats* by Mary Ednig.

STRATEGY 59
Refrigerate or freeze your nuts and seeds

Most people don't realize that nuts go bad just like fruits and vegetables do. It's assumed that because nuts are seeds, they will last a long time like they do in nature. However, this is not the case when we buy shelled nuts. In fact, shelled nuts have a much shorter life span than unshelled nuts because their fats are exposed to heat, humidity, and air. This is especially true of nuts sold in bulk bins.

An easy way to store nuts and seeds is to refrigerate or freeze them. Keeping nuts cold will protect them from rancidity and prolong their freshness. Refrigerated nuts and seeds will stay fresh for up to 4 months, depending on the nut, whereas nuts kept in the freezer will stay fresh for as long as a year.

Also, be careful when buying your nuts. Many of the nuts sold in stores are already rancid! Yuck! We just don't know it because we are used to eating rancid nuts. When buying nuts in bulk, try to purchase them from a store whose bulk bins have a quick turnover and are well sealed. An easy way to find out if a store's bins have a high turnover is to see how often people frequent them. If there are a lot of people using the bins, this is a good sign; however, if you don't see anyone visiting the bins during your shopping trip, then I would avoid them like the plague. It's likely these bulk bins contain nuts that have gone rancid. Very oily nuts like macadamia nuts, pine nuts and hemp seeds are often sold in bulk while they are rancid, so try to buy them from a store that keeps them refrigerated. An easy way to avoid rancid hemp seeds is to buy them prepackaged from brands like Nutiva. In addition, look for nuts that are uniform in color and not shriveled. The best way to tell if a nut is rancid is to taste it. Although this can be hard because most of us are accustomed to eating rancid nuts, by using these tips to find fresher nuts, you will get used to eating fresh nuts and after a while, you will be able to identify the rancid ones immediately.

STRATEGY 60
Regularly check your produce

It's so easy to lose track of the produce we have in our kitchens. I can't tell you how many times I have found rotten fruit beneath a pile of apples or spoiled lettuce in the back of my refrigerator! Loosing track of our food is an easy way to waste food. This is why it's important to monitor or regularly check your produce. And I will admit, it's kind of fun. It's like rediscovering the food you already have!

There are several easy ways to keep tabs on your produce. One way is to keep a list of the produce you have on your refrigerator, and cross the items off as you eat them. This tip was mentioned in chapter 7 as a way to help you eat all that you have, and it's equally useful in helping you to monitor your produce. Or you can do quick weekly checks. Simply, clean out your fridge and fruit bowls to see what you have and what should be tossed. The downside of this method is that some veggies and fruits will have already begun to spoil before you do your weekly check. Another strategy is to keep everything visible. When you have a clean fridge and are only buying what you need, then it's a lot easier to see and keep track of the foods you have.

STRATEGY 61
Immediately freeze produce that will spoil

If you have produce that will spoil immediately and you don't plan on using it in the near future, just freeze it. Maybe you are going on vacation and you have some fresh kale in the refrigerator, or maybe you are simply tired of kale. A good option is to freeze it and then to use it in green smoothies. You will be surprised at how many fruits and veggies you can successfully freeze. All you need is an airtight, freezer-ready plastic bag and you are ready to go! In the past I have frozen basil and parsley and used it in flatbreads and pestos. I have also frozen the pulp from almond milk and used it to make cookies.

Keep in mind that freezing does cause some changes to the cellular structure of fruits and vegetables because of their high water content. Water expands when frozen and actually breaks the cellular walls of the fruit or vegetable, thereby altering the physical look of it. This is why previously-frozen strawberries are limp and look nothing like fresh strawberries. Despite these cellular changes, very little nutrition is lost when fruits and vegetables are frozen.

FUN Activities

ACTIVITY 1:

Create a food monitoring system

This week, create a simple food monitoring system. This may be as easy as listing all of the foods you currently have in your refrigerator and cupboards, and then crossing them off as you eat them. You may also find it useful to list the date you purchased each item. This will help you remember how long you have had each food. When I first made my list, I was amazed that I already had 2-3 weeks worth of food! I had no idea! And I won't tell you how many medjool dates I found in my freezer!

In creating your list, decide what types of food you want to have on your list. I would not recommend putting spices on the list because it takes a long time to eat them all. You may want to stick to the more perishable foods like fruits and vegetables, oils, and nuts. However, it's really up to you!

Another way to monitor your food is to check on your food once or twice a week. Simply go through all of your cupboards, produce bowls, and the refrigerator and freezer to make sure none of your food is going bad. The benefit to using this strategy is that you are always aware of what state your fruits and vegetables are in, and it will remind you what produce you currently have in your kitchen. The disadvantage is that it is easy to forget about these checks when you're busy.

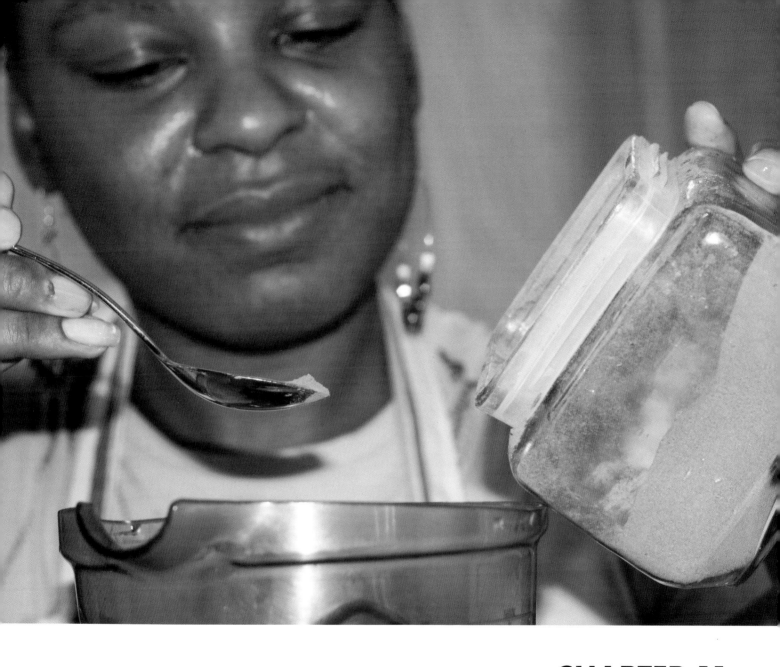

CHAPTER 11

Improve How You **PREPARE** Food!

Have you ever marveled

at the pictures of delicious recipes in popular raw food books? I know I have! Did you also become discouraged after reading the ingredients required to make these recipes? So many of us have been there! This is why I only open the few raw food books I own 1-2 times per year. The dishes in most raw food recipe books use very expensive ingredients, which makes them impractical for everyday living.

This chapter will present several strategies for lowering the costs of raw food recipes you make at home, including the ones you find in popular recipe books. This way you can get more out of these raw food recipe books that have been gathering dust on your shelves. But before we jump into the strategies, let's see what our friend Impulsive Ida has been up to!

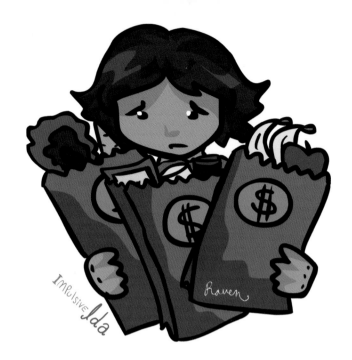

On a Saturday night, Ida dined at a fancy raw food restaurant in New York City. She had an amazing meal and was convinced that if she could eat this way every day, she could be 100% raw vegan. She joyfully held onto this belief until she received her bill, which diminished all her hopes of eating out at this restaurant in the near future. Then she noticed that the restaurant had its own raw food recipe book for sale, so she decided to buy it. She figured that if she could make the recipes at home, the costs of the meals would be cheaper, right? However, she soon learned that this was not the case...AT ALL. The recipes in the book required a lot of fancy, expensive raw food ingredients like Thai coconuts, macadamia nuts, specialty oils, and tropical produce. Despite the pricey ingredients, Ida decided to power through and make the recipes anyway! She selected 3 recipes for each meal of the day, and prepared her shopping list. After a long day of grocery shopping, Ida finally returned home with all of her ingredients and over $100 in grocery bills!

This is a common scenario. Almost everyone I know who has experimented with raw foods has gone through this experience. In fact, the pricey recipes in many raw food books may be one of the reasons why this diet is considered an expensive lifestyle. The truth is that *this* type of raw foods is an expensive lifestyle, and it's different than the budget-loving raw food lifestyle that I'm advocating in this book. The good news is that there are four simple strategies that you can use to keep recipe costs low.

STRATEGY 62
Substitute traditional sweeteners with low-cost sweeteners

This is one of my favorite strategies in the whole book! When I thought of it, it was like I had discovered the missing key to eating raw foods. This strategy even helped me tame one area of my budget! The strategy is to partially (or fully) substitute your traditional raw food sweeteners like agave, honey, and dates with more low-cost sweeteners like green stevia powder, raisins, and dried fruit.

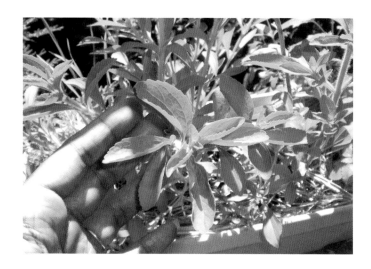

Green stevia powder. Also known as sweet leaf, stevia is a shrub (shown on top right) native to Paraguay that has been used for centuries as a sweetener in herbal and medicinal teas. Though less common in the United States, stevia is used in Asia, South America, and some European countries. It even accounts for 40% of all the sweeteners sold in Japan. In addition, stevia is unlike many sweeteners in that it doesn't promote dental cavities or raise blood glucose levels (University of Nebraska-Lincoln Extension). Yay!

Personally, I love using stevia in my own raw vegan recipes because it has a long-lasting sweetness that is useful in frozen recipes like ice cream and sorbet. Freezing temperatures reduce the sweet taste of many sweeteners including agave and honey, so you end up using a lot. In fact, this is why all of my ice cream and sorbet recipes have a little green stevia in them.

Stevia also does a good job of extending the amount of agave you already have. For example, last winter I drank a lot of tea lattes. The problem was that I would put 3 teaspoons of agave in each 12 ounce cup of my tea latte. This quickly became very expensive since I would drink 3-4 cups a day.

So, I came up with the idea that maybe I could add stevia to my tea latte in addition to agave to reduce my overall agave usage. Given that I wasn't a big stevia lover, I didn't know what to expect. Boy, was I surprised! The green stevia powder helped me reduce my agave usage by 66%! Now, I only use 1 tsp of agave in my tea lattes and it tastes the same! Plus, now I only buy agave every once 1-2 months, whereas I used to buy it every 1-2 weeks. Try your own "stevia" experiment at home! Make a cup of lemonade and measure the amount of honey or agave you add it to. Then make another cup of lemonade and add several pinches of stevia before adding honey or agave. Now compare how much traditional sweetener you used in both lemonades.

You may be resistant to the idea of using stevia in your recipes because you have tasted it before and didn't like it. However, keep a few things in mind. I am recommending that you use green stevia powder and not the white stevia that is sold most often at health food stores. Stevia that is green is just ground up stevia leaves, whereas stevia that is

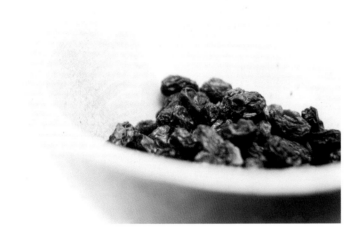

white has been processed and often contains other ingredients. In my experience, white stevia tastes more bitter than green stevia, although they both can taste bitter when used in large amounts. In most of my recipes, I use no more than 1/8 teaspoon because stevia is so sweet. In addition, I recommend that you use partial substitution when it comes to stevia. Unless you really like stevia, you will find that stevia has a different kind of sweetness, compared to traditional sweeteners. This is because stevia does not contain any sugars like fructose or glucose and lacks the ability to add texture to a recipe in the way that dates, agave, and honey do. For these reasons, stevia does not work well alone. However, it works wonders when used in combination with traditional sweeteners. Sometimes, I even pour stevia into my agave bottles so that it's already mixed in and ready to use.

Raisins. This is my second favorite sweetener. Honestly, I like them more than agave and dates because raisins are sweet, fruity, and very moist. They complement fruity desserts better than agave and dates, and they give desserts a more well-rounded flavor.

I got the idea to use raisins in my desserts from one of my favorite restaurants in New York City. I couldn't figure out why their fruit pies tasted so much more fresh and flavorful than the pies served at other raw food restaurants. Then, my waiter told me that raisins were used to sweeten the desserts, and I couldn't believe that raisins made that much of a difference. It took me a while to start experimenting, but when I did, I was shocked. The recipes I was creating were amazing!

When substituting raisins for other sweeteners, it's useful to consider the level of sweetness and type of texture that raisins will add to the recipe. Raisins are sweeter than dates and many other dried fruits, so you may need less of them when using them as a substitute. Raisins also add a fruity flavor to desserts, so if that's not what you are going for, then raisins may not be a great substitute. In addition, raisins help to increase the creamy texture and moistness of your desserts. I love using raisins in crusts because it makes them so succulent. You will find that many of the dessert recipes in this book include raisins such as the Creamy Plum Sorbet (on page 253) and Sweet Glory Nectarine Pie (on page 220).

Additional dried fruits. This is where substitution becomes a lot of fun! Try using a variety of dried fruits to sweeten your green smoothies and desserts. In the past, I have used dried currants and plums (or prunes) to sweeten green smoothies, and dried figs to sweeten pie crusts and cookies. And the great thing is that most dried fruits are cheaper than dates and agave. However, be careful when buying dried fruits. Make sure that no sweeteners or other ingredients have been added.

Substituting traditional sweeteners is an art form that becomes easier the more you do it. To help you get started, refer to the quick Sweetener Substitution Guide below! In the guide I do not mention the amount of sweeteners recommended in these substitutions. This is because it really varies by recipe. However, when substituting a sweetener I have found that relying on my intuition does the trick. For example, when I am using stevia, I rarely use more than 1/4 teaspoon. In fact, most of the time I only use 1/8 teaspoon because stevia is so sweet. So here is how my sequence goes: I add a small amount of stevia (about 1/8 tsp or a pinch or two), a tiny bit of agave, and then I taste the recipe. If I can barely taste the stevia and there is no weird aftertaste, which is caused by adding too much stevia, I add a little bit more

SWEETENER SUBSTITUTION GUIDE

Traditional Sweetener	Substitution Sweetener	Notes
Dates	*Combinations of:* dates and raisins raisins and green stevia dates and green stevia	Dates are tricky to substitute because they not only add sweetness, they also add texture to a recipe. In fact, they add more texture than sweetness. So, any type of substitution will need to add both of these dimensions to the recipe.
Agave	*Combinations of:* agave and green stevia raisins and green stevia	Agave is pretty easy to substitute. I have found that a combination of stevia and agave is a nice substitute and you can't even tell the difference. However, the combination will really depend on your recipe. If it looks like the recipe needs agave to add both sweetness and liquid content (e.g. when making syrups) to the recipe, you may need to increase the other liquid portions of the recipe or add water.
Honey	*Combinations of:* agave and green stevia honey and green stevia	Honey is a little hard to substitute because there are very few sweeteners that taste like honey. However, adding a little stevia in addition to honey will decrease the amount of honey you need.

NUT SUBSTITUTION GUIDE

Traditional Nuts	Substitution Nuts	Notes
Macadamia nuts	*Combinations of:* 2-3 parts cashews/1 part walnuts	Macadamia nuts are used in many raw food recipes because they add a creamy, oily texture and are bland in flavor. For example, macadamia nuts are often used to prepare buttery pie crusts. When I have substituted macadamia nuts, I have used cashews and walnuts. Walnuts add an oily texture, and cashews are very creamy and bland.
Almonds	*Combinations of:* Sunflower seeds, walnuts, cashews Sunflower seeds, cashews Shredded coconut, sunflower seeds, walnuts Shredded coconut, sunflower seeds, cashews	Almonds may be the most difficult nut to mimic because they taste like nothing. Almonds have very little flavor, which is why people like to use them. You can do whatever you want with almonds; they are like a white canvas. So, when I substitute almonds, I accept at the beginning that the flavor of the crust will be different. But that is okay with me because I like creating awesome new recipes. You can really have fun here and experiment. Sometimes I just create my own crust by thinking of the type of flavors that will complement the pie filling, and I go from there.
Cashews	**For cashews in pie crusts:** *Combinations of:* Cashews and walnuts **For cashews in ice creams and pie filling:** *Combinations of:* 1 part cashews/1 part meat from a young coconut Arrowroot and cashews Lecithin and cashews	How you substitute cashews will ultimately depend on the type of recipe you are making. When a recipe asks for a pie crust primarily composed of cashews, I substitute some of the cashews with walnuts. Sometimes I even create a whole new crust. Also when using cashews in ice creams, I have found that using ½ of the amount cashews and 1-2 tbsp of arrowroot or lecithin is a nice substitution. A combination of cashews and Thai young coconut meat is probably the best substitution because the coconut meat adds a nice creamy, fluffy filling. However, young coconuts can be difficult to find in some locations.

stevia and taste the recipe again. Finally, I sweeten the recipe with agave until it reaches the sweetness I like. The same technique applies when you are using raisins or other dried fruits as substitutions. You just add a little to the recipe and then taste it, and then you add a little bit more.

When doing substitutions, allow yourself to create new flavors. Using a substitute is an opportunity to experience a new variation on an existing recipe. Most substitutions will not perfectly reproduce the taste of traditional sweetener; however, more often than not, you will create something new and delicious!

STRATEGY 63
Substitute expensive nuts with low-cost nuts

This is one of my favorite things to do with nuts, primarily because I love working with inexpensive nuts like sunflower seeds, pumpkin seeds, and walnuts. And when I do use pecans, almonds, or cashews, they are in very small amounts. So rather than using multiple cups of cashews in one recipe, I use enough to achieve the texture that I want and then I concentrate on using less expensive nuts to create the flavor I want. It's important to remember that expensive nuts like cashews and macadamia nuts do not add flavor to a recipe, rather they add a creamy texture. So, I only use them to add texture. The interesting thing about walnuts is that they are just as expensive as pecans and more expensive than cashews, but I like to use them because a little goes a long way. Walnuts add a creamy texture to the recipe that doesn't overwhelm it, and they are less expensive than their creamy alternatives like macadamia nuts.

To help you substitute expensive nuts like macadamia nuts, cashews, and almonds, take a look at the Nut Substitution Guide on page 106. I personally use these nut combinations when I want to reduce the cost of a recipe without losing the flavor. Note that I do not indicate the portions for most of the substitutions because it really depends on the recipe you are preparing. So, you will have to use your own judgment here. Be playful with it and have fun!

STRATEGY 64
Keep your recipes simple

The more ingredients you add to a recipe, the more expensive it gets. It's really that simple. Plus, when there are too many ingredients, it's difficult to enjoy the flavors of the individual ingredients, and often, we end up preparing something that tastes too complex.

Consider taking a complex recipe and making it simple. A friend of mine is a pro at this. She likes to take raw food recipes that require fancy ingredients like Irish moss and lecithin, and not use them. This, of course, changes the texture of the recipe because these ingredients are used as thickeners; however, I have found that the recipe tastes just as good. So the next time you are looking through your raw recipe books, ask yourself if you can make these recipes simpler.

STRATEGY 65
Keep most of your meals simple

An easy way to keep your food costs low is to prepare a lot of simple meals. Simply eating one or two apples for breakfast is a lot cheaper than eating granolas and breakfast bars. This doesn't mean that you shouldn't eat complex meals; instead, consider saving the more complex meals for lunch and dinner and leaving your breakfast and snack recipes very simple. This may be difficult at first for people who are used to eating a heavy breakfast; however, as you progress on our raw foods journey, you may find that your breakfast meals naturally lighten up! Also, drinking green smoothies is a nice way to prepare a hearty breakfast that is both quick and incredibly nutritious!

FUN Activities

ACTIVITY 1:
Practice substituting nuts or sweeteners

Choose a favorite raw food recipe that you know how to make really well. If you can't think of one, try something simple like lemonade or a cookie recipe from one of your raw food books. Now, take one ingredient like agave, honey, dates, cashews, macadamia nuts, or pecans, and either fully or partially substitute it with less expensive ingredient(s).

Refer to the Sweetener and Nut Substitution Guides on pages 105-106 for ideas.

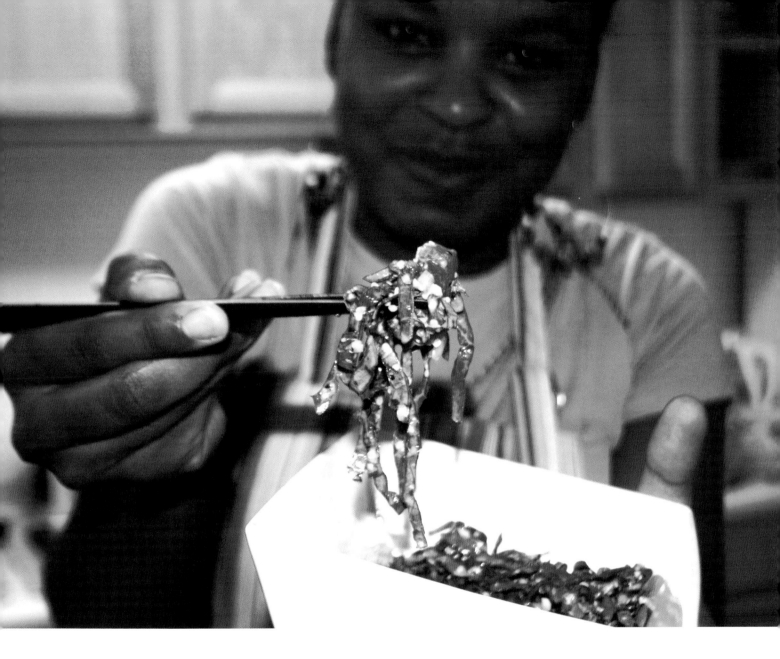

CHAPTER 12
Improve How You **EAT** Food!

If we eat wrongly, no doctor can cure us; if we eat rightly, no doctor is needed.

- Dr. Victor G. Rocine

We live in the era of unconscious eating.

In fact, we have it down to a complete science. We eat while watching TV or talking on the phone; we eat until our plates are clean instead of responding to internal signals of fullness; we eat so quickly that our food doesn't digest properly; we eat late at night when our digestive forces are naturally slow; and we eat when we're stressed, sad, nervous, in pain, and even happy! In fact, it's rare that we eat in response to real hunger and without distractions. Unfortunately, when we engage in unconscious eating, we lose the opportunity to fully experience the flavors in our food and benefit from its nutrients. In addition, because these poor eating habits are hard on the body, they diminish the benefits of a raw food diet. I have found this to be true in my own experience and amongst other raw vegans that I know. In the past, I have eaten while working on my computer, inhaled food late at night, and eaten while stressed. In all of these cases, I woke up the next day feeling wretched and bloated. What a way to start the day! Over time, these poor eating habits can slow down your weight loss and even promote weight gain, encourage moodiness and irritability, and may contribute to digestive problems like Candida overgrowth.

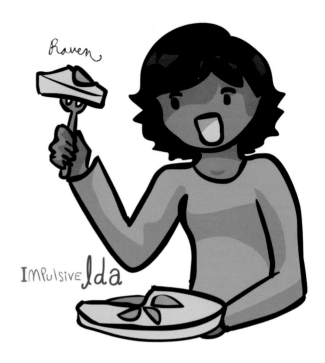

So, what exactly is unconscious eating? Well, let's first consider what conscious eating looks like:

Conscious Eating is the awareness of how the food we eat affects our body, emotions, mind, and spiritual life. It is understanding how what we eat directly affects the planetary ecology and the degree of peace we have with the human and animal life on this planet...

The art of conscious eating is learning how to eat just the right amount of food to maximize every aspect of our lives. It is not a deprivation or minimal-eating diet. It is a pattern of eating that adds to our wholeness."

- Gabriel Cousens

This is conscious eating and, as you can guess, unconscious eating is the complete opposite! And don't feel bad; we all have engaged in unconscious eating at some point in our lives. We grew up learning that it was normal to eat this way. As children, we were taught to be good eaters, which meant cleaning our plates, eating what was given to us, and eating it quickly. But now we are adults and it's our responsibility to get rid of these old habits and exchange them for new ones that nurture our bodies and enhance our experience in the world.

Unconscious eating takes a negative toll on our wallets as well. For example, when we eat too fast or while watching TV, we end up eating more just to feel nourished and satisfied, but this is food that could have been saved for another meal. The same applies to when we eat to cope with negative emotions such as stress and sadness. Even though the food makes us feel good, it doesn't remove the event that actually caused the stress! In the end, we spend extra money to feed our unhealthy eating habits. For example, let's take our friend, Impulsive Ida:

It's Friday night and Ida is celebrating the end of the week by making herself a delicious nectarine cream pie (recipe on page 234). The pie fits within her budget and will make use of the nectarines ripening on her counter. She figures that she could eat one slice tonight after her dinner and eat the rest of the pie throughout the week. After she makes the pie, she helps herself to a big slice, which was actually the equivalent of 2 servings. Then an hour later, she finds herself wandering into the refrigerator for another slice. Unfortunately, all hell breaks loose and she ends up eating half the pie for dinner. She had planned on making a salad for dinner, but at some point she lost control and couldn't break herself away from the pie. Even though the pie was raw vegan, eating one-half of a pie did not sit well with her stomach and she woke up the next day feeling wretched and like her food was still sitting in her stomach.

It's obvious that Ida ate too much, but what could she have done to make herself stop eating? All the pie she ate could have lasted her the whole week, but instead, she ate half of it in one night. Ida didn't know it, but she was setting herself up to eat too much! First, Ida gave herself too large of a portion. Research shows that we eat what's on our plates; so, when we serve ourselves a lot, we eat a lot. Second, Ida should have eaten her dinner first and her dessert second. This way, she could have filled up on veggies and had less room in her tummy for dessert. Third, Ida ate so fast that she didn't give herself a chance to savor her food. By chewing her food slowly, she could have allowed her gastric hormones to do their work and reduce her hunger levels.

In this chapter, I will show how small changes to the way you eat can get you more bang for your buck. It's my hope that this chapter will give you the tools you need to begin your conscious eating journey. But please keep in mind that conscious eating is a HUGE topic that can't be covered in one chapter. For this reason, I have provided multiple resources on page 118 to support and empower you as you continue on your conscious eating path.

Know When to Eat

Thou shouldst eat to live; not live to eat.

- Marcus Tullius Cicero

I love this quote because it's a simple reminder that *what* and *when* we eat should support our lives. Often, when we consume food while bored, stressed, sad, or in the absence of hunger, we turn *eating* into our end-goal instead of our goal being an enriched, energized life. Even when we eat according to a schedule (e.g. it's 12pm, so it's time for lunch) instead of listening to our internal signals for hunger, we make eating our ultimate goal. In fact, so many external factors and events determine when we eat that many of us don't know what real hunger actually feels like. The question then becomes: how do we know when to eat?

The following two strategies will give you guidance in knowing when to eat as well as helping you to save money!

STRATEGY 66
Eat when you are hungry

Yes, I know...this is easier said than done. But it will save you money, keep your digestive system happy, enhance the health benefits of a raw foods diet, promote weight loss, reduce aging, strengthen your mind-body-nature connection, and keep you energized all day long so that you can do the activities you want to do! Eating when you're hungry requires that you know when you experience biological hunger and fullness. The good news is that our bodies come equipped with biological signals that tell us when we are hungry and full; the bad news is that we have been ignoring these signals

for so long that many of us don't know what they feel like. In fact, most of us were taught by our parents and other adults to ignore these signals. As children, we were taught to clean our plates and eat at specific times of the day like lunch and dinner time (i.e. eat on demand). In addition, our role models were not conscious eaters themselves and we adopted their poor eating habits. Thus, it's not surprising that many of us confuse stress, boredom, or other emotions with hunger, experience a loss of control while eating, and continue to clean our plates. We rely on cues like a cleaned plate or filled-to-capacity stomach to know when we are full, when in fact we were biologically full long before we took the last bite. So how do we break these habits and sensitize ourselves to our biological cues for hunger and fullness? The key is to become more conscious or mindful before and while we eat.

To determine when you should eat, ask yourself the following questions BEFORE YOUR EAT:

- Am I really hungry or am I feeling bored, stressed, depressed, etc.?

- Are there other activities that I can do (e.g. go for a walk) instead of fulfilling this desire to eat? Real hunger cannot be distracted but fake "feelings" of hunger can.

- Am I actually thirsty? Often we eat when we are actually thirsty! Drink a glass of water first and if your hunger persists, then eat.

To determine when to stop eating, ask yourself the following questions WHILE YOU EAT. These questions will help you focus on your food and the eating process, and make it easier to determine when you are biologically full:

- Am I eating too fast?

- Am I chewing my food?

- Am I distracted? Am I doing other activities while I eat?

- Am I listening for my internal sensations for fullness? You may not feel anything at first. Stay persistent and repeatedly ask yourself, "Am I full?" Eventually, the sensation will become stronger and you will get an answer.

- Am I eating because I am still hungry or because the food tastes good?

- If I stopped eating right now, would I be comfortably full?

These are a lot of questions, so bring them to the table with you! Write them down on a piece of paper, put the paper in your wallet, and pull it out whenever you want to eat. You may even want to put this list on your refrigerator. Every time you go to the refrigerator for food, ask yourself these questions. The more you do it, the easier it will get, and the more connected you will feel to your biological signals for hunger and fullness.

Also, consider keeping a food diary. Traditionally, a food diary is a small book in which you write down when and what you ate throughout the day. For the purposes of learning when to eat (and to stop eating), I recommend that you expand upon the traditional food diary and write down your answers to the previous questions before and after you eat. By doing this, you will notice trends in how you eat. For example, you may crave more junk foods when you are stressed or depressed (I know, I do!). Refer to the Worksheet "Keep A Food Diary" on page 119 for more guidance in creating your food diary.

STRATEGY 67
Follow your digestive cycle

According to Ayurvedic medicine, our bodies naturally go through a daily, three-point digestive cycle of cleansing, absorption, and assimilation. Cleansing occurs from night to mid-morning; absorption (i.e., when your body digests and absorbs nutrients) occurs from mid-morning to mid-afternoon; and assimilation (i.e., when nutrients are distributed throughout your body) occurs from mid-afternoon to the evening. This means that the bulk of your meals should be eaten during the absorption period, and very little should be eaten during the cleansing and assimilation period. This means that your biggest meal should be eaten at high noon, when your digestive fires are strongest. Although this timing may slightly differ depending on your constitution (e.g., for some, their digestive fires may be highest in the mid-morning), this general guideline applies to most people.

As usual, our cultural norms completely clash with our natural digestive cycle. We eat our biggest meal at night, when our digestive fires are their weakest. It's not surprising that we wake up feeling sluggish and wretched the next morning. Plus, when we eat at night, it becomes more difficult to do activities that require a more quiet state of mind such as meditation, yoga, and prayer.

Following your digestive cycle will also save you money! By eating less in the mornings and evenings, you will naturally buy less food. Plus, because most of your meals will occur around noon, the assimilation of nutrients will be greatly enhanced and you will, subsequently, get more from your food!

So where do you start? Because we have trained our bodies to eat throughout the day, you will now have to train yourself to eat according to your digestive cycle. This may be difficult at first because you may be used to eating at night and, as a result, may feel hungry in the evening. So start the transition slowly. Begin by "lightening" your evening and morning meals, and eating more in the mid day. Also, consider eating earlier in the evenings such as 5 or 6pm. And don't try to rush the process. When we go too fast, it's so easy to fall off the wagon and eat everything in sight (believe me, I have been there). This process will also be easier if you utilize the recommendations from the previous strategy about eating when you are hungry. Think of it this way: if you were to cut out all of the evening meals and snacks where you ate in the absence of real hunger, you will naturally lighten your meals.

Can you guess how many calories are in today's portions?

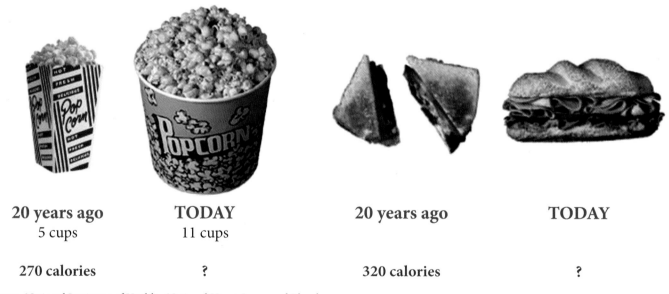

20 years ago	TODAY	20 years ago	TODAY
5 cups	11 cups		
270 calories	?	320 calories	?

Source: National Institutes of Health - National Heart, Lung, and Blood Institute (http://hp2010.nhlbihin.net/portion/)

Answers are on page 116.

Lastly, when learning to follow your digestive cycle, consider adopting the habit of going to bed early. Many of us experience a second-round of hunger when we stay up late at night. This obviously makes it difficult to follow your natural digestive cycle. So go to bed before 10pm! Plus, as you go to bed earlier, you will become more attuned to your natural sleep cycle and begin to experience more energized and creative mornings.

Get Off the Overeating Roller Coaster

Overeating is a way of numbing oneself to life.

- Gabriel Cousens

Overeating is so common that it has become the norm. And when we try to break this habit, we find that it's a lot like riding a roller coaster. Sometimes we successfully avoid it and other times we unleash the beast and binge. Unfortunately, these overeating habits have a numbing effect on our lives by keep us from experiencing the richness of life, the sensuality and magic of raw foods, and weight loss. Plus, to top it off, overeating can stir up feelings of guilt and shame as we punish ourselves *for* overeating.

In this section, I will show you how to break the vicious cycle of overeating through the art of portion control. Yes, I said portion control. Now I know, no one likes to be restricted, which is the image that most people conjure up when they hear those two words; however, all portion control means is to eat an amount of food that supports your life rather than an amount that takes away from it. Call it "happy portions" or "joyful portions" if it helps!

STRATEGY 68
Serve yourself smaller portions

As food portions have increased in size over the last 2 decades, we have responded by eating more. It's now the norm for people to place great mounds of food on their plates and eat foot-long sandwiches. For example, on page 114 are pictures of food portions that were served 20 years ago and portions that are served today. Can you guess how many calories are in today's portions?

Today's huge portion sizes are wreaking havoc on our waistlines and wallets! Research shows that the more food we put on our plates, the more we will eat! Therefore, when I place the equivalent of 1 ½ raw food meals on my plate, I will consume all of it. This happens because we are more sensitive to the amount of food on our plates than the nutrient density of this food. Plus, the extra food that we are eating is food that we could have saved for later! Just imagine if you saved one-quarter of your food everyday, three times a day. That would amount to at least one free meal a day without making any other changes to your budget! That's 30 free meals a month or 10 days worth of meals! Now, I know what you may be thinking: "What if I am still hungry?". Well, research tells us that when people are served 25% less food on their plates, they don't report any difference in hunger or fullness. This is great news! Try this experiment for a day and see what happens! Serve yourself your normal portion and then remove 1/4 of the food from your plate. Do this all day and see how you feel! Use the worksheet on pages 124-125 for this experiment.

Consider trying the more subtle experiment of eating on smaller plates. As portion sizes have increased, so have plate and bowl sizes to accommodate them. It's very easy to notice that you are giving yourself less food when you use a large plate, but you barely notice the difference when you use a smaller plate (on right). I tried this a few years ago when I replaced all my 12" plates with 8" plates. And guess what? I overate less!

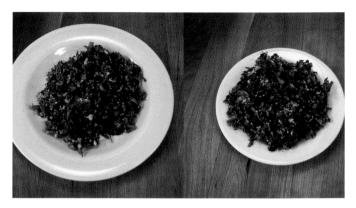

11-inch plate   **8-inch plate**

STRATEGY 69
Eat 1-2 mono meals a day

To minimize overeating, try eating at least one mono-meal a day. Mono meals are composed of only one food, making them the true fast food! For example, a mono-meal for breakfast could be 1-2 pears or apples. Because of their simplicity, they work great for breakfast or snacks. Plus, you will notice that it's very difficult to overeat when you are only eating one food. A few years ago, I had the habit of eating mono meals for breakfast. I always found that it was impossible for me to overeat. When I was done eating pears, I was done and had no interest in them for hours. At the time, I didn't understand why this occurred; however, recent studies suggest that as we consume one food, we habituate to that food and our intake decreases. But, as soon as we are provided with a different food, we start eating again. In other words, having too much variety in one meal can increase the likelihood that we will just keep on eating.

STRATEGY 70
Savor your food

Many of us have the habit of eating our food too fast. We put food on our plates and 5 minutes later it's gone. But then we are still hungry! It's easy to do this when we are distracted by other activities like watching television or talking to a group of friends, and before we know it, our food is gone. Unfortunately, a 5-10 minute meal is barely enough time for our brains to register that we are full! It's no wonder we still feel hungry after eating a meal. Plus, we never gave ourselves a chance to savor our food! For example, one afternoon, I was talking to a friend on the phone while eating my dinner: homemade walnut pesto spread onto Italian flax crackers, topped with sun-baked tomatoes. It was exquisite, but I was so busy talking that I barely noticed. Then, at some point my friend interrupted me and told me to focus on what I was eating. So I did, and I could barely peel myself off the couch as I began to experience the magnificent flavors of my meal. Try this activity for yourself: pick a meal today and

Answers: large popcorn = 630 calories, large sandwich = 820 calories

savor it. Make an event out of it by removing all distractions (including your very talkative pal), lighting a candle, and/or saying a prayer. These small changes will help you slow down and focus on the food right in front of you! Plus, you will feel more nourished, your food will taste more flavorful, and your meals will digest better. For more guidance on learning to savor your meals, see the worksheet on pages 126-127.

STRATEGY 71
Eat lower energy-dense foods first

Energy-density refers to the amount of energy (e.g. calories) that is in a given mass or volume of food. Low energy-dense foods like fruits and vegetables weigh a lot but have relatively fewer calories, whereas, high energy-dense foods like nuts, seeds, and oils weigh very little but contain a lot of calories. Because low energy-dense foods have a lot of volume, they quickly fill our stomachs. In contrast, it would take a lot more high energy-dense foods to get that prized full feeling. Therefore, when we focus on eating low energy-dense foods first, we experience a HUGE savings in calories! And given that energy-dense, processed foods like prepackaged raw crackers, chips, and chocolates are more expensive than their raw ingredients, you will also experience a HUGE savings in your wallet.

Impulsive Ida could have used this strategy. She ate her high energy-dense dessert first and found that it was difficult to tear herself away from it. In fact, she lost interest in the salad she had planned on preparing for dinner. To prevent this from occurring in the future, Ida could make it a rule to eat her meal first and dessert second. Like us, Ida's stomach can only hold so much food, so if she would have filled up on voluminous, low energy-dense, raw food, she would have naturally eaten less of the energy-dense pie.

STRATEGY 72
Bring your goals to the dinner table

Research shows that when dieters are reminded of their weight loss goals, they eat less than when they are not reminded. This has the same effect as placing an old picture of your "healthy-self" on the refrigerator in order to prevent grazing on unhealthy foods. When we are reminded of our goals, it's easier to make healthy decisions. We can quickly see that the long-term goal of happiness (or in the former case, weight loss) dramatically outweighs the short-term gratification of a slice of pizza. And the cool thing is that our brains were made for this! Some argue that our ability to practice self-control is like a muscle--the more you exercise it, the stronger it gets, and the less work it takes to exercise it next time!

STRATEGY 73
Eat at home

We eat out at restaurants more than ever before. Given that it's cheaper to make food at home, eating out can quickly weigh heavy on our budget. Plus, the typical raw food restaurant is more expensive than the average cooked restaurant, thereby making eating out an expensive venture for the average raw foodie. For example, whenever I go to a raw vegan restaurant, I expect to spend between $20-$30 on a meal, which is a lot of money for a student like me. That's 10% of my food budget for the whole month! Or, think of it this way: that's 2-3 days worth of food spent on one meal! Plus, over the years, I have turned into my favorite cook and no restaurant can spice the food exactly how I like it. So, not only am I paying a lot for the food itself, but I am paying for food that doesn't taste exactly how I like it.

The next time you are at a restaurant, justify the money you are about to spend. Typically, you can get more mileage out of your money at a grocery store or farmers market than at a raw food restaurant. Ask yourself: how much in groceries can I buy with the money I am about to spend on one meal? Could I make a better version of this recipe at home? How many servings of this recipe can I make for the same price? This doesn't mean that you should never eat out. Rather, eating out should be something special. It's an opportunity to enjoy a meal that you wouldn't ordinarily make for yourself. For example, whenever I go out to eat, I make a huge event out of it! I am super excited and already know what I want to order days and even weeks in advance. And if they serve large portions, I have already planned to save it for later meals. In short, if you can justify spending the money, then go for it. If not, head for the farmers market!

More Resources for Conscious Eating

- *Mindful Eating: A Guide to Rediscovering a Healthy and Joyful Relationship with Food* (2009), by Jan Chozen Bays, MD

- *Conscious Eating* (2000), by Gabriel Cousens, MD.

- *Breaking Free from Emotional Eating* (1984), by Geneen Roth.

- The Camp System: http://www.mindfuleating.org

- The Center for Mindful Eating: http://www.tcme.org

- Dr. Susan Alber's website for Eating Mindfully: http://www.eatingmindfully.com

KEEP A FOOD DIARY

It's amazing what a food diary can reveal! We eat for so many different reasons that don't involve hunger and it has become normal to eat beyond what our bodies actually need. This translates to a lot of money being spent on food that our bodies don't even want. Through this activity, you will learn *why you eat* and *why you keep on eating*.

In order to see trends in your behavior (e.g. how often you *feel* hungry vs. how often you are *actually* hungry), it's also important to complete this worksheet in the moment when you experience hunger, and before and after you eat. Otherwise you may be guessing at how you felt when you ate a couple of hours ago. Lastly, before you begin, remember that this is a process. The goal is not to be perfect. Rather, the goal is to LEARN. Through learning we give ourselves the opportunity for real, meaningful change.

PART 1: DETERMINE IF YOU ARE HUNGRY!

Complete this part of the worksheet every time you have the urge or desire to eat. Ask yourself the following questions and write your responses on pages 120-121:

- **How hungry am I?** On a scale of 1 (not hungry) to 10 (very hungry), rate how hungry you are.

- **How do I feel? Am I nervous, sad, depressed, stressed, bored, or happy?** Often, we eat as a way to cope with difficult situations. Think about how you feel and write it down.

- **Am I thirsty?** Often we eat when we are actually thirsty. Try drinking a glass of water when you feel hungry. If you are still hungry or if your hunger quickly returns, then you are truly hungry.

- **Can I do another activity like going for a walk?** The truth is that if you could do another activity instead of eating, then you were never hungry in the first place. Hunger cannot be distracted.

- **What would I like to eat?** Write down what you would like to eat right now. Answering this question will help you understand why you eat what you eat (e.g. I eat chips in response to stress).

Date & Time	How hungry am I? (10=very hungry, 1=not at all)	How do I feel? Am I nervous, sad, depressed, stressed, or happy?	Am I thirsty?	Can I do another activity like go for a walk? If so, what?	What would I like to eat right now?
5/30 - 12 pm	6	I am writing and am kind of bored. So I want to eat.	No	I could go for a walk or just do anything to leave my apartment	I want to finish my breakfast of chia seeds soaked in nut milk
5/30 - 1 pm	9	I feel okay. Kind of neutral	No	No, I am hungry!!!	I still want to finish my breakfast

Date & Time	How hungry am I? (10=very hungry, 1=not at all)	How do I feel? Am I nervous, sad, depressed, stressed, or happy?	Am I thirsty?	Can I do another activity like go for a walk? If so, what?	What would I like to eat right now?

PART 2: DETERMINE IF YOU ARE FULL!

As you continue this activity, you may find that your urge to eat occurs more often than when you actually eat. When you decide to eat, complete this second part of the worksheet to help you determine when you are biologically full:

- **Did I eat too fast?** It takes 20 minutes for our brains to register that we are full, so give your brain a fighting chance by eating slowly and chewing your food. Plus, this will improve the digestion of your food. Think of it this way, you can either pay for supplements or you can chew your food!

- **Did I eat while distracted?** We eat more food when we are distracted with watching TV or talking to friends. Make it your goal to focus on your food in the absence of distractions.

- **Did I listen for internal cues for fullness?** Many of us don't know what fullness feels like. One way to find out, is to just keep asking yourself "Am I full?". Eventually, you will hear that little voice saying, "Yes, you are full. Thank you for asking".

- **Did I eat more than I needed because the food tastes good?** This is one of the biggest reasons for overeating. The food just tastes so good that you couldn't stop eating.

- **How full am I (comfortable, uncomfortable, nauseated)?** When you are done eating, ask yourself how full you are. Your goal is to eat until you are comfortably full (i.e. being full without feeling physically bloated, tired, or in pain).

	Did I...				
Date/Time	...eat slowly?	...eat while distracted?	...listen for internal cues for fullness?	...eat more than I needed because the food tastes good?	How full am I? (comfortable, nauseated, un-comfortable)
5/30 – 1 pm	Yes. One spoonful at a time.	A tiny bit. The TV was on in the background	Yes!!!! I kept asking myself, "Am I full"!	I did eat 2 extra spoonfuls	very comfortable

SERVE YOURSELF LESS TO GET MORE FROM LIFE

In this experiment, you will serve yourself less food for one whole day. Simply serve yourself as usual and then remove 1/4 of the food from your plate. You can either give this food to someone else or place it in the refrigerator or freezer to save for later. If you feel that this will be a very difficult exercise for you, then do anything (but eat) to get rid of the food such as placing it in the freezer or throwing it away. Consider serving your food on smaller plates so that you don't notice the decrease in food.

Be sure to do this activity for every meal and snack you eat! It won't work if you eat less during a meal but then overeat your next meal. The objective of this experiment is to see how you feel when you reduce your portion sizes. In this worksheet, you will record how you feel after every meal and snack. Ask yourself these questions:

- **What did I eat?** Simply write down what you ate.

- **Do I still feel hungry?** When you finish your meal or snack, simply ask yourself if you still feel hungry. Remember that this is how you feel. It doesn't have to be biological hunger, although the two will (hopefully!) begin to coincide as you practice more conscious eating.

- **If I were to eat more, would it be because 1) the food tastes good, 2) I am hungry, or 3) it just feels right?** This question will help you understand why you feel the need to eat a certain amount of food, irregardless of hunger.

Meal & Time	What did I eat?	Do I still feel hungry?	If I were to eat more, would it be because 1) the food tastes good, 2) I am hungry, or 3) it just feels right?
Lunch 11:31 am	2 slices of Spring Pizza	A little	I would keep on eating because the pizza tastes so good.

IT'S TIME TO SAVOR YOUR FOOD

Every meal is an opportunity to experience the amazing flavors of fresh, nutritious foods. Unfortunately, when we gobble down our food, we miss out on this experience. Plus, there is an added advantage to savoring our food. When we focus on our food, it can actually help us stay raw vegan. Unlike cooking, raw food preserves the dynamic flavor of fruits and vegetables, and when you give yourself an opportunity to savor these flavors, it's hard to go back to the dull flavors of cooked foods. Cooked foods just don't compare.

PART 1: GET SOME PRACTICE!

In the first part of this activity, you will choose to savor 1-3 of your meals. The meals can all be in one day or across several days. It's up to you. But try to make an event out of your meals so that you will remember to do it. All too often we intend to change how we eat, but when it comes down to actually doing it, we forget. So, write it in your planner or schedule. When you are ready to eat the meal, return to this worksheet and write down what you are about to eat. During the meal, make a commitment to focus on the food. Don't attempt to read or do another activity while you eat. Instead, chew slowly and savor every bite. You will find that it will take you longer to eat, so make sure you have planned for this extra time. After the meal, think about what you just ate and how it made you feel. Do you feel full? How does your tummy feel? If you ate a meal that you previously ate in the past, did it taste differently? And last, but not least, give yourself a gold star by coloring in an empty gold star in the table below! When you have practiced savoring a few meals, move on to the second part of this activity!

Meal	What did you eat?	If you savored your meal, give yourself a Gold Star!
Breakfast	2 Fiesta Bars + 1 Honeycrisp apple	★
		☆
		☆
		☆

PART 2: TURN IT INTO A HABIT!

Now that you have practiced savoring several meals, it's time to turn this behavior into a habit. Using the table shown below, make a commitment to savor all of your meals for 5 days. This may seem overwhelming, but the more you do it, the easier it will become and eventually it will turn into a habit. Habits take time to develop, so give yourself the space and time to turn this behavior into a habit. If you stick with it, you will find that it will dramatically change your relationship with food by making you more present during your meals. And every time you savor your food, be sure to commemorate your success by coloring in a gold star!

	Breakfast	Snack	Lunch	Snack	Dinner
Day 1	☆	☆	☆	☆	☆
Day 2	☆	☆	☆	☆	☆
Day 3	☆	☆	☆	☆	☆
Day 4	☆	☆	☆	☆	☆
Day 5	☆	☆	☆	☆	☆

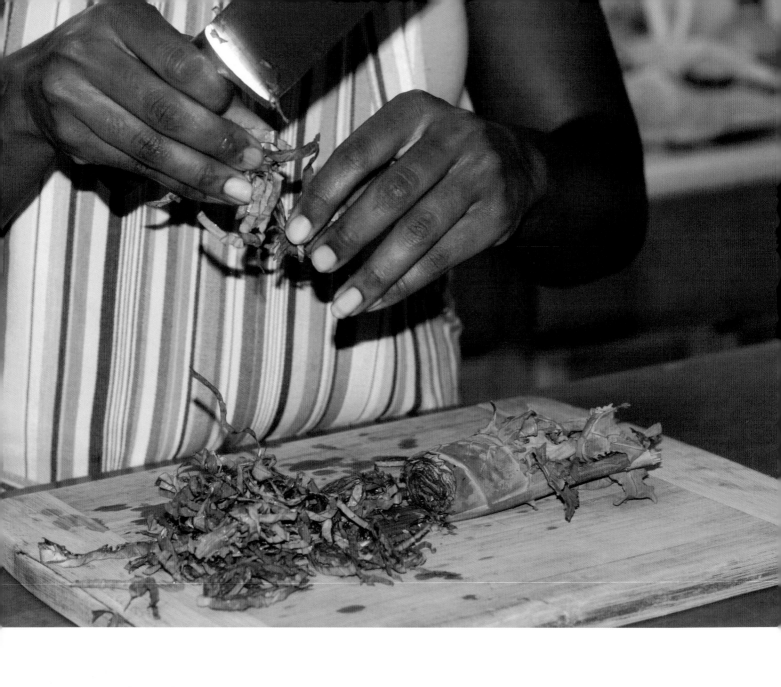

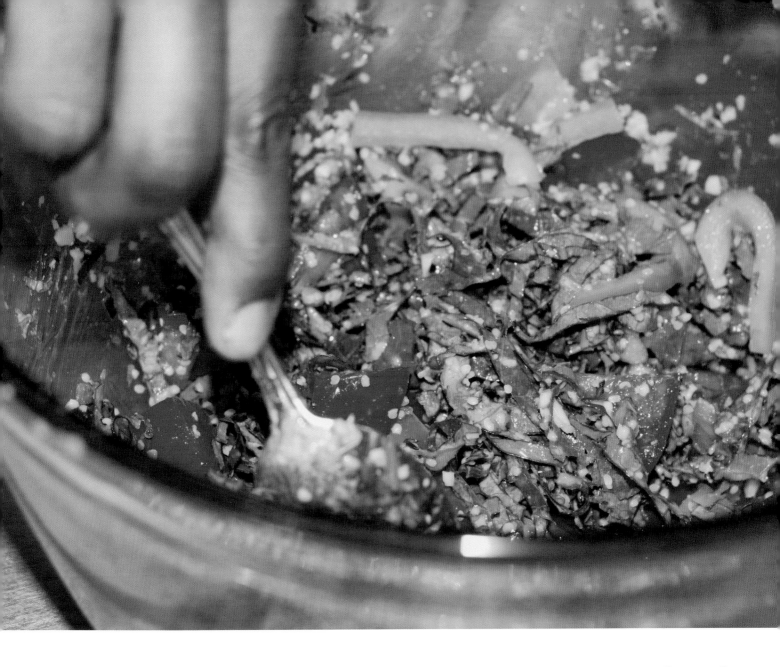

SECTION 3
Raw Start-Up Costs

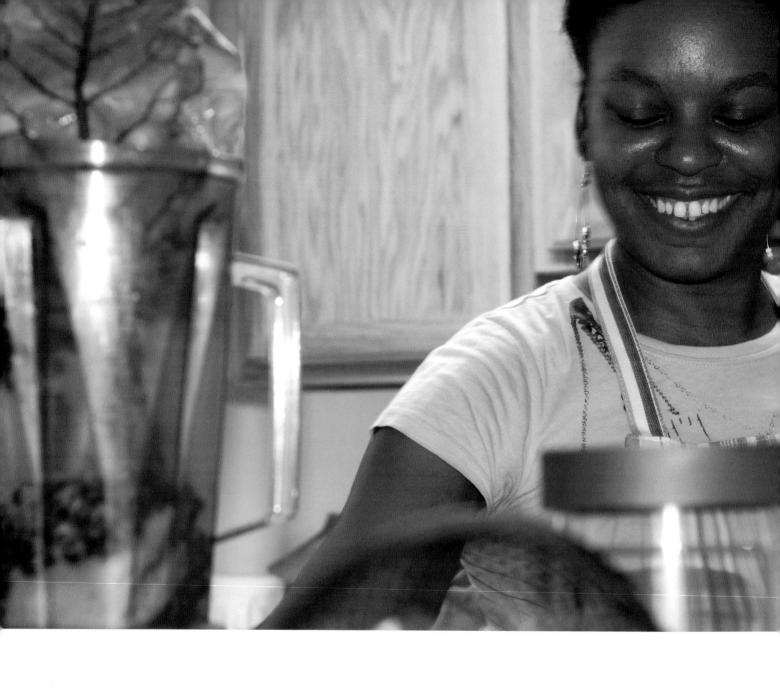

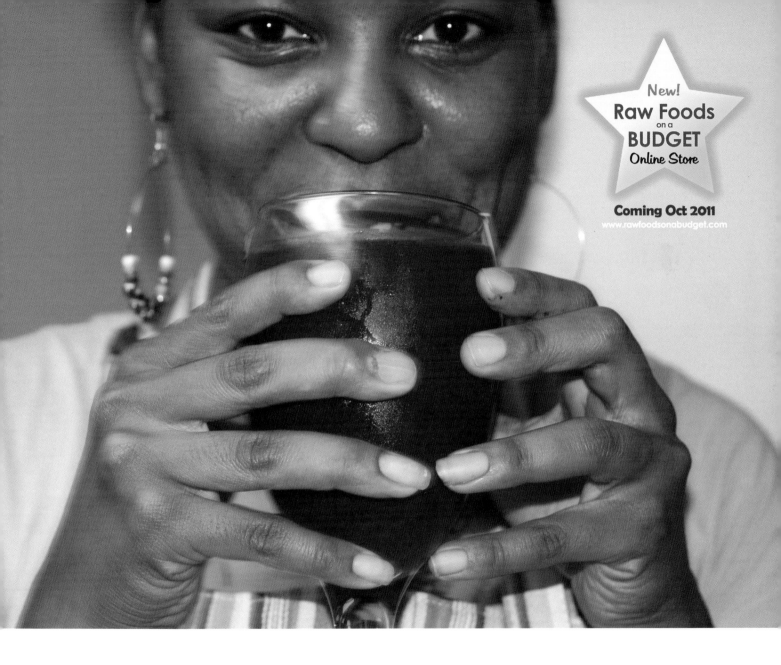

CHAPTER 13

Raw FOOD Start-Up Costs

In this chapter, you will find a list of ingredients that are commonly eaten in the raw foods diet and used in the recipes in this book. Each ingredient includes a description and information on the type of raw food category it falls under (i.e. simple, moderate, or fancy, see pages 28 for definitions), estimated costs, low-cost sources to buy, and recommended storage methods. Note that fruits and vegetables have not been included in this list because there are just too many types and varieties to list.

Coconut

Coconut is a versatile nut that deserves a section of its own. It grows on palm trees in tropical climates and is sold dried, fresh, or as a butter or oil.

(M) Coconut Butter or Cream is the "cream" that rises to the top when coconut milk is allowed to sit. It has a thick paste-like consistency and is often used in raw food desserts. When buying coconut cream, make sure it smells very fragrant and is raw. My favorite brands of coconut cream or butter are Tropical Traditions™, Artisana™, and Let's Do Organic™.

Organic: $6-12 /16 oz bottle
Low-Cost Sources: Buy at health food stores or online. Let's Do Organic™ is a low-cost brand that sells 7 oz. boxes of coconut cream for $2-4. It can sometimes be found in grocery stores.

Storage: Store in a dark, cool place.

(M) Coconut Oil is produced from the meat of mature coconuts. Due to its fragrance and taste, coconut oil is often used to make raw cookies and cheesecakes. This oil has a very long shelf life and can be stored for 2+ years. When buying coconut oil, make sure it's smells very fragrant and has been extracted using low-heat methods such as centrifuge extraction or cold-press.

Organic: $6-20 /16 oz jar
Low-Cost Sources: Buy at health food stores or online.

Storage: Store in a dark, cool place.

(S) Shredded or Flaked Coconut comes from the meat of mature coconuts. The meat is scraped from the coconut and allowed to dry in the sun. Shredded coconut is often used to prepare raw cookies, and dehydrated bars and granolas. When buying shredded coconut, make sure it smells very fragrant and that no additional ingredients have been added.

Organic: $2-3 /1 lb
Conventional: $2-3 /1 lb
Low-Cost Sources: Buy from bulk bins at your local health food store.

Storage: Store in a dry container or refrigerate.

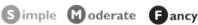

S **Young Coconuts (meat and water)**, also referred to as Thai coconuts, are coconuts that have been harvested before they reach maturity. They are sold encased in a cream-colored fibrous husk that is easy to break open with a large knife. In raw food preparation, Thai coconuts are used for their water and soft meat to prepare ice creams, cookies, soups, drinks, and other fantastic recipes. When buying, choose young coconuts that feel heavy and have no soft or moldy spots. Although organic young coconuts would be ideal, they are difficult to find and conventional coconuts share the same taste and health benefits as organic ones.

Organic: $2-5 per coconut
Conventional: $1-5 per coconut
Low-Cost Sources: Buy from Asian and international markets. They are no different than the ones sold at health food stores.

Storage: Refrigerate.

Nuts and Seeds

S **Almonds** are sold in many different forms: raw shelled and unshelled, sliced, slivered, blanched, roasted, salted, as a flour, and so on. As with any nut or seed, it's best to buy almonds in their raw form (shelled or unshelled). Almonds are the most common nut used in the raw foods diet; however, due to current legislation in California (the biggest producer of almonds), most of the almonds labeled as 'raw' are actually pasteurized.

Organic: $6-15 /1 lb
Conventional: $4-8 /1 lb
Low-Cost Sources: Buy from the bulk bins at your local health food store. Or if you are lucky, get them from your local farmers market.

Storage: Refrigerate or freeze.

 F ancy **M** oderate **S** imple

S **Almond and Cashew Nut Butters** are nuts that have been ground into a thick paste. The most common nut butters that are used in raw food recipes are cashew, coconut, and almond. When buying these butters, make sure that they are raw and no additional ingredients have been added (e.g. sugars, salts). The butter should smell nutty and not have large amounts of oil floating at the top as this may indicate prolonged storage. Raw food enthusiasts use nut butters to add a creamy texture to recipes like pates, desserts, sushi rolls, etc. Because these butters can be expensive, try to make them at home, use the whole nut form instead, or buy them from bulk bins.

Organic: $6-20 /16 oz bottle
Conventional: $6-12 /16 oz bottle
Low-Cost Sources: Buy from health food and grocery stores (from bulk bins, if possible).

Storage: Refrigerate or freeze.

S **Buckwheat Groats** are three-cornered seeds that were first cultivated in prehistoric China. Buckwheat groats are often used in raw food recipes to make breads, crackers, and granolas. Buy groats that are hulled (i.e. shell removed) and untoasted.

Organic: $2-3 /1 lb
Conventional: $1.50-3.00 /1 lb
Low-Cost Sources: Buy from bulk bins at your local health food store.

Storage: Store in a dry-container or refrigerate.

S **Cashews** are native to the tropics and widely used to add a creamy texture to raw food dishes and desserts (e.g. cheesecakes and cookies). Because high temperatures are used to remove cashews from their hard caustic shells, most cashews sold in grocery stores are not actually raw (even though they are labelled 'raw'). The best way to find truly raw cashews is to buy from companies like Nativas Naturals™. Due to the high costs of truly raw cashews, they are only used in limited quantities in the recipes in this book.

Organic: $8-15 /1 lb
Low-Cost Sources: Buy in bulk from online stores like www.pangaia.cc and Amazon.com.

Storage: Refrigerate or freeze.

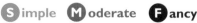 **S** imple **M** oderate **F** ancy

(S) **Flaxseeds** are shiny, oval-shaped, brown or golden seeds that taste nutty and are a rich source of omega 3s, fiber, magnesium, and folate. Flaxseeds are commonly sold in their whole or ground state, or as an oil. It's best to buy whole flaxseeds and then grind them yourself as needed with coffee grinder or blender. Brown and golden flaxseeds have a similar nutritive quality, though golden flaxseeds have a more buttery flavor. Flaxseeds are typically used in raw bread and cracker recipes to help bind ingredients.

Organic: $1-3 /1 lb
Conventional: $1-3 / 1 lb
Low-Cost Sources: Buy from bulk bins at your local health food store.

Storage: Refrigerate or freeze.

(M) **Macadamia Nuts** are rich and fatty nuts that grow in the South Pacific. Because of their buttery texture, macadamia nuts are often used to make raw food desserts like ice creams, pie crusts, and cheesecakes. Due to their high fat content, macadamia nuts can quickly become rancid (i.e. < 1 month), so it's ideal to purchase them from retailers that keep them refrigerated or sell them unshelled.

Organic: $15-20 /1 lb
Conventional: $10-15 /1 lb
Low-Cost Sources: Buy in bulk from online stores like www.pangaia.cc or from local health food stores.

Storage: Refrigerate or freeze.

(S) **Pecans** are a soft, rich nut produced in the United States. The nuts are 70% fat and provide some calcium, iron, magnesium, potassium, and selenium. Pecans are often used in raw food cuisine to make desserts and pie crusts. It's okay to buy pecans from bulk bins, however, keep them refrigerated or in the freezer until you are ready to use them.

Organic: $10-15 /1 lb
Conventional: $8-13 /1 lb
Low-Cost Sources: Buy from bulk bins at your local health food store.

Storage: Refrigerate or freeze.

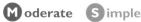 **F**ancy **M**oderate **S**imple

Pumpkin Seeds are an inexpensive, nutritious snack that have been eaten for centuries. Most of our pumpkin seeds come from Mexico, however, some are grown in the United States. Pumpkin seeds are high in protein, iron and phosphorus, and do contain some calcium, vitamin A, and B-complex vitamins. Pumpkin seeds make a wonderful chocolate nut milk and are typically used in raw food recipes to make pates, breads, and salads.

Organic: $3-8 /1 lb
Conventional: $3-5 /1 lb
Low-Cost Sources: Buy from bulk bins at your local health food store.

Storage: Refrigerate or freeze.

Sunflower Seeds are derived from the magnificent sunflower, which can grow up to 17 feet tall! Sunflower seeds are a great survival food that is high in protein and a wonderful source for calcium, iron, magnesium, phosphorus, potassium, several b-complex vitamins, and vitamin A. Sunflower seeds are normally sold in the seed form; however, you can also buy sunflower sprouts and sunflower seed oil and butter in many health food stores. Sunflower seeds are typically used to make raw pates, breads and crackers, and are used in salads; however, you will find that I use them in a wide range of recipes due to their versatility and flavor.

Organic: $2.50-4 /1 lb
Conventional: $1-2 /1 lb
Low-Cost Sources: Buy from bulk bins at your local health food store.

Storage: Refrigerate or freeze.

Walnuts are native to Persia, and are grown in many parts of the world. Walnuts are a creamy, versatile nut that adds a buttery texture to raw food recipes. Walnuts are a good source of iron, magnesium, phosphorus, potassium, and zinc. When buying walnuts, look for nuts that are brittle and will snap if broken. Avoid nuts that are shriveled, rubbery, or have mold.

Organic: $8-11 /1 lb
Conventional: $6-8 /1 lb
Low-Cost Sources: Buy from bulk bins at your local health food store.

Storage: Refrigerate or freeze.

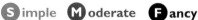

Simple **M**oderate **F**ancy

Oils

(S) Olive Oil comes from the fruit of the olive tree, an evergreen that is known to live for 1,500 to 2,000 years. When purchasing olive oil, be sure to buy extra virgin oil as this is the only form of olive oil that is truly cold pressed. Olive oil is one of the most common ingredients in raw food recipes. Purchase olive oil that is sold in dark bottles and, if possible, buy it in small quantities (e.g., 1-2 bottles).

Organic: $7 & Up /16 oz bottle
Conventional: $4 & Up /16 oz bottle
Low-Cost Sources: Buy from discount stores like TJ Maxx™, or in bulk cans from health food stores.

Storage: Refrigerate or store in a dark, cool place.

(M) Sesame Seed Oil is pressed from sesame seeds and is one of the oldest vegetable oils used today. Cold-pressed raw sesame seed oil can be difficult to find, however, Eden™ makes a wonderful oil. Sesame seed oil has a wonderful nutty and mild flavor, and should be purchased in dark bottles. This oil can be used to make salad dressings, crackers, Asian-flavored dishes, and anything else you can think of!

Organic: $10 & Up /16 oz bottle
Low-Cost Sources: Buy it from health food stores or online.

Storage: Refrigerate.

Seaweeds

(S) Dulse is a red seaweed that grows in the North Atlantic Ocean near Maine, Scotland, and Wales. Its use as a food dates back to the 18th century in the British Isles. Dulse has a salty taste and chewy texture, and is often used in place of salt. Dulse can be cut into small pieces and sprinkled on top of salads and soups, and used to make breads and crackers. When purchasing dulse make sure that it's untoasted.

Organic: $4-7 /4 oz bag
Conventional: $2-4 /4 oz bag
Low-Cost Sources: Buy in bulk from health food stores or online.

Storage: Can be stored indefinitely in air-tight moisture proof bags and containers.

(M) **Kelp** is the fastest growing plant in the world. It can grow 2 feet a day and reach over 100 feet in length. Kelp grows along the east and west coasts of the United States. Kelp is used in many raw food recipes in the form of 'Kelp Noodles'. Kelp noodles make delicious recipes like Pad Thai, seaweed salads, and Chow Mein (page 207). These noodles can be expensive or unavailable in some areas, so consider looking for them in your local Asian markets or online.

Organic: (dried strips) $5-7 /4 oz bag
Conventional: (noodles) $3-5 /1 lb bag
Low-Cost Sources: Buy in bulk from health food and grocery stores, or from online stores like www.seaveg.com.

Storage: Refrigerate kelp noodles; dried kelp can be stored indefinitely in air-tight moisture proof bags and containers.

(S) **Laver Nori and Nori Sheets** are produced from the laver seaweed, a tender seaweed found off the coasts of Hawaii, Japan, Europe, California, and along the North Atlantic. 'Laver nori' refers to laver that is sold in its sea vegetable form, whereas 'nori sheets' refers to laver that has been pressed into paper-thin sheets. Laver nori and nori sheets are wonderful to use in soups, noodle dishes, salads, or as a quick snack. And, of course, nori sheets are great for making sushi! When purchasing, be sure to buy raw, dried, or untoasted nori. Toasted nori is green in color whereas raw nori tends to be purple-black.

Organic: (laver nori) $4-6 /1 oz, $20 /1 lb; (nori sheets) $4-6 /10 sheets, $12-30 /50 sheets
Conventional: (nori sheets) $1-4 /10 sheets, $10-15 /50 sheets
Low-Cost Sources: Buy in 50 or 100 sheet packages online at www.pangaia.cc or www.seaveg.com, or at health food stores. The price for nori sheets can range dramatically, so be sure to look around before purchasing.

Storage: Can be stored indefinitely in air-tight moisture proof bags and containers.

 imple ancy

Spices

(M) Chinese Five Spice is a beautiful combination of five spices that provide all the five flavors: sweet, salty, sour, bitter, and pungent. It's one of my favorite spices and an easy way to add a multidimensional flavor to a recipe. You can find this spice at most grocery and health food stores, and Asian markets. Try to make your own Chinese five spice by using equal parts of ground cinnamon, ground clove, ground peppercorns, ground fennel seed, and ground anise seed.

Organic: depends on amount purchased
Conventional: depends on amount purchased
Low-Cost Sources: Buy from bulk or spice bins at your local health food store. Bottles of this spice can range from $2-6.

Storage: Store in moisture proof containers or bags.

(S) Italian Spices: basil, thyme, and oregano are herbs that should be kept in the pantry at all times. They can be used to make beautiful raw marinara sauces and are quite yummy when sprinkled on salads and into salad dressings. Try growing these herbs in your indoor and outdoor garden, and using them fresh or drying them for later use.

Organic: depends on amount purchased
Conventional: depends on amount purchased
Low-Cost Sources: Buy from bulk or spice bins at your local health food store. Bottles of this spice can range from $2-6.

Storage: Store in moisture proof containers or bags.

(S) Mexican or Hot Spices: cumin, chipotle, chili powder, and coriander are all amazing seasonings that are easy to use. They work well together and a little sprinkle goes a long way. You can find these spices at most grocery and health food stores. If you grow cilantro in your garden, try saving the seeds and drying them to make your own home-grown coriander.

Organic: depends on amount purchased
Conventional: depends on amount purchased
Low-Cost Sources: Buy from bulk or spice bins at your local health food store. Bottles of this spice can range from $2-6.

Storage: Store in moisture proof containers or bags.

(S) **Sea Salt** comes in so many varieties from so many parts of the world that it's really up to you to decide which kind you want to use. Sea salt is unlike regular salt in that it contains small amounts of minerals and has a deeper salty flavor, which means you use less. Popular sea salts consumed by raw vegans are Celtic Sea Salt, Red (or Real) Sea Salt, and Himalayan Sea Salt. Personally, I like Celtic Sea Salt because it's both delicious and affordable.

Sea Salt: $2 & Up / 1 lb
Low-Cost Sources: Buy in bulk from a health food store.

Storage: Store in moisture proof containers or bags.

(S) **Sweet Spices: cinnamon, clove, nutmeg, and pumpkin pie spice** are wonderful spices to use in desserts. In fact, they are used in most of the desserts in this book. Plus, they are easy to find at grocery and health food stores.

Organic: depends on amount purchased
Conventional: depends on amount purchased
Low-Cost Sources: Buy from bulk or spice bins at your local health food store. Bottles of this spice can range from $2-6.

Storage: Store in moisture proof containers or bags.

(S) **Vanilla** is used to enhance the flavor of recipes such as ice creams, cakes, pies, and granolas. It's sold in many different forms including the whole pod, powder (i.e. pods that have been ground up), and as an extract (in an alcohol or glycerol solution). My favorite brand of vanilla is Frontier's™ Vanilla Flavor, which is composed of vanilla beans, glycerin (to extract the flavor from the beans), and water. It has no alcohol, so the flavor is sweet and clean.

Organic: (glycerin-based) $9 & Up / 4 oz bottle; (alcohol-based) $7 & Up / 4 oz bottle
Conventional: (alcohol-based) $2 & Up/ 4 oz bottle
Low-Cost Sources: Buy bottles from local health food and groceries stores; vanilla powder can be found online at websites like www.pangaia.cc.

Storage: Store in an air-tight bottle or container in a cool, dry place.

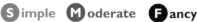
(S)imple   (M)oderate   (F)ancy

Sweeteners

(S) **Agave Syrup** comes from the nectar of agave plants and has been traditionally used to flavor foods and drinks. Agave is processed at low temperatures, making it a great sweetener in raw food recipes. However, more recently, raw experts have begun to question whether agave is truly a raw food.

Organic: $5 & up /16 oz bottle
Conventional: $4 & up /16 oz bottle
Low-Cost Sources: Buy in bulk from health food stores or online. Bottles can also be found in many grocery stores.

Storage: Store in a cool place.

(S) **Dates** are the candy that grows on trees. There are more than 100 different varieties of dates; however, you will most likely see only 1-2 varieties in your local store. Most of the dates produced in the United States are of the Deglet Noor variety, which makes them the cheapest dates to buy. Medjool dates are larger, meatier dates, but they are also more expensive. You can use either variety when preparing raw food recipes. If a recipe calls for medjool dates, and you only have Deglet Noor dates, use 1.5 Deglet Noor dates for every 1 medjool date.

Organic: (Deglet Noor) $3-4 /1 lb; (Medjool) $6-8 /1 lb
Conventional: (Deglet Noor) $3-4 /1 lb; (Medjool) $5-7 /1 lb
Low-Cost Sources: Buy from bulk bins at your local health food store.

Storage: Store in moisture proof containers or bags.

(S) **Honey** is one of the oldest sweeteners known to man. It's manufactured by honeybees and depending on the type of pollen collected by the bees, honey can take on many subtle flavors. When purchasing honey, be sure to buy RAW honey. Most of the honey found in grocery stores has been pasteurized and filtered. Try to find locally produced raw honey at a local farm, farmers market, or health food store.

Organic: $6 & up /1 lb
Conventional: $4 & up /1 lb
Low-Cost Sources: Buy in bulk from health food stores, local farms, or farmers markets.

Storage: Store in moisture proof containers.

(S) Raisins are the most popular dried fruit in the United States. Most of the raisins sold are of the Thompson Seedless variety and are allowed to naturally dry in the sun. Raisins are amazing as a sweetener in recipes because they are both very sweet and moist. Note that golden seedless raisins are artificially dried with sulfur dioxide gas and should be avoided.

Organic: $2-5 /1 lb
Conventional: $2-4 /1 lb
Low-Cost Sources: Buy from bulk bins at your local health food store.

Storage: Store in moisture proof containers.

(S) Green Stevia has been used for centuries as a sweeter. Green stevia is sold in leaf and powder form, though the latter form is easier to use in recipes. See page 103 for more information on stevia. Stevia enhances the sweetness of other sweeteners like agave and honey, which means that you use less of them. Green stevia can be difficult to find, however, you can buy it online or at many herb stores. Although the price of stevia is somewhat high, an 8 oz. bag (~$10-12) can last 1-2 years.

Organic: $10 & up /1 lb
Low-Cost Sources: Buy in bulk from online stores like www.pangaia.cc and amazon.com. May be available in bulk at your local herb stores.

Storage: Store in moisture proof containers.

Sauces and Vinegars

(S) Apple Cider Vinegar is a flavorful vinegar that is made from fermenting apples, and is used in salad dressings and to flavor leafy greens and vegetables. When buying apple cider vinegar, choose a brand that has fermented the vinegar in oak barrels. Two popular brands of apple cider vinegar are Braggs™ and Eden™.

Organic: $4-6 /32 oz bottle
Conventional: $3-6 /32 oz bottle
Low-Cost Sources: Buy from local health food and grocery stores. If you use great quantities of apple cider vinegar, purchase it by the gallon ($15-20).

Storage: Store in a dry, cool place.

S imple **M** oderate **F** ancy

(S) **Balsamic Vinegar** is made from pressed white grapes that have been boiled down and allowed to ferment. The older the vinegar, the more flavorful it is. Balsamic vinegar is often used in raw food recipes to flavor salad dressings, but it can also add a wonderful flavor to fruits and ice creams. When choosing a bottle of balsamic vinegar, avoid brands that have added colors, sulfites, and other additives.

Organic: $7 & up /16 oz bottle
Conventional: $3 & up /16 oz bottle
Low-Cost Sources: Buy from local health food and grocery stores.

Storage: Store in a dry, cool place.

(M) **Brown and White Rice Vinegars** are light, sweet vinegars that have been made from cooked rice that has been allowed to ferment. These vinegars are wonderful for adding a subtle sweet flavor to recipes and are a staple in Chinese and Japanese dishes. These vinegars are used throughout this book, however, they can be easily substituted with apple cider vinegar. For the best tasting vinegar, try to purchase an organic brand.

Organic: (brown) $5-7 /10 oz bottle; (white) $4-5 /24 oz bottle
Conventional: (brown) $3-5 /10 oz bottle; (white) $2-4 /24 oz bottle
Low-Cost Sources: Buy organic brands from local health food and grocery stores; buy conventional brands from grocery stores and Asian markets.

Storage: Store in a dry, cool place.

(S) **Nama Shoyu** is a non-pasteurized type of soy sauce that is produced from fermented soy beans, grains, and enzymes. Like soy sauce, nama shoyu is used as a dipping sauce or to add a meaty flavor to vegetable recipes. When purchasing a brand of nama shoyu, make sure that no sugars or additive flavors have been added. The brands Oshawa™ and Eden™ make a wonderful-tasting nama shoyu.

Organic: $3-7 / 10 oz bottle
Low-Cost Sources: Buy organic brands from local health food stores.

Storage: Store in a dry, cool place.

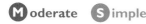 **F**ancy **M**oderate **S**imple

(M) **Ume Plum Vinegar** is a red color seasoning that is produced from ume plums and salt. It's not a traditional vinegar, although it does have sour and salty properties, which makes it a great addition to salad, soups, and even beverages. When using ume plum vinegar, remember that a little goes a very long way, as it is very salty. Eden™ makes a wonderful brand of ume plum vinegar.

Conventional: $2-5 /10 oz bottle
Low-Cost Sources: Buy from local health food stores or Asian markets.

Storage: Store in a dry, cool place.

Other

(M) **Arrowroot Powder** is made from pulverized arrowroot tubers that have been strained and allowed to sun-dry. The powder is used as a thickener in many recipes. Traditionally, arrowroot powder is cooked to activate its thickening properties, however, it does have subtle thickening properties when uncooked. When purchasing arrowroot, make sure that it's pure arrowroot and no additional ingredients have been added.

Conventional: $0.35-1.00 /1 oz
Low-Cost Sources: Buy from spice or bulk bins at your local health food and grocery stores.

Storage: Store in moisture proof containers or bags.

(S) **Nutritional Yeast** is produced from culturing *Saccharomyces cerevisiae* (a yeast) on a mixture of sugarcane and beet molasses. The yeast is sold in its inactive form, and is a wonderful source of B-complex vitamins and protein. It's used in many vegetarian and raw food dishes to add a nutty, cheesy, or creamy flavor. When purchasing nutritional yeast, Red Star™ or Braggs™ are wonderful brands.

Organic: $4-7 /5 oz bottle
Conventional: $4-7 /5 oz bottle
Low-Cost Sources: If you can, purchase the brands, Red Star™ and Braggs™. You can find them at your local health food stores. You can also buy nutritional yeast from bulk bins.

Storage: Refrigerate or freeze.

Sources: The cost estimates are based on pricing data I collected from several health food, grocery, and online stores and my own experience of visiting many health food and grocery stores across the United States.

Roehl, Evelyn. (1996). *Whole Food Facts: The Complete Reference Guide*. Rochester: Healing Arts Press.

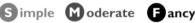 imple oderate **(F)** ancy

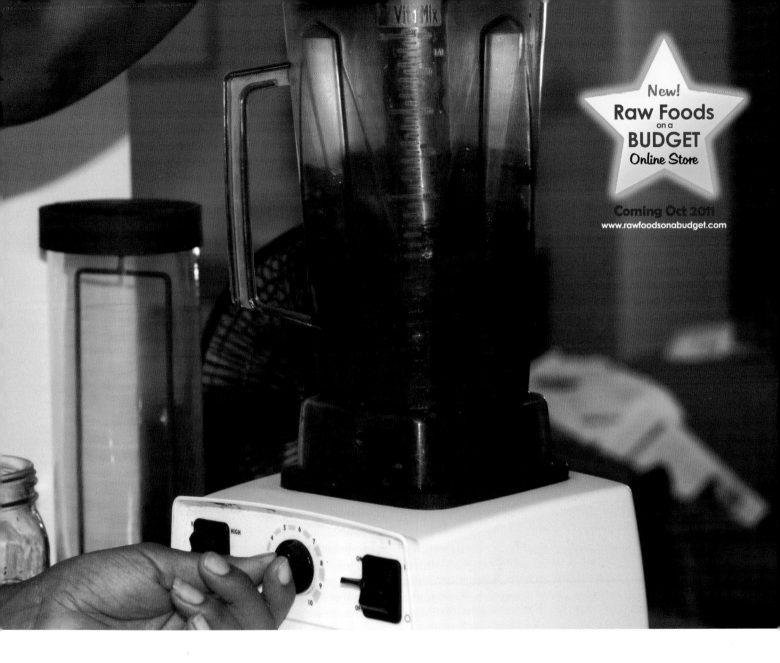

New!
Raw Foods
on a
BUDGET
Online Store

Coming Oct 2011
www.rawfoodsonabudget.com

CHAPTER 14

EQUIPMENT Start-Up Costs

In this chapter, you will find a list of equipment that are commonly used to prepare raw food recipes. Each piece of equipment includes a description and information on the type of raw food category it falls under (i.e. simple, moderate, or fancy, see pages 28 for definitions), estimated costs, and low-cost sources to buy.

(S) (M) (F) **Blenders** are an essential part of the raw food kitchen. If you are looking to make smoothies, sauces, cheesecakes, and creamy pies, then you will want to invest in a blender. Blenders come in different shapes and sizes, and the best blender is the one that fits your budget and needs. If you are looking to make smoothies and easy-to-blend sauces, then a $20 blender will do the trick! Just make sure that the blade is sharp. If you have an old blender, then invest in a new one or replace the blade (many manufacturers sell their blades online). If you want to make creamier recipes like cheesecakes and creamy pies, then a high-speed blender is ideal. The most popular high-speed blenders are the Vitamix™ and Blendtec™, which can cost $400-600. I personally have a Vitamix™ and given that it will last me 20-30 years, it's worth every penny; however, it still may be too expensive for most people. Consider purchasing refurbished and used models from these manufacturers on their websites. Because these blenders have long warranties and are meant to last decades, a used model will still have a lot of life in it. Alternatively, you can invest in personal high-speed blenders like the Tribest™ or Magic Bullet™, which can cost $30-100.

Basic: $15-100
High-Speed (personal): $35-100 (e.g. Tribest)
High-Speed (large): $350 & up (e.g. Vitamix)
Low-Cost Sources: You can find basic blenders at discount stores like Ross™, TJ Maxx™, and Ollies™, and online at www.amazon.com. Shop around so that you will find the best price. The best source to buy high-speed personal blenders is online. Sometimes you can find a great deal locally, but these blenders are not sold in many stores. Shop online to find the best deals on large high-speed blenders. Sometimes you can find used blenders on websites like www.craigslist.org. For information on shopping at Craigslist, see page 90.

(S) **Casserole Bowl with Lid (Clear Glass).** This comes in handy when you want to bake dishes in the sun. Because the bowl and lid are glass, all of the food gets exposed to the sun. Plus, it keeps all of the curious insects and small animals out.

Costs: $3-10
Low-Cost Sources: Buy from discount stores like TJ Maxx™ and Ross™.

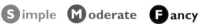

(S)imple **(M)**oderate **(F)**ancy

(S) Coffee Grinders are useful for grinding small batches of spices and nuts. For example, many of the cracker and bread recipes in this book call for ground flaxseeds. With a coffee grinder you can do this in seconds. A simple coffee grinder will do the job... there is no need to get fancy here.

Costs: $10-30
Low-Cost Sources: Buy online from stores like www.amazon.com or your local kitchen supply store.

(S) Cutting Board. This is an essential part of any kitchen. A cutting board can be made of bamboo, wood, or plastic, and the cost will depend on the type of wood and size. A bamboo cutting board will be slightly more expensive, but it's much kinder to your knives and has anti-bacterial properties.

Costs: $3 & up
Low-Cost Sources: Buy from discount stores like Ross™ and TJ Maxx™, or online from stores with free shipping like www.amazon.com.

(M) (F) Dehydrator and Texflex Sheets. A dehydrator is used to make crackers and breads, and even to warm raw food dishes like soups. When buying a dehydrator, purchase one with an adjustable thermostat because most dehydrators are automatically set to run at 145 degrees Fahrenheit. Excalibur™ makes a fantastic dehydrator that will last for 10 years, however there are less expensive brands like Nesco™. Texflex sheets are plastic sheets that are used to line dehydrator trays so you can prepare recipes like fruit roll ups and crackers. However, you can use parchment paper instead to line dehydrator trays if necessary. Note that your foods will dehydrate faster with parchment paper.

Costs: $50 & up
The costs of a dehydrator will depend on the size and brand. Be sure to buy what you need and avoid being extravagant.

Low-Cost Sources: Buy online from stores like www.amazon.com, and be sure to shop around for the best price.

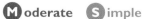
(F) ancy **(M)** oderate **(S)** imple

(S) (M) Food Processor. This is an essential part of the raw food kitchen. A food processor is used for making pie crusts, pates, breads, crackers, and some sauces. When purchasing a food processor, if possible, buy a good quality one that will last you 10+ years. However, there are cheaper brands that will also get the job done. Because many people have food processors they don't use, consider asking a relative or friend for their food processor (that's how I got mine).

Costs: $20 and up
The cost of a food processor will vary depending on the quality, brand, and size. A small food processor may run you $15, but a large one may cost $30 & up (some sell for $100+).

Low-Cost Sources: Buy online from stores like www.amazon.com, and be sure to shop around for the best price.

(M) (F) Frother. This is not an essential part of the raw food kitchen, but it's a fun piece of equipment that will take your tea lattes to the next level. The frother "froths" up the milk portion of your latte to create a creamy foam. It's like having a raw Starbucks™ in your kitchen!

Costs: $10-20
Low-Cost Sources: Buy online from stores like www.amazon.com or your local kitchen supply store.

(S) (M) (F) Ice Cream Maker. If you would like to easily make ice creams and sorbets, an ice cream maker is a must have! It's a great investment and if you take care of it, it will last for many years. When buying an ice cream maker, there is no need to get fancy. A basic model will work. An ice maker is great for making impromptu sorbets and ice creams. During the summer, I like to keep my ice cream maker ready because I never know when I will find a quart of super-ripe plums or peaches at a local farm.

Costs: $25 & up
The cost depends on the size and brand. A 1.5 quart ice cream maker will make enough to feed 3-4 people. The brand doesn't really matter as long as you take care of it. And just so you know, I got my ice cream maker for $30 at Ollies™ discount department store.

Low-Cost Sources: Buy from discount stores like Ollies™ and TJ Maxx™, or online from stores like www.amazon.com.

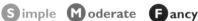

Japanese Mandoline. This is a useful tool when you want to create noodles, thinly sliced vegetables, or match-stick vegetable strips for your sushi. I like to use mine for making yam chips, thinly sliced onions for my flatbreads, and for creating noodles. When buying a mandoline, I recommend purchasing one from an Asian market. They are sharper and sturdier than many of the American versions sold today, and will last 2+ years.

Costs: $15-20
Low-Cost Sources: Buy from your local Asian market or, if you have to, get them online from stores like www.amazon.com.

Julienne Peeler. I love this tool! It's affordable, easy to use, and makes noodles within seconds. Use this peeler when you want to create noodles using cucumbers, zucchini, and winter squash.

Costs: $8-20
Low-Cost Sources: Buy from discount stores like Ross™ and TJ Maxx™, from your local kitchen supply store, or online from stores like www.amazon.com.

Juicer. If you want to create lovely raw juices, then a juicer is a must have. When buying a juicer, it's useful to consider the type of juices you would like to make. If you want to juice wheatgrass, fibrous leafy greens, and fruits, then a low-speed juicer will do the job. If you plan to juice a lot of carrots and less fibrous fruits and vegetables, then a high-speed blender like the Champion Juicer™ will work. I recommend a low-speed juicer like a Samson™, Omega™, or Greenstar™. Because these juicers last 20+ years, consider buying one that is used or refurbished. You can find used juicers for sale on websites like Craigslist. I purchased my juicer on Craigslist when it was about 5 years old, and now it's over 10 years old and still working like new. When purchasing a juicer, also consider how easy it is to clean. You don't want this to stand in the way of you creating yummy juices everyday!

Costs: $75 & up
The cost depends on the quality of the juicer. Juicers that cost less that $100 typically don't do a good job of extracting all of the juice and will only last you a year or two. Ideally, you will purchase a juicer that will last 20+ years.

Low-Cost Sources: Buy online and be sure to shop around. The prices will vary by website.

  Fancy **M**oderate **S**imple

S M F **Knives.** Raw food involves a lot of chopping and it's worth the investment to buy a sharp knife. Not only is a sharp knife safer, it's easier on your wrist. When purchasing a new knife, wonderful brands are J.A. Henckels™, Chicago Cutlery™, and even Cuisinart™. It may be tempting to purchase a big knife set, but all you really need is one good chef's knife. In addition, invest in a knife sharpener so that your knife will last for many years to come.

Costs: $20 & up
Low-Cost Sources: You can find low-priced, high-quality knives from discount stores like Tuesday Morning™, TJ Maxx™, and Ross™, or from online stores like www.amazon.com.

S **Nut Milk Bag.** This is a must have if you plan on making nut milks. Basically, the bag is used to separate the nut pulp from the nut milk. These bags can also be used for sun baking (i.e. to cover a glass bowl while keeping insects away), sprouting seeds, and keeping fruit flies away from your precious fruit.

Costs: $4-15
Low-Cost Sources: Buy online from stores like www.pangaia.cc and www.amazon.com, or your local health food store.

S **Pie Plate.** This is a must have if you want to make pies. Although pie plates are inexpensive, in some cases you can get away with using a dinner plate instead.

Costs: $2-4
Low-Cost Sources: Buy from your local grocery store.

S **Salad Spinner.** This is one of my favorite pieces of equipment in the whole kitchen. A salad spinner removes excess water from your lettuce. The costs of a salad spinner can vary from $3 to $20; however, stores like Target™ (where I got my $3 salad spinner), Ross™, and TJ Maxx™ will have them for less. If you buy a cheap one, like I did, be sure to take care of it so that it will last a long time.

Costs: $3 & up
Low-Cost Sources: Buy from discount stores like Target™, Ross™, or TJ Maxx™.

  S imple **M** oderate **F** ancy

M Spiralizer. This piece of equipment is used to create beautiful noodles for raw food dishes.

Costs: $15-40
Low-Cost Sources: Buy online from stores like www.amazon.com or your local kitchen supply store.

M Spring Pan. This is a useful piece of equipment that is great for making cheesecakes, cakes, and pies.

Costs: $2-5
Low-Cost Sources: Buy from discount stores like Target™, Ross™, or TJ Maxx™.

S Sprout Tray. A sprout tray is useful for growing your own sprouts right on your kitchen counter. Sprouts are a wonderful addition to the raw food diet and a great source of protein, vitamins, and minerals.

Costs: $10-30
Low-Cost Sources: Buy online from stores like www.amazon.com, or from your local health food store.

S Wire Sieve. I am a big fan of the wire sieve. It comes in handy when you need to filter a tea, make watermelon juice, or even sprout seeds. These sieves come in all sizes, so I would recommend buying a large and small one if possible. They can range in costs, so be sure to buy one that fits within your budget. In addition, try your best to take care of it because if you clean and store properly, it will last for years.

Costs: $2-10
Low-Cost Sources: Buy from discount stores like Target™, Ross™, and TJ Maxx™, or your local kitchen supply store.

Sources: The cost estimates are based on pricing data I collected from several health food, grocery, and online stores and my own experience of visiting many health food and grocery stores across the United States.

 Fancy   **M**oderate   **S**imple

I tried the Lemon Green Yum Kale salad tonight and it was so good! It was the last one of the three in the book for me to try and all of them are tremendous.

-Linda

I just made the raw walnut pesto!! Love it!!

-Shasta

Yum Yum!

-Scott

My family and I adore your "Oatmeal" recipe. I served it for breakfast one day this week, and it stuck to their ribs the whole morning. Yum!

-Ida

Great Recipes

-Helene

LOVE the kale recipe!!! Thanks :-)

-Sarah

I can say the recipes are easy and delicious first hand. My meat and potato man loves them too.

-Teresa

Okay, for the record, girlIIIIIIIIIIIIIIIIIII - that corn salad was GOOD!

-Rufiena

I tried and love the vegetable pate.

-Damianna

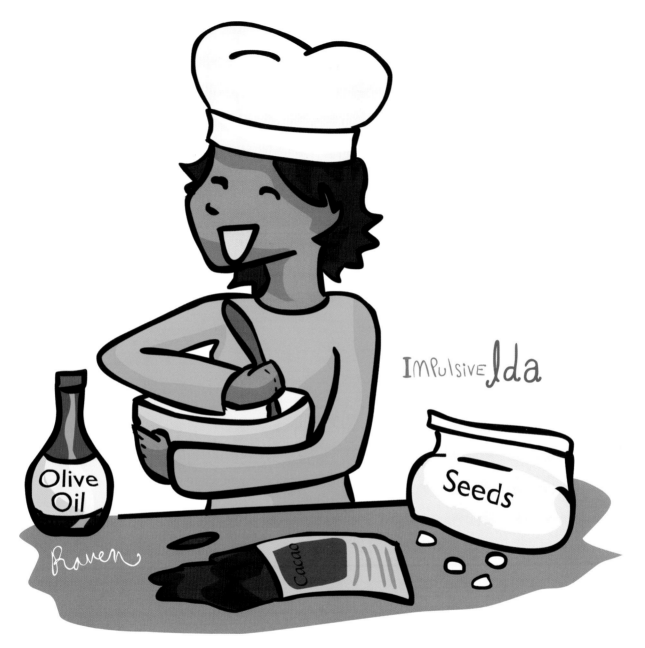

IMPULSIVE Ida

Olive Oil

Seeds

Cacao

Raven

SECTION 4

Recipes

My Un-Cooking Philosophy

Every recipe has the potential to be an awesome experience. Yet, often, when we prepare raw foods, we offer feelings of self-doubt and uncertainty into our food rather than joy and abundance. Unfortunately, when we feel uncertain while preparing a recipe, our food comes out tasting uncertain (i.e. it kinda tastes like something is missing).

Try this: Right before you prepare your next meal, light a candle, say a prayer or affirmation, and/or think positive thoughts. This will help you relax, release any doubts or worries, and make you more present. For example, When I prepare food, I think positive and reassure myself that whatever I create will be a beautiful experience. And it is! Why wouldn't it…I made it! And I figure, I could either radiate positive, negative, or uncertain thoughts, so why not choose positive ones. It's simply a choice. It may be difficult at first, but as your dishes begin tasting better, you will develop greater confidence in your ability to prepare raw food recipes and thinking positive will be as easy as one…two…and three!

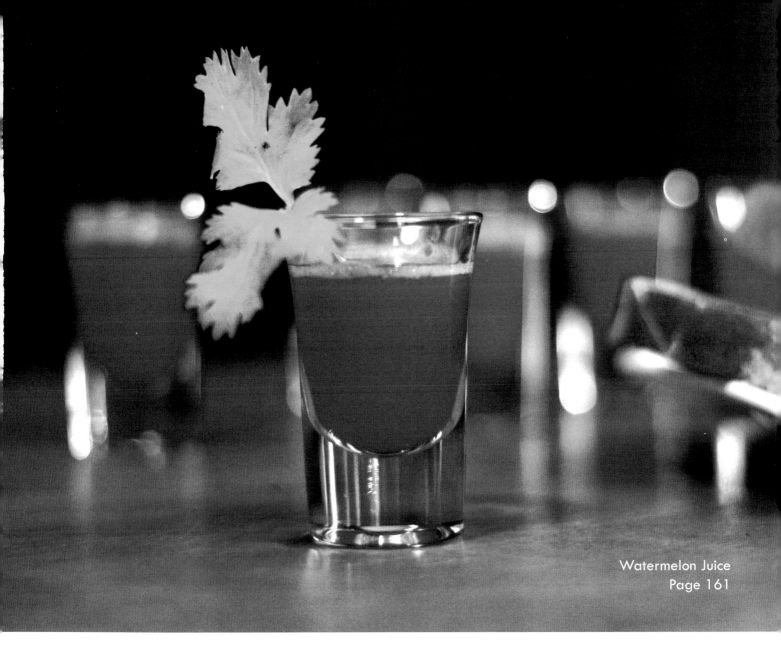

Watermelon Juice
Page 161

Drinks

Smoothies

Glorious Green Smoothie

This is such a beautiful smoothie! It's cold and perfect after a hard workout.

Makes 2 Cups | 1 Serving

2 cups (packed) red Russian kale	$1.00
1/2 cup blueberries	$0.50
1/2 cup strawberries, whole	$0.50
1/2 cup water	$0.00
1/4 cup currants, dried	$0.25
green stevia powder to taste	<$0.05
Total estimated cost	$2.30
Estimated cost per serving	$2.30

Tips to reduce the cost:
- Grow the kale and berries yourself, or purchase them from a local farm.
- If you can't find dried currants, use raisins instead!

Preparation
Equipment needed: Blender

1 Blend all ingredients until smooth.

Nutrition Information Per Serving (based on 2,000 calorie daily intake): calories 224, protein 6g, total fat 1g, carbohydrate 54g, dietary fiber 8g, total sugars 35g, calcium 33%, iron 32%, sodium 4%, potassium 31%, zinc 6%, vitamin A 84%, vitamin E 5%, thiamin 13%, riboflavin 11%, niacin 15%, vitamin B6 24%, folate 16%, vitamin B12 0%, vitamin C 380%

Apple-Collard Green Smoothie

This is a wonderful winter smoothie! The sweet taste hits the spot while the collards keep you warm for hours!

Makes 3 Cups | 1 Serving

2 medium apples	$0.75
1 medium banana	$0.20
5 leaves of collard greens	$1.00
1 date	$0.20
1/4 tsp green stevia powder	<$0.05
1/4-1/2 cup water	$0.00
Total estimated cost	$2.20
Estimated cost per serving	$2.20

Tips to reduce the cost:
- Make this recipe during the cooler months when collards are their least expensive.
- If you don't have green stevia, use raisins or another dried fruit instead.

Preparation
Equipment needed: Blender

1 Blend all ingredients until smooth.

Nutrition Information Per Serving (based on 2,000 calorie daily intake): calories 369, protein 7g, total fat 2g, carbohydrate 93g, dietary fiber 18g, total sugars 60g, calcium 30%, iron 7%, sodium 2%, potassium 34%, zinc 4%, vitamin A 245%, vitamin E 31%, thiamin 13%, riboflavin 24%, niacin 14%, vitamin B6 45%, folate 84%, vitamin B12 0%, vitamin C 144%

Smoothies

Strawberry Ambrosia Green Smoothie

This is the drink of the gods! The ingredients work together to bring out the rich and sensuous flavor of strawberries. What a celebration!

Makes 4 Cups | 1 Serving

2/3 lbs spinach (~4-5 cups, packed)	$2.00
1/2 cup water	$0.00
1 1/2 cups strawberries, whole	$1.50
1 1/2 medium bananas	$0.30
1/3 cup raisins	$0.30
1/4 tsp vanilla	<$0.05
Total estimated cost	$4.15
Estimated cost per serving	$4.15

Tips to reduce the cost:
- Make this recipe when spinach and strawberries are in season.
- Buy strawberries from your local farms in bulk.

Preparation
Equipment needed: Blender

1 Blend all ingredients until smooth.

Nutrition Information Per Serving (based on 2,000 calorie daily intake): calories 471, protein 14g, total fat 3g, carbohydrate 113g, dietary fiber 18g, total sugars 66g, calcium 37%, iron 59%, sodium 11%, potassium 89%, zinc 16%, vitamin A 570%, vitamin E 47%, thiamin 27%, riboflavin 49%, niacin 24%, vitamin B6 76%, folate 171%, vitamin B12 0%, vitamin C 396%

Strawberry and Banana Green Smoothie

Amazingly, this smoothie tastes like strawberries and bananas even though it has 3 cups of chard in it.

Makes 4-5 Cups | 1 Serving

3 chard leaves (~3 cups, packed)	$1.00
1 medium banana	$0.20
1 1/2 cups strawberries, whole	$1.50
1 medium peach	$0.50
3 medium apples	$1.50
Total estimated cost	$4.70
Estimated cost per serving	$4.70

Tips to reduce the cost:
- Buy apples from your local farms in bulk.

Preparation
Equipment needed: Juicer • Blender

1 Juice the apples and pour it into the blender.

2 Blend the juice and remaining ingredients until smooth.

Nutrition Information Per Serving (based on 2,000 calorie daily intake): calories 450, protein 7g, total fat 2g, carbohydrate 111g, dietary fiber 13g, total sugars 82g, calcium 14%, iron 36%, sodium 13%, potassium 56%, zinc 9%, vitamin A 189%, vitamin E 47%, thiamin 14%, riboflavin 22%, niacin 19%, vitamin B6 42%, folate 26%, vitamin B12 0%, vitamin C 712%

Smoothies

Beet Greens Smoothie

This smoothie is perfect for people who are new to green smoothies! You can't even detect the greens! Plus, it's red!

Makes 4 Cups | 1 Serving

3 cups (packed) beet greens	$1.00
2 cups strawberries, whole	$2.00
1/2 cup mangos	$0.50
1/2 cup blueberries	$0.50
2 medjool dates	$0.40
3 medium apples	$1.50
Total estimated cost	$5.90
Estimated cost per serving	$5.90

Tips to reduce the cost:
- Save your beet tops for this smoothie!
- Freeze your own strawberries at the height of strawberry season when they are less expensive.

Preparation
Equipment needed: Blender

1 Juice the apples and pour it into the blender.

2 Blend the juice and remaining ingredients until smooth.

Nutrition Information Per Serving (based on 2,000 calorie daily intake)**:** calories 559, protein 6g, total fat 2g, carbohydrate 140g, dietary fiber 16g, total sugars 115g, calcium 27%, iron 47%, sodium 15%, potassium 70%, zinc 9%, vitamin A 209%, vitamin E 48%, thiamin 22%, riboflavin 33%, niacin 16%, vitamin B6 33%, folate 23%, vitamin B12 0%, vitamin C 822%

Coolers

White Peach - Raspberry Cooler

This cooler tastes like peach and raspberry clouds. Use sweet, ripe white peaches for a sweet, fluffy cooler.

Makes 2 Cups | 2 Servings

2 medium white peaches	$1.00
1/2 cup raspberries	$1.25
2 medjool dates	$0.40
4 cubes ice	$0.00
1/8 tsp vanilla	<$0.05
1 tsp raw agave	<$0.10
Total estimated cost	$2.80
Estimated cost per serving	$1.40

Tips to reduce the cost:
- Make this recipe in the late summer when white peaches are in season and their least expensive.
- Use an inexpensive variety of dates like Deglet Noor dates.

Preparation
Equipment needed: Blender

1 Peel the peaches using a knife or vegetable peeler.

2 Cube the peaches and add them to the blender.

3 Add the remaining ingredients and blend until smooth and fluffy.

Lemon-Lime Cooler

This is a great flavorful cooler for a warm day! It's simple to prepare and makes use of that lemon balm or lemon verbana you have growing in your garden. If you don't have access to these herbs, just leave them out.

Makes 1 Serving

1 medium lemon	$0.35
1 medium lime	$0.35
1 cup ice	$0.00
1 cup water	$0.00
4-6 leaves lemon balm/verbana	<$0.20
agave to taste	<$0.25
stevia to taste	<$0.05
Total estimated cost	$1.20
Estimated cost per serving	$0.30

Tips to reduce the cost:
- Buy lemons and limes in bulk; just be sure to use them all before they spoil!

Preparation
Equipment needed: Blender

1 Juice the lemon and lime, and pour it into the blender.

2 Add the remaining ingredients and blend until smooth.

Juices

Celery Rejuvenation

This is a wonderful, refreshing drink! The ginger and grapefruit add a nice zing! It's the perfect after workout drink. Enjoy!

Makes 2 1/2 Cups | 1 Serving

3 stalks celery	$0.25
2 medium apples	$1.00
1-inch piece of ginger root	<$0.20
1 handful parsley	$0.25
1 large grapefruit	$0.75
Total estimated cost	$2.45
Estimated cost per serving	$2.45

Tips to reduce the cost:
- Buy apples in bulk from a local farm.
- Buy inexpensive ginger at Asian markets.
- Buy grapefruit in bulk bags; just be sure to use them all before they spoil!

Preparation
Equipment needed: Juicer

1 Juice all ingredients and enjoy!

Carrots Rejoice!

This juice is the perfect after-workout drink! It's simple to make and tastes delicious!

Makes 2 Cups | 1 Serving

3 stalks celery	$0.25
2 medium apples	$1.00
2 large carrots	<$0.15
1/2-inch piece of ginger root	<$0.10
1/2 lemon with rind	<$0.20
Total estimated cost	$1.70
Estimated cost per serving	$1.70

Tips to reduce the cost:
- Buy carrots in bulk from your grocery store.
- Buy inexpensive ginger at Asian markets.
- Buy lemons in bulk bags; just be sure to use them all before they spoil!

Preparation
Equipment needed: Juicer

1 Juice all ingredients and enjoy!

Juices

Watermelon Juice

Watermelon juice is cool, fruity, subtle, and smooth, and it's the perfect summer drink on a hot day. This juice is super easy to make and tastes amazing.

Makes 3 Servings

5 cups fresh watermelon	$2.00
Total estimated cost	$2.00
Estimated cost per serving	$0.67

Tips to reduce the cost:

- In my experience, small health food stores tend to sell the best tasting, most inexpensive watermelon; however, be sure to shop around.

Preparation
Equipment needed: Blender • Wire sieve

1 Blend the watermelon (with seeds) on low to medium speed until all of the juice is released from the pulp.

2 Pour the watermelon pulp into the wire sieve over a large bowl. Use a spoon to press any remaining juice out of the pulp.

If you don't have a wire sieve, just leave the pulp in. Just be sure to remove all of the watermelon seeds before blending. Also, try adding a few cubes of ice and some agave for a watermelon shake.

Homemade Spiced Apple Cider

Spiced apple cider is a wonderful combination of freshly pressed apples and mulling spices (a beautiful blend of cinnamon, cloves, ginger, orange peel, and lemon peel).

Makes 2 Cups | 2 Servings

4 medium apples	$2.00
1 tea bag mulling spices	<$0.25
Total estimated cost	$2.25
Estimated cost per serving	$1.13

Tips to reduce the cost:

- You can find mulling spices in bulk or tea bag form during the fall season when apples are in season. A box of 15-20 tea bags will cost you $2-3 dollars.

Preparation
Equipment needed: Juicer • Wire sieve • Blender

1 Juice the apples and pour the juice into a blender.

2 Empty the packet of mulling spices into the blender and blend until frothy (15-30 seconds).

3 Strain the juice using a wire sieve and serve.

Juices

Flu-Be-Gone Remedy Cocktail

This is my favorite remedy for the flu or cold. It feels and tastes so good, plus it will keep you warm and help you heal faster!

Makes 1 Cup | 1 Serving

2 medium apples	$1.50
1 to 3-inch piece of ginger root	$0.30
1/2 whole lemon	<$0.20
Total estimated cost	$1.50
Estimated cost per serving	$1.50

Tips to reduce the cost:

- Buy inexpensive ginger at Asian markets.
- Omit the lemon!

Preparation
Equipment needed: Juicer

1 Juice all ingredients and enjoy!

Luscious Pink Cocktail

This juice is beautiful and it tastes pretty amazing too!

Makes 2 Cups | 1 Serving

2 medium apples	$1.00
2 medium celery stalks	<$0.20
1 large carrot	<$0.10
1/2 lemon	<$0.20
1 thumb-sized piece of ginger	$0.30
1 1/2 cups red cabbage	$0.75
Total estimated cost	$2.55
Estimated cost per serving	$2.55

Tips to reduce the cost:

- This recipe uses small portions of each ingredient. So, to get the most for your money, make this recipe several times this week.

Preparation
Equipment needed: Juicer

1 Juice all ingredients and enjoy!

Milks

Almond Milk

I love to make my own almond milk. It's much cheaper and it tastes a whole lot better when you make it yourself!

Makes 2 1/2 Cups | 2 1/2 Servings

1 cup raw almonds	$2.30
Total estimated cost	$2.30
Estimated cost per serving	$0.92

Tips to reduce the cost:
- Buy almonds in bulk.

Preparation
Equipment needed: Blender • Nutbag

1 Soak the almonds in 2 cups of water for at least 8 hours or overnight. After the almonds have soaked, remove the water and rinse the soaked almonds several times.

2 Pour the soaked almonds into the blender and add 2 cups of fresh water (add 2.5-3 cups if you are really on a low budget). Blend the soaked almonds until they are completely broken down into a pulp.

3 Let the mixture sit in the blender for 5 to 10 minutes; this helps to make the milk richer.

4 Strain and squeeze the milk into a large bowl using a nutbag, cheesecloth, or juicer. Enjoy!

Sunflower Seed Milk

This was one of the first nut milks I made when I started my raw foods journey, and I'm always amazed at how creamy and flavorful it tastes.

Makes 4 Cups | 4 Servings

1 cup raw sunflower seeds	$1.20
4-6 tbsp raw agave	$0.75
1 medium banana	$0.20
1/4 tsp vanilla	<$0.05
Total estimated cost	$2.20
Estimated cost per serving	$0.55

Tips to reduce the cost:
- None! This is a freakin' cheap recipe!

Preparation
Equipment needed: Blender • Nutbag

1 Soak the sunflower seeds in 2 cups of water for at least 8 hours or overnight. After the seeds have soaked, remove the water and rinse the soaked seeds.

2 Pour the soaked seeds into the blender and add 3 cups of fresh water. Blend the soaked seeds until they are completely broken down into a pulp. Let the mixture sit in the blender for 5 to 10 minutes

3 Strain and squeeze the milk into a large bowl using a nutbag, cheesecloth, or juicer. Rinse the blender.

4 Blend the milk, agave, banana, and vanilla until the milk is completely smooth. Enjoy!

Warm Drinks

Tea Latte

Tea lattes are one of my favorite drinks to make during the winter. You can make a latte out of any tea! I have made lattes using nettle tea, chamomile tea, roobios tea, and the list goes on.

Makes 1 Cup | 1 Serving

1 cup hot tea	<$0.25
1/3 cup nut milk	$0.30
1/8 tsp green stevia powder	<$0.05
1 tbsp raw agave	<$0.25
Total estimated cost	$0.85
Estimated cost per serving	$0.85

Tips to reduce the cost:
- Buy tea leaves in bulk. They are always cheaper!

Preparation
Equipment needed: Frother (optional)

1 Make a cup of your favorite hot or sun tea and set aside.

2 Pour the nut milk (e.g. almond milk, sunflower seed milk) into a large mug and add the sweeteners. If you have a frother, use it to froth up your nut milk.

3 Pour the tea into the milk and stir.

To make your tea latte a beautiful experience, use a frother. They cost ~$15 and will last years if you take care of it.

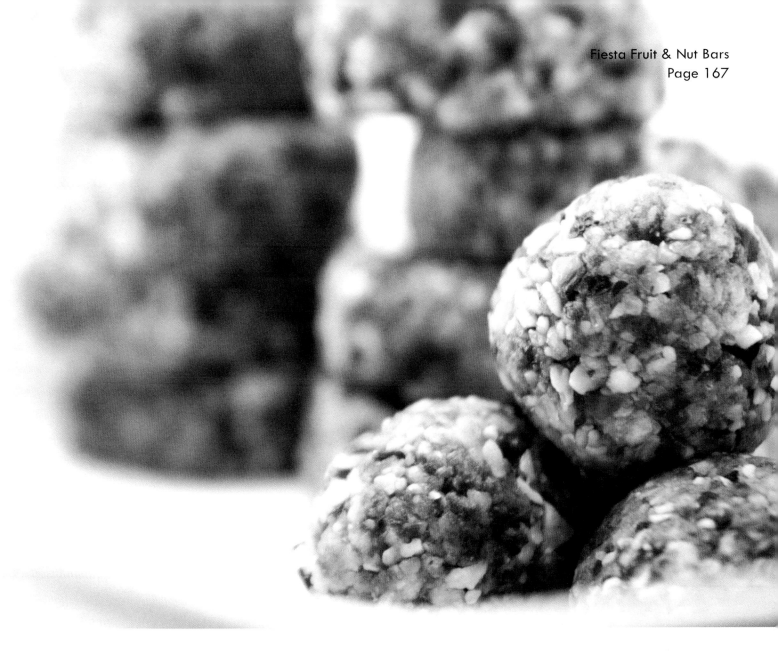

Fiesta Fruit & Nut Bars
Page 167

Breakfast

DEHYDRATING IN YOUR OVEN

Some of the recipes in this section call for a dehydrator; however, if you don't have one, consider drying the fruit or bars in your oven. Simply line a baking sheet with parchment paper and place on top the food you would like to dry. Set the oven on its lowest temperature and keep the oven door ajar. You can even buy a thermometer to place inside the oven to make sure the temperature doesn't rise above 115 degrees!

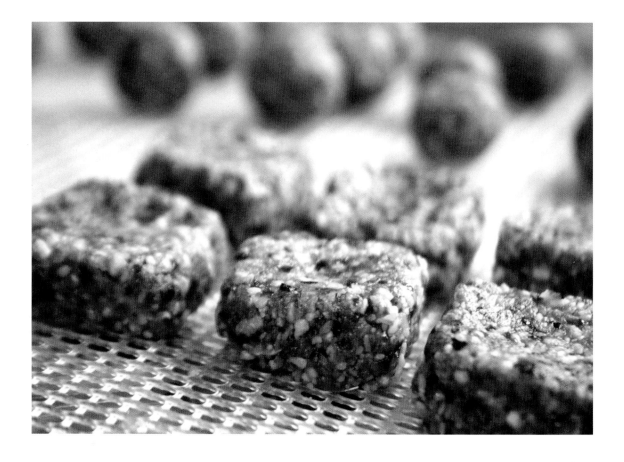

Fiesta Fruit & Nut Bars

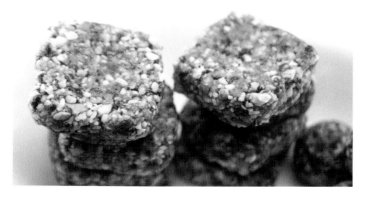

These bars are better than the fruit and nut bars sold at the store! Plus, they are super simple to make! Try using a variety of different fruits in this recipe like strawberries and bananas.

Preparation
Equipment needed: Food processor • Dehydrator

1 Peel and core the apples and pear, and cut them into 1/4-inch slices. Slice the peaches into ¼-inch slices. Dehydrate the fruit slices for 24 hours at 105-degrees. After the fruit slices have dehydrated, prepare the rest of the recipe.

2 In a food processor, process the coconut flakes until the oils begin to come out of the coconut (about 30 seconds). Add the sunflower seeds, pumpkin seeds, sea salt, and vanilla and process until the seeds are well broken down. Add the raisins, dates, and dried fruit slices, and process until they are broken down into small pieces. Lastly, add the agave to taste and process until the dough begins to clump.

3 To form the 1-inch square bars, take a small amount of dough (about 1 tbsp) and roll it into a ball with the palms of your hands. Next, flatten the ball and shape it into a square with your fingers. You will create 20 1-inch squares.

4 Dehydrate the bars for 8-12 hours in your dehydrator at 105-degrees or in your oven (see tip on page 166).

When stored in an airtight container, these bars will keep for 3-4 days. If you would like to store the bars longer, keep them in the refrigerator or freezer.

2 medium apples (baking)	$1.00
1 medium pear	$0.50
1 medium peach	$0.50
1/2 cup raw shredded coconut	$0.25
1/4 cup raw sunflower seeds	$0.30
1/4 cup raw pumpkin seeds	$0.30
1 pinch sea salt	<$0.05
1 tsp vanilla	<$0.25
1/3 cup raisins	$0.30
3 dates	$0.60
1-2 tsp agave	<$0.25
Total estimated cost	$4.30
Estimated cost per serving	$0.43

Tips to reduce the cost:
- Use whatever fruits you have in your kitchen! These are called fiesta bars for a reason!
- Buy the apples from a local farm.

Nutrition Information Per Serving (based on 2,000 calorie daily intake): calories 185, protein 3g, total fat 11g, carbohydrate 22g, dietary fiber 5g, total sugars 15g, calcium 3%, iron 8%, sodium 1%, potassium 8%, zinc 5%, vitamin A 2%, vitamin E 10%, thiamin 8%, riboflavin 4%, niacin 3%, vitamin B6 6%, folate 4%, vitamin B12 0%, vitamin C 6%

Creamy Apple Pie Breakfast Bars

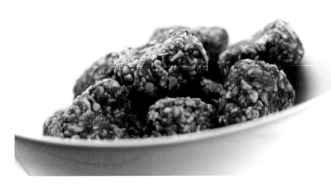

5 medium apples	$2.50
1/2 cup raw shredded coconut	$0.25
1/4 cup raw walnuts, whole	$0.50
1 pinch sea salt	<$0.05
1 tsp vanilla	<$0.20
1/2 tsp cinnamon, ground	<$0.05
2 pinches nutmeg, ground	<$0.05
1/4 tsp green stevia powder	<$0.05
2 dates	<$0.40
1-2 tbsp raw agave	<$0.50
Total estimated cost	$4.50
Estimated cost per serving	$0.45

Tips to reduce the cost:

- Try to buy all of the dry ingredients from bulk bins. This way you can buy the amounts you need.
- Buy the apples from a local farm.

These quick apple bars are the best I have ever tasted. They are truly a treat that celebrates the apple season! Enjoy!

Preparation
Equipment needed: Food processor • Dehydrator

1 Peel and core the apples, and cut them into 1/4-inch slices. Dehydrate the apple slices for 24 hours at 105-degrees. After the apple slices have dehydrated, prepare the rest of the recipe.

2 In a food processor, process the coconut flakes until the oils begin to come out of the coconut (about 30 seconds). Add the walnuts, sea salt, vanilla, cinnamon, nutmeg, and stevia, and process until the walnuts are well broken down. Add the dates and dried apple slices, and process until they are completely broken down into small pieces. Finally, add the agave and process until the dough begins to clump.

3 To form the 1-inch square bars, take a small amount of dough (about 1 tbsp) and roll it into a ball with the palm of your hands. Next, flatten the ball and shape it into a square with your fingers. You will create 20 1-inch squares.

4 Dehydrate the bars for 8-12 hours in your dehydrator at 105-degrees or in your oven (see tip on page 166).

When stored in an airtight container, the bars will keep for 3-4 days. If you would like to store the bars longer, keep them in the refrigerator or freezer.

Nutrition Information Per Serving (based on 2,000 calorie daily intake): calories 149, protein 2g, total fat 10g, carbohydrate 17g, dietary fiber 4g, total sugars 11g, calcium 2%, iron 4%, sodium 1%, potassium 5%, zinc 3%, vitamin A 1%, vitamin E 2%, thiamin 2%, riboflavin 2%, niacin 1%, vitamin B6 5%, folate 1%, vitamin B12 0%, vitamin C 6%

Apple and Banana Granola

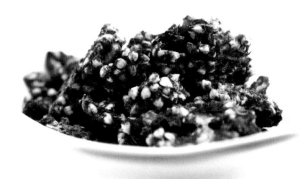

This granola is crunchy, chewy, and sweet! Make this granola when you are making almond milk, so you can use the almond pulp to make the granola and eat the granola with the milk!

Preparation

Equipment needed: Food processor or high-speed blender • Dehydrator • Sprout tray, colander, or nut bag to sprout buckwheat

2 cups buckwheat groats	$2.00
6 medium apples	$3.00
7 medium bananas	$1.40
1 1/2 cups raisins	$1.50
1/2 cup almond pulp	<$1.00
1 1/2 tsp vanilla	<$0.30
2 tsp cinnamon, ground	<$0.20
1/4 tsp nutmeg, ground	<$0.05
2 pinches clove, ground	<$0.05
1/4 tsp green stevia powder	<$0.05
1 tbsp coconut oil	<$0.25
Total estimated cost	$9.80
Estimated cost per serving	$1.23

1 First, sprout the buckwheat. This usually takes 2-3 days; however, the sprouts will grow faster in warmer climates. To sprout the buckwheat groats, soak them overnight. Next, drain the buckwheat and rinse the groats 2-3 times. Place the buckwheat in a sprouting tray, colander, or nut bag, and rinse it 2 times per day until the sprouts are 1/2 inch long. Rinse the buckwheat groats before using them.

2 Peel and core the apples and set aside. Using a food processor or high-speed blender, blend 3 of the apples, 3 bananas, and 1/2 cup of the raisins until liquefied. Pour the mixture over the buckwheat sprouts and mix well. Add the almond pulp, vanilla, cinnamon, nutmeg, clove, and green stevia powder, and mix. Add the coconut oil and mix well.

3 Cut the remaining apples and bananas into ¼-inch slices, and fold the cut fruit and raisins into the buckwheat.

4 Pour the mixture onto two dehydrator trays and spread. The layer will be 1/2-inch thick. Dehydrate the granola for 24 hours in your dehydrator at 105-degrees or in your oven (see tip on page 166).

Tips to reduce the cost:

- Check with your grocer to see if they sell overripe bananas. They are usually half-priced.
- Make this recipe when apples are in season and/or least expensive.

Nutrition Information Per Serving (based on 2,000 calorie daily intake): calories 392, protein 8g, total fat 4g, carbohydrate 90g, dietary fiber 11g, total sugars 40g, calcium 4%, iron 11%, sodium 0%, potassium 25%, zinc 9%, vitamin A 2%, vitamin E 2%, thiamin 8%, riboflavin 19%, niacin 20%, vitamin B6 28%, folate 10%, vitamin B12 0%, vitamin C 24%

Quick Succulent Granola

1 cup raw sunflower seeds	$1.20
1 cup raw walnuts, whole	$2.00
1 1/2 tsp vanilla	<$0.30
1/2 tsp sea salt	<$0.05
1 1/2 tsp cinnamon, ground	<$0.05
3 heavy pinches nutmeg, ground	<$0.05
1/4 tsp green stevia powder	<$0.05
3 dates	$0.60
2 1/2 cups raw slivered almonds	$1.90
4-5 tbsp maple syrup, agave, or honey	$1.00
Total estimated cost	$7.20
Estimated cost per serving	$1.44

Tips to reduce the cost:
- Try to buy all of the dry ingredients from bulk bins. This way you can buy the amounts you need.

This is one of the best granolas I have ever tasted. It's so simple and decadent.

Preparation
Equipment needed: Food processor • Dehydrator

1. In a food processor, process the sunflower seeds until they are broken down into a nutty flour. Add the walnuts, vanilla, sea salt, cinnamon, nutmeg, and stevia, and process until the walnuts are completely broken down into a nutty flour. Finally, add the dates and process until they are broken into small pieces. Pour the nut mixture into a large bowl.

2. Sprinkle the slivered almonds onto the nut mixture and mix.

3. Pour on the maple syrup and stir. The granola should clump together into nutty clusters.

4. Pour the granola onto a dehydrator tray (no lining needed) and dehydrate for 24 hours (at 105 degrees).

When stored in an airtight container, the granola will keep for 1 week. If you would like to store the granola longer, keep it in the refrigerator or freezer.

Nutrition Information Per Serving (based on 2,000 calorie daily intake): calories 526, protein 17g, total fat 39g, carbohydrate 37g, dietary fiber 8g, total sugars 24g, calcium 13%, iron 23%, sodium 10%, potassium 18%, zinc 26%, vitamin A 1%, vitamin E 102%, thiamin 49%, riboflavin 16%, niacin 12%, vitamin B6 22%, folate 20%, vitamin B12 0%, vitamin C 2%

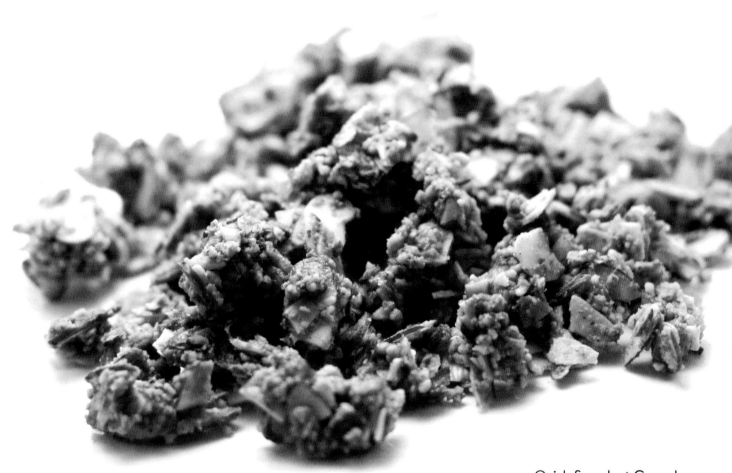

Quick Succulent Granola

Oatmeal

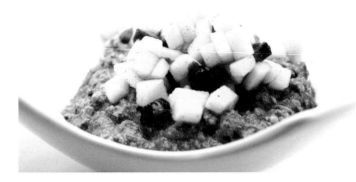

1 cup raw nuts	$1.00 +
2 tbsp chia seeds	<$0.25
1/2 cup coconut or nut milk	$0.50 +
3 dates (or raisins)	$0.65
Total estimated cost	$2.40 +
Estimated cost per serving	$2.40 +

Tips to reduce the cost:

- The price of this recipe depends on the type of nuts you use. For a lower price, use less expensive nuts like sunflower seeds and walnuts.
- Use a cheaper variety of dates like Deglet Noor dates or substitute the dates with dried fruits like raisins.
- Leave out the chia seeds if you don't have them.

This is one of my favorite meals to make in the winter. It fills me up like oatmeal, but it tastes so much better. For this recipe you can use whatever nuts you have on hand. In the past, I have used sunflower seeds, pumpkin seeds, and walnuts together. You can also make a dessert-like oatmeal by using pecans, macadamia nuts, or cashews. Just trust your instincts and go with it.

You can replace the coconut milk with a nut milk. Create your own nut milk on the spot by blending 4-6 nuts with 1/2 cup of water until liquefied, and then adding the remaining ingredients and blending until the desired texture is reached.

Top the oatmeal with fresh fruits and raisins. In the picture, the oatmeal is topped with chopped pears and raisins.

Preparation

Equipment needed: Food processor or high-speed blender

1 Soak nuts overnight.

2 Blend the soaked nuts and remaining ingredients until the desired consistency is reached (it can be smooth or chunky).

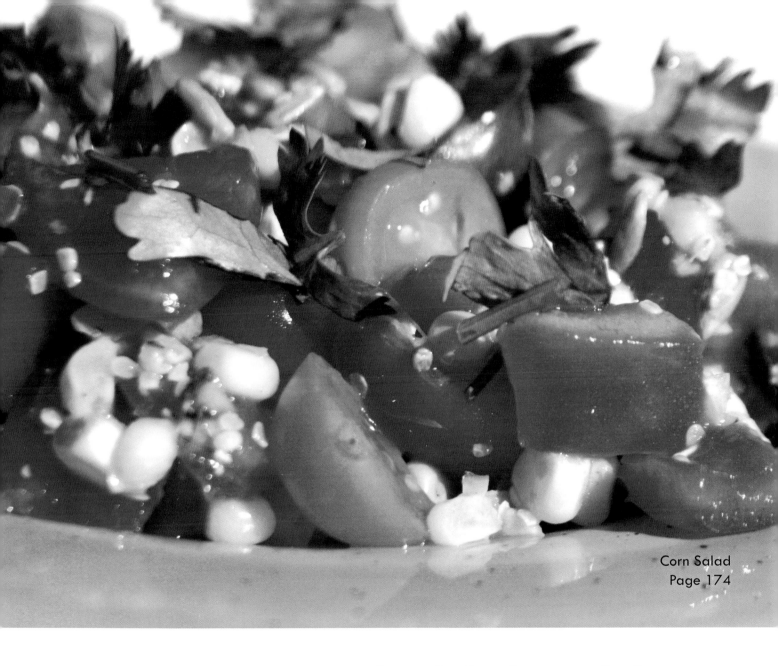

Corn Salad
Page 174

Light Salads and Soups

Corn Salad

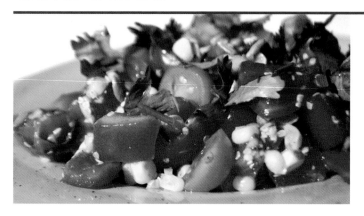

1 ear corn	$0.50
2 medium red tomatoes	$1.00
1 handful fresh cilantro	<$0.25
1 handful cherry tomatoes	$0.50
1 clove garlic	<$0.10
1 small scallion	<$0.20
1 pinch cayenne pepper	<$0.05
sea salt to taste	<$0.05
1 tbsp extra virgin olive oil (optional)	$0.25
Total estimated cost	$2.85
Estimated cost per serving	$2.85

Tips to reduce the cost:

- Get the main ingredients from local farms, farmers markets, CSA programs, or grow them yourself!

This salad is one of the reasons why I love the summer! Consider making this salad during the middle to late summer when tomatoes and corn taste amazing.

Preparation
Equipment needed: Just a knife and cutting board!

1 Remove the corn from the cob using a knife. Place the corn into a large bowl.

2 Chop the tomatoes and cilantro, slice the cherry tomatoes in half, and mince the garlic and scallion. Add to the corn.

3 Add the cayenne pepper and mix well.

4 Salt to taste and mix. Lastly, add the olive oil and mix. Enjoy!

Nutrition Information Per Serving (based on 2,000 calorie daily intake): calories 310, protein 8g, total fat 16g, carbohydrate 42g, dietary fiber 8g, total sugars 14g, calcium 5%, iron 11%, sodium 14%, potassium 35%, zinc 9%, vitamin A 68%, vitamin E 27%, thiamin 28%, riboflavin 10%, niacin 23%, vitamin B6 20%, folate 30%, vitamin B12 0%, vitamin C 92%

Winter Salad & Sweet Mustard Dressing

Makes 2 Servings

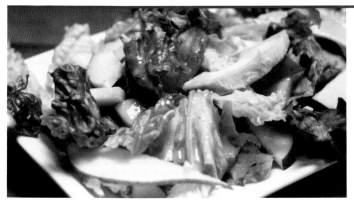

SALAD

1 large head of lettuce	$2.00
1 medium pear (any variety)	$0.50
1 medium apple (any variety)	$0.50
1 medium avocado	$1.25
1 clove garlic	<$0.10

DRESSING

1 tbsp stone ground mustard	<$0.20
1/4 tsp balsamic vinegar	<$0.05
1 1/2 tbsp extra virgin olive oil	<$0.40
2 1/2 tbsp water	$0.00
1/2 tsp lemon juice (optional)	<$0.10
agave or stevia to taste	<$0.10
1 pinch sea salt	<$0.05
Total estimated cost	$5.25
Estimated cost per serving	$2.63

This salad is pure s-e-n-s-u-a-l-i-t-y! It celebrates winter fruits and is loaded with fresh fruit and lettuce flavor! This is a very versatile recipe that can be adapted to any locale. If you don't have access to avocados, then use another fruit instead. Consider replacing the pears and apples with mandarins, grapefruit, persimmons, etc. The dressing can be prepared ahead of time.

Preparation
Equipment needed: Just a knife and cutting board!

SALAD

1 Chop the lettuce, slice the pear, apple, and avocado, and mince the garlic. Combine into a large bowl, mix well, and set aside.

DRESSING

2 Mix all of the ingredients in a small cup or bowl. Pour the dressing over the salad and enjoy.

Nutrition Information Per Serving (based on 2,000 calorie daily intake): calories 365, protein 5g, total fat 25g, carbohydrate 35g, dietary fiber 11g, total sugars 17g, calcium 11%, iron 20%, sodium 6%, potassium 28%, zinc 7%, vitamin A 351%, vitamin E 26%, thiamin 17%, riboflavin 19%, niacin 11%, vitamin B6 25%, folate 17%, vitamin B12 0%, vitamin C 37%

Tips to reduce the cost:
- Substitute fruits with in-season, local fruits.
- Substitute balsamic vinegar with apple cider vinegar or lemon juice.

Simple Savory Salad

1 head lettuce	$2.00
1-2 cloves garlic	<$0.20
sea salt to taste	<$0.05
1 pinch cayenne powder	<$0.05
4 tbsp hemp seeds	$1.00
2-4 sheets nori seaweed	<$1.20
1 tbsp extra virgin olive oil	$0.25
Total estimated cost	$4.75
Estimated cost per serving	$2.38

Tips to reduce the cost:
- Buy the hemp seeds and nori seaweed in bulk to keep the costs of these ingredients low.

This is my staple salad. I can't get enough of it! It's easy to make, it tastes so good, and my body just loves it! Enjoy!

Preparation
Equipment needed: Just a knife and cutting board!

1 Wash and chop the lettuce, and place it into a large bowl. If you have one, use a salad spinner to remove excess water.

2 Mince the garlic and add to the lettuce.

3 Sprinkle the salt, cayenne, and hemp seeds onto the lettuce, and mix well. Tear the seaweed into small pieces and sprinkle onto the lettuce. Mix well.

4 Drizzle the olive oil onto the lettuce, mix, and serve.

Nutrition Information Per Serving (based on 2,000 calorie daily intake): calories 316, protein 13g, total fat 24g, carbohydrate 16g, dietary fiber 10g, total sugars 4g, calcium 14%, iron 33%, sodium 14%, potassium 34%, zinc 14%, vitamin A 384%, vitamin E 28%, thiamin 29%, riboflavin 36%, niacin 5%, vitamin B6 14%, folate 106%, vitamin B12 0%, vitamin C 152%

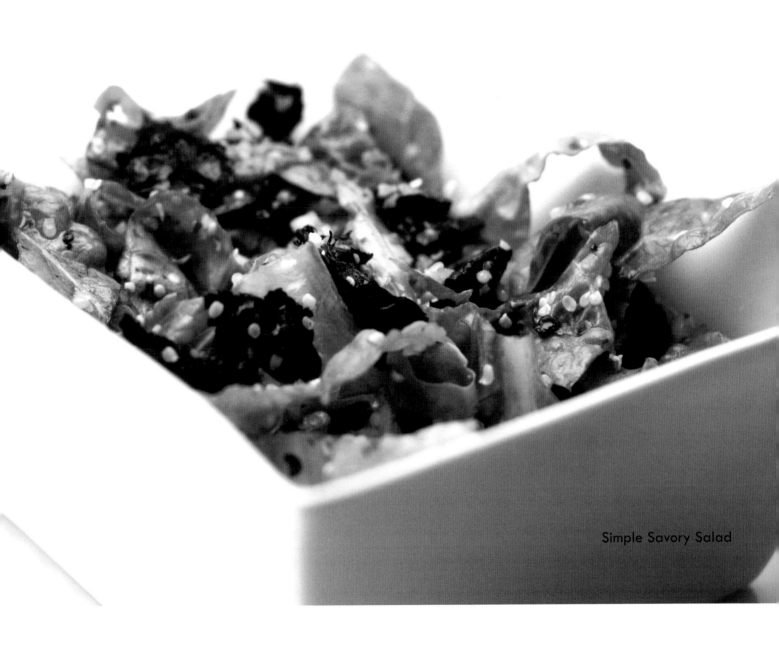

Simple Savory Salad

Summer Parsley Salad

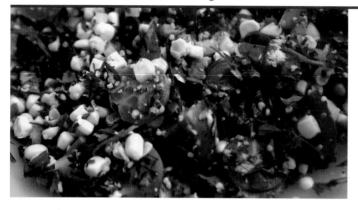

This salad harmoniously combines fresh corn, tomatoes, and parsley to create the perfect summer celebration!

When buying parsley, try to select bunches that don't have dry leaves. How can you tell? Feel the leaves - they should feel succulent and water dense.

Preparation
Equipment needed: Just a knife and cutting board!

1 Chop the parsley and add the vinegar and salt. Mix well. Allow the parsley to marinate while you prepare the remaining ingredients.

2 Remove the corn from the ear using a knife, slice the cherry tomatoes, and chop the tomatoes, pepper, and spring onion. Add to the parsley. Mince the garlic and add.

3 Finally, add the hemp seeds and olive oil. Mix well and enjoy!

1 bunch parsley	$1.00
1 tsp brown rice vinegar	<$0.10
1/4 tsp salt	<$0.05
1 ear of corn	$0.50
1 handful of cherry tomatoes	$0.50
1 small tomato	$0.50
1 small sweet pepper	$1.00
1/4 cup spring onion	<$0.25
1 clove garlic	<$0.10
2-3 tbsp hemp seeds	<$0.75
1 tbsp extra virgin olive oil (optional)	$0.20
Total estimated cost	$4.95
Estimated cost per serving	$2.48

Nutrition Information Per Serving (based on 2,000 calorie daily intake): calories 264, protein 10g, total fat 15g, carbohydrate 27g, dietary fiber 7g, total sugars 8g, calcium 13%, iron 37%, sodium 14%, potassium 28%, zinc 15%, vitamin A 142%, vitamin E 26%, thiamin 27%, riboflavin 18%, niacin 15%, vitamin B6 16%, folate 40%, vitamin B12 0%, vitamin C 243%

Tips to reduce the cost:
- Make this recipe during in summer when the costs of tomatoes are low.
- Try to purchase most of these ingredients from your local farmers market (s).

Herb Italian Salad

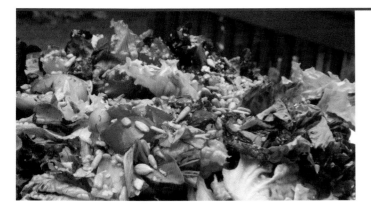

This salad is one of my summer favorites! The lettuce is crisp and light, the tomatoes are juicy, the sun-dried tomatoes and herbs are super flavorful, and the nuts add a nice savory touch!

Try using your own homemade 'sun-dried' tomatoes (page 270) in this recipe.

Preparation
Equipment needed: Just a knife and cutting board!

1 Wash and prepare the lettuce, placing it in a large bowl.

2 Tear the seaweed into small pieces and sprinkle it over the lettuce. Mix well.

3 Chop the tomatoes and add to the salad.

4 Mince the sun-dried tomatoes, basil, oregano, and thyme and add to the salad.

5 Add the sunflower and hemp seeds, balsamic vinegar, and salt, and mix well.

6 Lastly, pour the olive oil onto the salad and mix. Serve!

Ingredient	Cost
1 large head red leaf lettuce	$2.00
2 sheets nori seaweed	$0.60
1-2 medium tomatoes	<$1.00
4-5 pieces sun-dried tomatoes	<$0.50
1 handful fresh basil	<$0.25
1 tsp fresh oregano	<$0.10
1/2 tsp fresh thyme	<$0.10
3 tbsp hemp seeds	<$0.75
1 handful raw sunflower seeds	$0.30
1 tbsp balsamic vinegar	<$0.15
1 tbsp extra virgin olive oil	$0.25
sea salt to taste	<$0.05
Total estimated cost	$6.05
Estimated cost per serving	$3.03

Nutrition Information Per Serving (based on 2,000 calorie daily intake): calories 330, protein 14g, total fat 24g, carbohydrate 19g, dietary fiber 8g, total sugars 8g, calcium 13%, iron 38%, sodium 13%, potassium 33%, zinc 18%, vitamin A 270%, vitamin E 64%, thiamin 49%, riboflavin 28%, niacin 13%, vitamin B6 21%, folate 17%, vitamin B12 0%, vitamin C 54%

Tips to reduce the cost:
- Grow the fresh herbs yourself or get them from a friend who has an herb garden.
- Buy the salad ingredients from local farms, farmers markets, and/or CSA programs.

Strawberry - Rhubarb - Citrus Dressing

Makes 2 Cups | 8 Servings

1 stalk rhubarb	<$0.25
juice from 1/2 lime	<$0.20
1 cup of juice from 1 large orange	$0.75
1 cup strawberries, whole	$1.00
3 tbsp extra virgin olive oil	$0.75
1/4 cup raisins	$0.25
1 tbsp apple cider vinegar	$0.10
Total estimated cost	$3.30
Estimated cost per serving	$0.41

Tips to reduce the cost:
- Try to buy all of the ingredients in bulk.
- Buy the strawberries from a local farm.
- If rhubarb is out of season, consider using raspberries instead.

This dressing is strawberry-li-cious! It's so fresh, sweet, and tart! Enjoy this dressing with spring lettuce and sweet granola croutons! Yummy!

Preparation
Equipment needed: Blender

1 Chop the rhubarb and add to the blender.

2 Juice the lime and orange, and pour into the blender.

3 Add the remaining ingredients and blend until smooth. If you are using a regular blender, soak the raisins for 4 hours before blending.

Pour the dressing into a jar and keep refrigerated.

Nutrition Information Per Serving (based on 2,000 calorie daily intake): calories 78, protein 1g, total fat 5g, carbohydrate 9g, dietary fiber 1g, total sugars 6g, calcium 2%, iron 1%, sodium 0%, potassium 4%, zinc 0%, vitamin A 1%, vitamin E 6%, thiamin 2%, riboflavin 1%, niacin 1%, vitamin B6 2%, folate 3%, vitamin B12 0%, vitamin C 42%

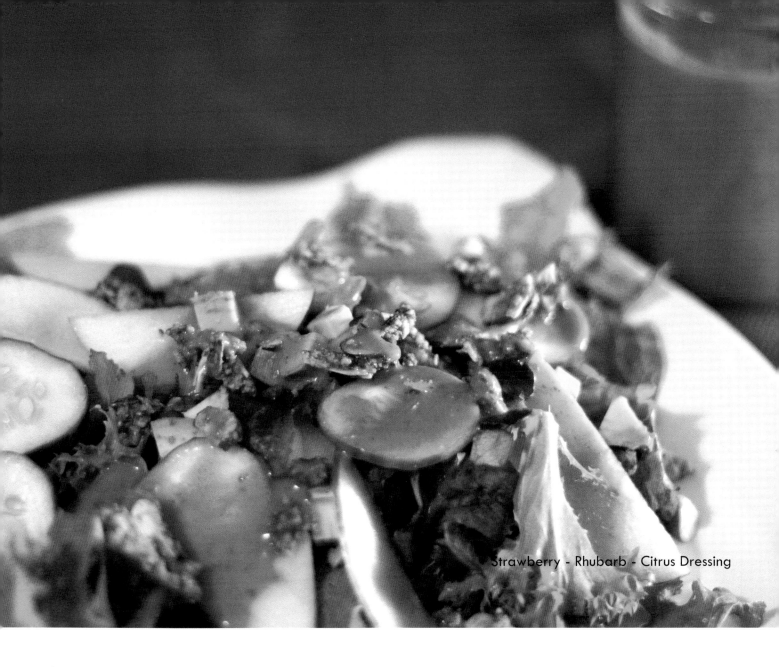

Strawberry - Rhubarb - Citrus Dressing

Creamy Carrot-Beet Soup

1 medium apple	$0.50
1/4 cup water	$0.00
1/2 medium beet	$0.25
1 medium carrot	$0.10
1 tsp apple cider vinegar	<$0.05
2 dates	$0.40
5-6 raw cashews, whole	$0.25
1 pinch sea salt	<$0.05
1 tsp extra virgin olive oil	<$0.10
Total estimated cost	$1.70
Estimated cost per serving	$1.70

Tips to reduce the cost:
- Replace the cashews with another creamy nut that you already have in your kitchen (e.g., walnuts, Brazil nuts, pecans, or coconut butter).

I first made this magnificent soup when I was running low on a lot of ingredients and wanted to try something new! Little did I know that I was going to create an amazing soup that takes advantage of winter produce!

You can easily warm the soup by blending it extra long or warming it on the stove (just keep you finger in the soup to prevent it from getting too hot).

You can use any type of high-speed blender to make this soup such as a Bullet™, Tribest™, Vitamix™, etc. You can also use a food processor and juicer combo, by processing the soup first and then feeding it into a masticating juicer (e.g. Champion juicer).

Preparation
Equipment needed: High-speed blender or a food processor and masticating juicer (e.g. Champion) combo

1 Peel and cube the apple, beet, and carrot.

2 Using a high-speed blender or food processor, blend the apple cubes and water until liquefied.

3 Add the remaining ingredients and blend until the soup is creamy (about 1-3 minutes in a food processor). If you are using a food processor, feed the soup (it will be slightly chunky) into a masticating juicer with a blank screen (the one with no holes). The juicer will chew up the small chunks. Enjoy!

Nutrition Information Per Serving (based on 2,000 calorie daily intake): calories 466, protein 5g, total fat 22g, carbohydrate 70g, dietary fiber 10g, total sugars 53g, calcium 8%, iron 12%, sodium 9%, potassium 26%, zinc 10%, vitamin A 208%, vitamin E 18%, thiamin 9%, riboflavin 9%, niacin 9%, vitamin B6 17%, folate 20%, vitamin B12 0%, vitamin C 20%

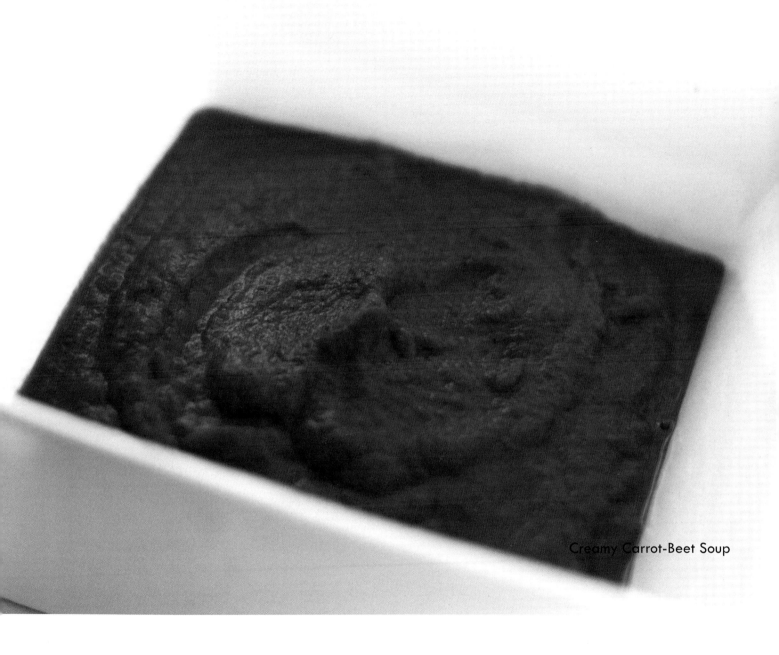
Creamy Carrot-Beet Soup

Creamy Miso Soup

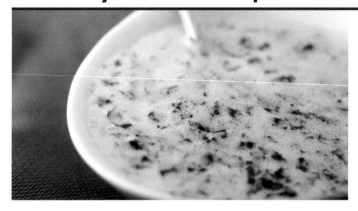

This is one of my favorite recipes. It's a staple during the winter months or whenever I can't figure out what to eat.

Plus, you only need to use a little bit of each ingredient, so one shopping trip makes a whole lot of miso soup.

For an extra thrill, add some cauliflower "rice". To create the rice, process chopped cauliflower in a food processor until a rice forms, and marinate it in the miso soup for 5 minutes. It's like eating rice soaked in miso soup. Yum!

Preparation
Equipment needed: High-speed blender

1 Blend the miso, vinegar, garlic, ginger, sunflower seeds, dulse, and water until liquefied (20-30 seconds).

2 Add the olive oil, salt, and laver seaweed, and blend until the seaweed is broken into small pieces. That's all! Enjoy!

1 tbsp white miso	<$0.25
1 tbsp brown rice vinegar	<$0.25
1 small clove of garlic	<$0.10
1/2 inch piece of ginger	<$0.05
1/4 cup raw sunflower seeds	$0.30
2 tbsp dried dulse seaweed	<$0.25
1 1/2 cups water	$0.00
1 tsp extra virgin olive oil	<$0.10
sea salt to taste	<$0.05
1/2 cup dried laver nori seaweed	$1.00
Total estimated cost	$2.35
Estimated cost per serving	$2.35

Nutrition Information Per Serving (based on 2,000 calorie daily intake): calories 381, protein 23g, total fat 19g, carbohydrate 31g, dietary fiber 17g, total sugars 2g, calcium 15%, iron 52%, sodium 56%, potassium 46%, zinc 27%, vitamin A 35%, vitamin E 83%, thiamin 72%, riboflavin 81%, niacin 21%, vitamin B6 252%, folate 21%, vitamin B12 120%, vitamin C 11%

Tips to reduce the cost:
- Though it may be tempting to buy cheap miso, try to buy medium or high-quality miso. And don't worry, a little miso goes a long way!
- Buy seaweed in bulk online. My two favorite websites are www.pangaia.cc and www.seaveg.com

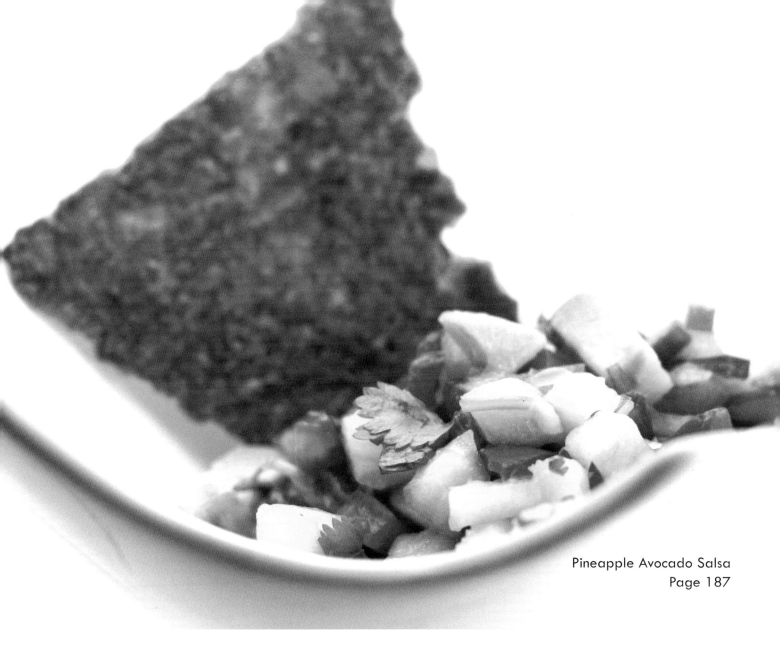

Pineapple Avocado Salsa
Page 187

Salsas and Spreads

Pear Tomato Salsa

Makes 4 Servings

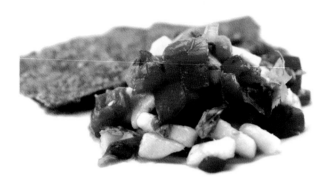

1 large pear	<$0.50
1/2 medium cucumber	<$0.25
2 medium red tomatoes	$1.00
2 tbsp fresh cilantro	<$0.25
1/2 whole jalapeno	<$0.15
1 clove garlic	<$0.10
juice from 1/2 lime	$0.20
sea salt to taste	<$0.05
Total estimated cost	$2.50
Estimated cost per serving	$0.63

Tips to reduce the cost:

- Prepare this recipe during the summer or early fall when the ingredients are in season and less expensive.

My roommate Sheena made this recipe for our annual Cinco de Mayo party! I couldn't believe how beautiful the pears tasted!

Be sure to use a ripe pear in this recipe. You may need to buy a pear several days in advance to give it time to ripen. This recipe goes well with any type of pear, but the light sweetness of Barlett pears tastes best.

Enjoy this salsa with South of the Border Flatbread (shown in the picture; page 263) or Sweet Summer Salsa Crackers (page 267).

Preparation
Equipment needed: Just a knife and cutting board!

1 Remove the skin from a large, ripe pear and dice the flesh. Pour the diced pears into a large bowl.

2 Chop the cucumber, and dice the tomatoes and cilantro. Add to the pears.

3 Remove the seeds from the jalapeno, mince the flesh, and add to the bowl of pears.

4 Mince the garlic and add to the pears. Mix the salsa very well.

5 Juice the lime and add the juice to the salsa. Then salt the salsa to taste and that's it! If you desire a hotter salsa, add some of the jalapeno seeds. Enjoy!

Nutrition Information Per Serving (based on 2,000 calorie daily intake): calories 45, protein 1g, total fat 0g, carbohydrate 11g, dietary fiber 2g, total sugars 7g, calcium 2%, iron 2%, sodium 12%, potassium 8%, zinc 2%, vitamin A 12%, vitamin E 3%, thiamin 3%, riboflavin 2%, niacin 3%, vitamin B6 5%, folate 4%, vitamin B12 0%, vitamin C 23%

Pineapple Avocado Salsa

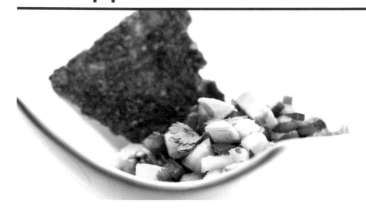

1 cup pineapple	$1.00
1 1/2 medium red tomatoes	$0.75
1/2 medium red onion	<$0.40
1 small sweet pepper	$1.00
1/2 medium avocado	$0.65
4 tbsp fresh cilantro	<$0.25
1 whole jalapeno	$0.25
juice from 1-2 limes	<$0.70
sea salt to taste	<$0.05
Total estimated cost	$5.05
Estimated cost per serving	$1.27

Tips to reduce the cost:

- Buy a non-organic pineapple to keep the recipe costs low. Organic pineapples are very expensive and typically don't taste any better than conventional ones.

This is a beautiful, tropical salsa that is super simple to make.

Enjoy this salsa with South of the Border Flatbread (shown in the picture; see page 263) or Sweet Summer Salsa Crackers (page 267).

Be sure to use a ripe pineapple and avocado in this recipe. When choosing a pineapple to buy, select one that has a yellow bottom and smells sweet. When choosing an Hass avocado, select one that has dark green skin and gives slightly to touch.

Preparation
Equipment needed: Just a knife and cutting board!

1 Take a fresh pineapple, remove the skin and core, and dice the meat. You will need about 1/4 to 1/3 of a whole pineapple. Pour the diced pineapple into a large bowl.

2 Dice the tomatoes, red onion, sweet pepper, avocado, and cilantro, and then add to the pineapple.

3 Remove the seeds from the jalapeno and mince the flesh. Add the minced jalapeno to the salsa and mix.

4 Juice the limes and add the juice to the salsa. Then salt the salsa to taste and that's it! If you desire a hotter salsa, add some of the jalapeno seeds. Enjoy!

Nutrition Information Per Serving (based on 2,000 calorie daily intake): calories 63, protein 1g, total fat 6g, carbohydrate 11g, dietary fiber 3g, total sugars 6g, calcium 2%, iron 2%, sodium 3%, potassium 7%, zinc 2%, vitamin A 16%, vitamin E 5%, thiamin 5%, riboflavin 4%, niacin 4%, vitamin B6 10%, folate 9%, vitamin B12 0%, vitamin C 79%

Sweet Tomato Melody

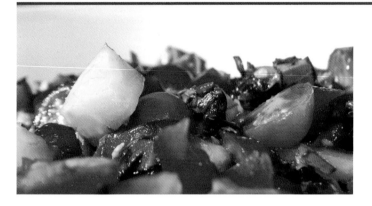

This recipe celebrates the best of the summer season! It contains fresh, juicy, ripe tomatoes and sun-dried tomatoes, and it's seasoned with fresh Italian herbs and a hint of balsamic vinegar! Try using your own homemade 'sun-dried' tomatoes in this recipe (see page 270).

This recipe is the perfect side to any salad, or it can be eaten with Italian flax crackers (see recipe on page 262) and pesto (see recipe on page 191).

Preparation
Equipment needed: Just a knife and cutting board!

1 Chop the whole tomatoes and slice the cherry tomatoes in half. Pour the tomatoes into a large bowl.

2 Mince the sun-dried tomatoes, oregano, thyme, garlic, and scallion, and add to the tomatoes.

3 Chop the basil and red bell pepper, and add to the tomatoes. Stir.

4 Add the olive oil and vinegar, and stir. Enjoy!

3 small tomatoes	$1.00
1 pint cherry tomatoes	$2.00
3 pieces sun-dried tomatoes	$0.30
1/4 tsp fresh oregano	<$0.10
1/4 tsp fresh thyme	<$0.10
1 clove garlic	$0.10
1 small scallion	$0.20
1 handful fresh basil	<$0.25
1/2 medium red bell pepper	<$1.50
2 tsp extra virgin olive oil	<$0.25
1 tsp balsamic vinegar	<$0.10
Total estimated cost	$5.90
Estimated cost per serving	$1.48

Nutrition Information Per Serving (based on 2,000 calorie daily intake): calories 57, protein 2g, total fat 3g, carbohydrate 8g, dietary fiber 2g, total sugars 5g, calcium 3%, iron 1%, sodium 2%, potassium 13%, zinc 2%, vitamin A 38%, vitamin E 9%, thiamin 5%, riboflavin 3%, niacin 6%, vitamin B6 9%, folate 8%, vitamin B12 0%, vitamin C 64%

Tips to reduce the cost:
- Get the main ingredients through a CSA program, which typically provides these ingredients during the summer season.

Mango Salsa

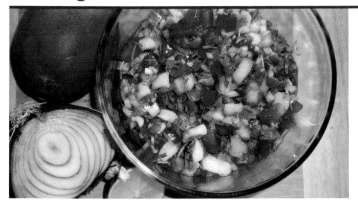

1 large fresh mango	$1.50
1 medium red tomato	$0.50
1/4 cup red onion	<$0.20
1/2 cup fresh cilantro	$0.50
1 medium jalapeno	$0.25
1/2 tsp sea salt	<$0.05
juice from 1 lime	$0.35
Total estimated cost	$3.35
Estimated cost per serving	$0.84

Tips to reduce the cost:

- Buy the mango from an Asian market or a store where you have access to ripe, juicy mangoes.

This is a great sweet salsa! Every time I make it, I receive rave reviews. It's simple, inexpensive, and tastes wonderful. It's always a crowd pleaser.

Be sure to use a ripe mango for this recipe. You may have to buy the mango several days in advance and allow the mango to ripen. I typically give my mangos a week to ripen before I make this recipe.

Enjoy this salsa with South of the Border Flatbread (see recipe on page 263) or Sweet Summer Salsa Crackers (see recipe on page 267).

Preparation
Equipment needed: Just a knife and cutting board!

1 Remove the flesh from a large ripe mango and dice. Place the diced mango into a large bowl.

2 Next, dice the tomato, red onion, and cilantro, and add to the bowl.

3 Remove the seeds from the jalapeno, mince, and add to the bowl.

4 Lastly, add the salt and lime juice, and stir. If you desire a hotter salsa, add some of the jalapeno seeds.

Nutrition Information Per Serving (based on 2,000 calorie daily intake): calories 47, protein 1g, total fat 0g, carbohydrate 12g, dietary fiber 2g, total sugars 9g, calcium 1%, iron 1%, sodium 0%, potassium 6%, zinc 1%, vitamin A 16%, vitamin E 6%, thiamin 4%, riboflavin 3%, niacin 3%, vitamin B6 7%, folate 4%, vitamin B12 0%, vitamin C 41%

Garlicky Pesto

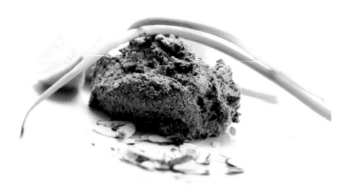

This is an amazing summer pesto. The under-used garlic scape (shown on top of the pesto) makes a wonderful pesto. You can find garlic scapes in the spring from many farms that grow garlic, and they are super inexpensive.

Preparation

Equipment needed: Food processor

1 Process sunflower seeds and walnuts in a food processor until they are well broken down into a nutty flour.

2 Add basil, garlic scapes, balsamic vinegar, and olive oil to the food processor, and process until creamy. Add 4-6 tbsp of water to help the mixture process.

3 Salt to taste and enjoy!

1/2 cup raw sunflower seeds	$0.60
1/2 cup raw walnuts, whole	$1.00
1/2 cup fresh basil leaves	$0.50
6 garlic scapes	<$0.75
2 tbsp balsamic vinegar	$0.30
3 tbsp extra virgin olive oil	$0.75
sea salt to taste	<$0.05
Total estimated cost	$3.95
Estimated cost per serving	$0.99

Nutrition Information Per Serving (based on 2,000 calorie daily intake): calories 308, protein 9g, total fat 28g, carbohydrate 9g, dietary fiber 4g, total sugars 3g, calcium 7%, iron 14%, sodium 6%, potassium 10%, zinc 11%, vitamin A 13%, vitamin E 54%, thiamin 30%, riboflavin 6%, niacin 6%, vitamin B6 13%, folate 18%, vitamin B12 0%, vitamin C 14%

Tips to reduce the cost:

- This is a pretty inexpensive pesto! What more could you ask for!

Simple Walnut Pesto

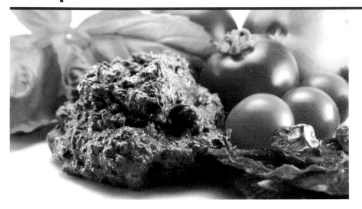

Okay, I will admit, this is not the best looking pesto. But, it's creamy, flavorful, and tastes great! Plus, it's simple to make and easy on your wallet. Traditional pesto is made with pine nuts, which are very expensive and often are sold rancid. An easy pine nut substitute are walnuts!

This pesto recipe tastes amazing when spread on top of Italian Flax crackers (recipe on page 262), and topped with fresh or sunbaked tomatoes.

Preparation
Equipment needed: Food processor

1 Process the walnuts and garlic in a food processor until they are well broken down. If you are adding sun-dried tomatoes, add them to the food processor now.

2 Add the basil to the food processor, and process until your pesto forms.

3 Add the remaining ingredients to the food processor, and process until you achieve the texture you desire. You want all of the ingredients to be well integrated (i.e. no chunky pieces) and for the pesto to be creamy. Enjoy!

1/2 cup raw walnuts, whole	$1.00
2 cloves garlic	$0.20
2-3 pieces sun-dried tomatoes (optional)	<$0.30
2 cups fresh basil	$2.00
1 tbsp extra virgin olive oil	$0.25
2 tsp nutritional yeast	<$0.25
1/8 tsp sea salt	<$0.05
1 tbsp chopped tomatoes (optional)	$0.50
Total estimated cost	$4.55
Estimated cost per serving	$1.14

Nutrition Information Per Serving (based on 2,000 calorie daily intake): calories 146, protein 5g, total fat 13g, carbohydrate 5g, dietary fiber 3g, total sugars 1g, calcium 5%, iron 1%, sodium 4%, potassium 9%, zinc 5%, vitamin A 27%, vitamin E 6%, thiamin 56%, riboflavin 50%, niacin 26%, vitamin B6 48%, folate 6%, vitamin B12 11%, vitamin C 13%

Tips to reduce the cost:

- Growing your own basil is the best way to reduce the cost of this recipe. Grow it in your kitchen or backyard! Or get some from a friend's garden!
- Prepare this recipe in the mid to late-summer when basil is less expensive.

The BEST Pate Ever!

1/3 cup raw sunflower seeds	$0.40
1/3 raw cashews, whole	$0.65
1/3-1/2 cup carrots	<$0.20
2 large celery stalks	<$0.25
1/3 medium apple	<$0.20
1 tbsp lemon juice (~1/4 lemon)	<$0.15
1/8 tsp sea salt	<$0.05
1 tbsp stone ground mustard	$0.20
Total estimated cost	$2.10
Estimated cost per serving	$0.70

Tips to reduce the cost:
- Buy the sunflower seeds and cashews from bulk bins so that you can buy the amounts you need.
- Buy a small bottle of mustard. It has a long shelf-life and a little bit goes a long way!

This is truly the best pate I have every tasted! It's so easy and tastes so fresh. It's also the perfect replacement for tuna salad.

Enjoy this pate with flax crackers, or slices of carrots or celery!

Avoid using Grey Poupon in this recipe. It makes the pate taste pretty bad. Trust me!

Preparation
Equipment needed: Food processor

1 Process the sunflower seeds in a food processor until the seeds turn into a nutty flour. This takes 20-30 seconds.

2 Add the cashews to the food processor and process until for 15 to 20 seconds.

3 Chop the carrots, celery, and apple. Add to the food processor and pulse until the mixture blends smoothly.

4 Juice the lemon and add to the food processor. Next, add the salt and mustard, and process until the mixture reaches the texture you prefer.

This recipe can be prepared ahead of time and it will stay fresh in the refrigerator for up to 3-4 days.

Nutrition Information Per Serving (based on 2,000 calorie daily intake): calories 207, protein 7g, total fat 15g, carbohydrate 14g, dietary fiber 4g, total sugars 5g, calcium 5%, iron 12%, sodium 9%, potassium 12%, zinc 12%, vitamin A 76%, vitamin E 40%, thiamin 29%, riboflavin 7%, niacin 7%, vitamin B6 12%, folate 17%, vitamin B12 0%, vitamin C 10%

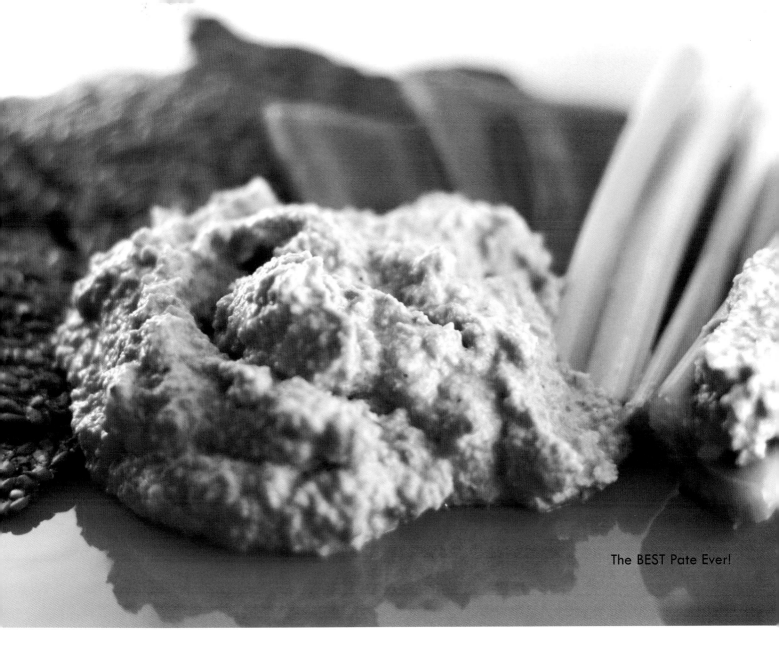

The BEST Pate Ever!

Better than Apple Sauce

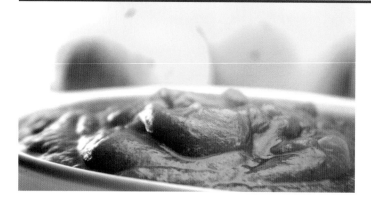

4 medium apples	$1.50
Total estimated cost	$1.50
Estimated cost per serving	$0.75

Tips to reduce the cost:

- For the most flavorful and inexpensive apples, buy them straight from a local farm.

I love, love, love raw apple sauce. It's so easy to make and tastes amazing! This recipe is great for children and adults, and it makes a nice late night snack.

You can prepare this apple sauce either with the peel on or without the peel. If you leave the peel on, you will make a sauce that has the consistency of regular apple sauce. However, if you leave the peel on, you will make a sauce that has the consistency of apple butter.

If you plan to use a food processor to prepare this recipe, I recommend peeling the apples first because they are easier to blend.

Use baking apples for this recipe. They have a softer flesh, which is perfect for blending. Crunchy apples will make a watery apple sauce.

Preparation
Equipment needed: High-speed blender or food processor

1 Peel the apples, remove the core, and chop into cubes. It's okay, if the apples are in big chunks.

2 If you are using a food processor, process the apples until they reach the texture you desire.

3 If you are using a high-speed blender, then process the apples on high speed, pressing the apples into the blade.

4 (Optional) For a more flavorful apple sauce, add 1/4 tsp of cinnamon, a pinch of nutmeg, and 1 tsp of honey or agave.

Nutrition Information Per Serving (based on 2,000 calorie daily intake): calories 144, protein 1g, total fat 1g, carbohydrate 38g, dietary fiber 7g, total sugars 29g, calcium 2%, iron 2%, sodium 0%, potassium 8%, zinc 1%, vitamin A 3%, vitamin E 3%, thiamin 3%, riboflavin 4%, niacin 1%, vitamin B6 6%, folate 2%, vitamin B12 0%, vitamin C 21%

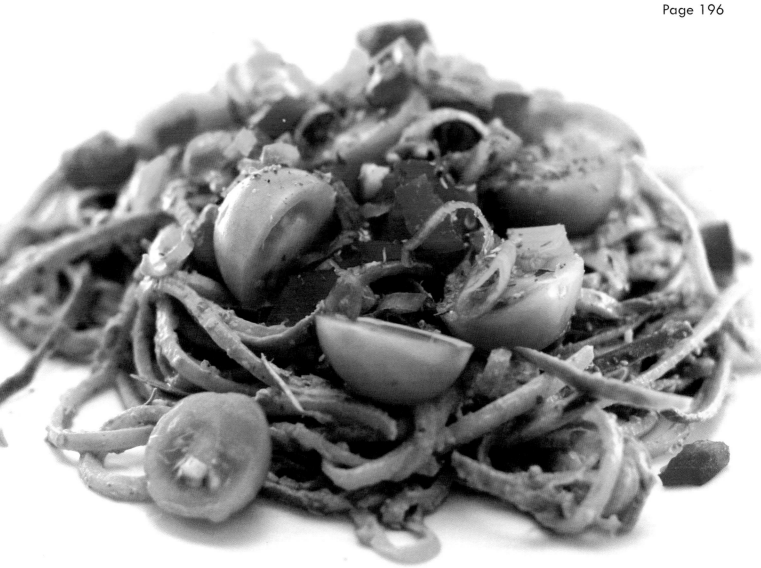

Garlicky Pesto with Cucumber Noodles
Page 196

Main Dishes

Garlicky Pesto with Cucumber Noodles

Makes 2 Cups | 1 Serving

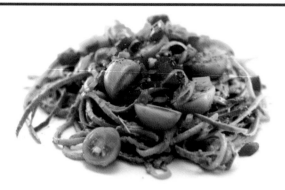

These noodles are delicious! The fresh garlic pesto (made with garlic scapes and basil) and sweet cherry tomatoes make this dish a rich delicacy! And it's super inexpensive!

Preparation

Equipment needed: Mandoline, spiralizer, or julienne slicer

1 Prepare the pesto recipe and set aside (see page 190 for recipe).

2 Create the cucumber noodles using a mandoline, spiralizer, or julienne peeler. Don't slice the center of the cucumber. It's too mushy (snack on it instead).

3 In a medium bowl, mix the pesto, noodles, and balsamic vinegar.

4 Place the pesto noodles on a plate and top with sliced cherry tomatoes, diced peppers, minced green onions, and dried Italian seasonings or fresh herbs. Enjoy!

1/4 recipe Garlicky Pesto Recipe (page 190)	$0.99
1 large cucumber	$0.75
1 tbsp balsamic vinegar	$0.15
1 handful sweet cherry tomatoes	$0.50
2 tbsp sweet peppers, diced	<$0.25
1 tbsp green onions, minced	<$0.10
1 pinch Italian spices/herbs	<$0.05
Total estimated cost	$2.79
Estimated cost per serving	$2.79

Nutrition Information Per Serving (based on 2,000 calorie daily intake): calories 378, protein 11g, total fat 28g, carbohydrate 25g, dietary fiber 7g, total sugars 10g, calcium 12%, iron 21%, sodium 8%, potassium 26%, zinc 15%, vitamin A 53%, vitamin E 57%, thiamin 37%, riboflavin 13%, niacin 10%, vitamin B6 23%, folate 31%, vitamin B12 0%, vitamin C 87%

Tips to reduce the cost:

• Make this recipe during the summer when all of the ingredients are inexpensive, flavorful, and easy to find.

Sweet Italian Herb Spaghetti

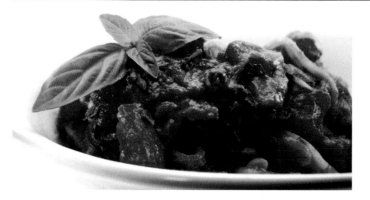

2 large zucchini	$0.50
sea salt to taste	<$0.05
3-4 medium red tomatoes	$2.00
1/2-3/4 cup sun-dried tomatoes	<$1.50
1/2 tsp fresh oregano	<$0.05
1/4 tsp fresh thyme	<$0.05
1/4 cup raw walnuts, whole	$0.50
1 clove garlic	$0.10
1/2 tsp balsamic vinegar	<$0.10
1 handful fresh basil	<$0.25
Total estimated cost	$5.10
Estimated cost per serving	$2.55

Tips to reduce the cost:

- Grow the main ingredients in your garden or buy them from a local farm, farmers market, or CSA program.

This is a wonderful recipe! The sauce is jam-packed with fresh tomatoes and Italian herbs. The secret is to use the best tomatoes you can find. If you can, make your own home-made dried tomatoes (see page 270 for recipe). They will make a sweeter marinara.

This recipe makes great leftovers! Enjoy!

Preparation

Equipment needed: High-speed blender or food processor • Mandoline, spiralizer, or julienne peeler

1 Create the zucchini noodles using a mandoline, spiralizer, or julienne peeler. Do not use the spongy zucchini core. Place the noodles in a large bowl and sprinkle the sea salt, and mix.

2 Blend 2 tomatoes, 1/2 cup of the sun-dried tomatoes, the oregano, thyme, walnuts, garlic, and vinegar until smooth. For a thicker sauce, add more sun-dried tomatoes.

3 Pour the sauce over the noodles and mix.

4 Chop the basil and remaining tomatoes, and pour on top of the noodles. Serve.

Nutrition Information Per Recipe (based on 2,000 calorie daily intake): calories 466, protein 24g, total fat 22g, carbohydrate 61g, dietary fiber 19g, total sugars 35g, calcium 23%, iron 44%, sodium 39%, potassium 115%, zinc 30%, vitamin A 125%, vitamin E 27%, thiamin 44%, riboflavin 70%, niacin 44%, vitamin B6 107%, folate 75%, vitamin B12 0%, vitamin C 311%

Italian Spaghetti Squash Bowl

Makes 3-4 Cups | 2 Servings

1/2 whole spaghetti squash	$2.00
1/4 cup sun-dried tomatoes	$0.50
2 leaves kale	$0.25
2 cloves garlic	$0.20
1 1/2 tbsp balsamic vinegar	<$0.25
2 tbsp hemp seeds	$0.60
1 1/2 tbsp nutritional yeast	<$0.40
1 tsp Italian spices	<$0.05
sea salt to taste	<$0.05
1 tbsp extra virgin olive oil	$0.25
Total estimated cost	**$4.55**
Estimated cost per serving	**$2.28**

Tips to reduce the cost:
- Organic spaghetti squash can be pricey ($4-6) at grocery stores, so purchase one from a local farm or farmers' market, or buy a non-organic one.

This recipe is one of my favorite winter dishes. It's the perfect combination of Italian seasonings, fresh kale, earthly flavor, and sun-dried tomatoes. And it's easy to make!

Preparation
Equipment needed: Dehydrator or warm oven (optional)

1 Prepare the spaghetti squash. Cut the squash in half along the long side with a sharp knife. You will only need 1/2 of the squash. The other half will stay fresh in the refrigerator for one week.

2 Take the squash and remove the "insides" (i.e. seeds). Using a fork, scrape the meat of the squash to remove the "spaghetti". Remove as much as you can. Because the squash is raw, the spaghetti will look more like rice. Pour the spaghetti into a medium size bowl.

3 Chop the sun-dried tomatoes into small pieces and add to the spaghetti. Remove the stalks from the kale, and thinly slice the leaves into strips. Add the kale to the spaghetti. Mince the garlic, add, and mix well. Add the balsamic vinegar, hemp seeds, nutritional yeast, and Italian seasonings to the squash, and mix well. Salt to taste and mix. Finally, add the olive oil and mix.

4 Allow the mixture to marinate for 5-10 minutes.

This recipe is best enjoyed when it's slightly warm. Try warming the recipe in a dehydrator or warm oven (see tip on page 166) for 10-20 minutes.

Nutrition Information Per Serving (based on 2,000 calorie daily intake): calories 220, protein 9g, total fat 13g, carbohydrate 21g, dietary fiber 4g, total sugars 4g, calcium 19%, iron 26%, sodium 17%, potassium 23%, zinc 9%, vitamin A 43%, vitamin E 12%, thiamin 228%, riboflavin 198%, niacin 105%, vitamin B6 175%, folate 9%, vitamin B12 43%, vitamin C 154%

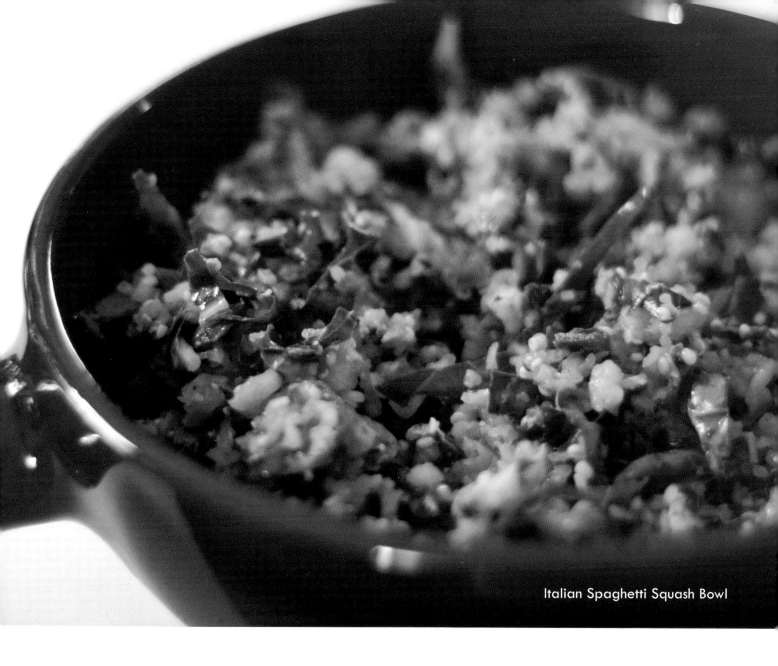

Italian Spaghetti Squash Bowl

Green Beans in Italian Marinara

Makes 2 1/2 Cups | 1 Large Serving

GREEN BEAN MIXTURE

5 oz of fresh green beans (~1/3 lb)	$0.50
1/3 medium red bell pepper	$1.00
4 crimini mushrooms	$0.75
1/2 medium spring onion	<$0.40
1 tbsp balsamic vinegar	$0.15

TOMATO MARINARA

2 medium tomatoes	$1.00
3-5 pieces sun-dried tomatoes	$0.50
1 tsp dried Italian spices	<$0.05
1/2 clove garlic	$0.05
sea salt to taste	<$0.05
Total estimated cost	$4.45
Estimated cost per serving	$4.45

Tips to reduce the cost:

- Make this recipe when green beans are in season, and are most flavorful and affordable.

This is a wonderful green bean recipe! It's incredibly flavorful and decadent without being oil or greasy. In fact, there no oil in the recipe at all!

Preparation

Equipment needed: Dehydrator or glass casserole dish with glass lid for sun-baking

GREEN BEAN MIXTURE

1 Remove the ends of the green beans and set aside in a large bowl.

2 Slice the red bell pepper, mushrooms, and spring onion, and add to the green beans. Add the balsamic vinegar and mix well.

3 Dehydrate or sun-bake the vegetables for 5-6 hours. If you are using a dehydrator, spread the vegetables on top of a texflex sheet. Dehydrate at 105 degrees or in your oven at the lowest temperature (see oven dehydrating tip on page 166). If you are sun-baking the vegetables, pour the vegetables into a glass casserole dish. Prepare the vegetables for sun-baking as described on page 218.

TOMATO MARINARA

4 Blend all of the ingredients in a food processor or blender until smooth. If you are using a food processor, soak the sun-dried tomatoes for 4 hours before using.

Once the green bean mixture has dehydrated, place it into a medium bowl. Add the marinara by the spoonful and mix. Set aside for 10 minutes and then serve.

This recipe stores well in the refrigerator and can be prepared 1-2 days ahead of time.

Nutrition Information Per Serving (based on 2,000 calorie daily intake): calories 204, protein 10g, total fat 1.4g, carbohydrate 45g, dietary fiber 12g, total sugars 25g, calcium 13%, iron 22%, sodium 9%, potassium 48%, zinc 11%, vitamin A 87%, vitamin E 17%, thiamin 27%, riboflavin 35%, niacin 32%, vitamin B6 38%, folate 31%, vitamin B12 0%, vitamin C 197%

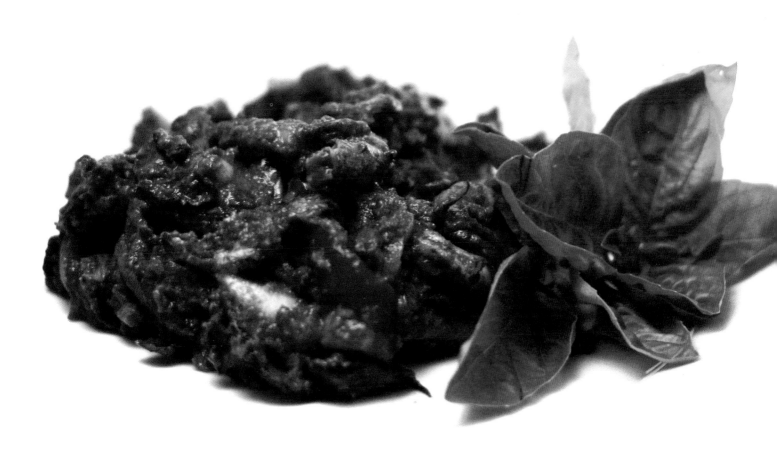

Green Beans in Italian Marinara

Winter Pizza

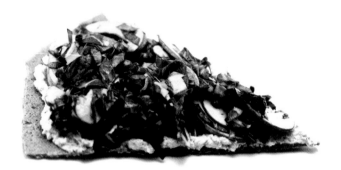

This pizza is incredible! Actually, it's more than a pizza because it celebrates the beauty of winter produce! There are 4 parts to this pizza, so there are a lot of ingredients; but the ingredients are common and you probably already have them in your kitchen! This recipe is very job-friendly because it can be prepared ahead of time and assembled by the slice on the spot.

Preparation
Equipment needed: High-speed blender or food processor • Dehydrator • Coffee grinder (optional)

CRUST

1 Peel and cube the apples and butternut squash. You will need 2/3 of a medium butternut squash for this recipe.

2 Blend the apples using a food processor or high-speed blender until liquefied. Add up to 1/4 cup of water to help the apples blend. Now, add the butternut squash, sea salt, and vinegar and blend until liquefied. This may take 1-3 minutes in a food processor and 20-30 seconds in a high-speed blender. Pour the mixture into a large bowl. Set aside.

3 Grind the flaxseeds into a powder using a coffee grinder or high-speed blender. Add the ground flaxseeds to the butternut squash mixture and mix well with a whisk or large spoon. Allow the mixture to sit for 5-10 minutes. Then add the oil and mix well.

4 Spread the butternut mixture onto one 14x14-inch Texflex sheet and dehydrate at 105 degrees. After 12 hours, turn the crust over and remove the Texflex sheet. Score the crust into 8 pizza slices with a sharp knife, and then return it back to the dehydrator to dry for 24 more hours. When the crust is done, break it into 8 slices and store it in an air-tight container or plastic bag.

CRUST

2 medium apples	$0.75
2 cups butternut squash	$2.00
1/2 tsp sea salt	<$0.05
2 tbsp apple cider vinegar	$0.20
3/4 cup golden flaxseeds, whole	$0.75
3 tbsp extra virgin olive oil	$0.75

WHITE SAUCE

1 1/2 cup raw cashews, whole	$3.00
7-9 tbsp water	$0.00
3 tsp lemon juice	$0.35
1-2 pinches cayenne powder	<$0.05
1 tsp extra virgin olive oil	<$0.10
2 pieces sun-dried tomatoes	$0.20
2 tsp Italian spices, dried	$0.20
2 tbsp nutritional yeast	$0.50

TOMATO SAUCE

1-2 medium tomatoes	$1.00
6 pieces sun-dried tomatoes	$0.60
1 tsp Italian spices, dried	$0.10
1 pinch sea salt	<$0.05
1 tsp nutritional yeast	<$0.10
1 clove garlic	$0.10

COLLARD TOPPING

10 large collard green leaves	$1.50
sea salt to taste	<$0.05
4 tbsp balsamic vinegar	$0.60
4 cloves garlic	$0.40
8 pieces sun-dried tomatoes	$0.80
10 crimini mushrooms	$1.90
1 tbsp extra virgin olive oil	$0.25
Total estimated cost	$15.35
Estimated cost per serving	$3.83

Tips to reduce the cost:

- Simply, leave out the tomato sauce and save $2-3!
- Substitute the collard topping with a vegetable topping of your own. Try replacing the collard greens with another hardy winter green like kale.
- Substitute the butternut squash for another winter squash variety, yam, or sweet potato. Even try adding carrots or beets.

WHITE SAUCE

5 Soak the cashews for 6-8 hours or overnight. After the cashews have soaked, blend them in a strong blender or food processor, adding water one tablespoon at a time to help it blend. Be careful not to add too much liquid. Blend until very smooth. Add the remaining ingredients and blend until smooth and creamy.

TOMATO SAUCE

6 Blend all of the ingredients until smooth in a food processor or blender.

COLLARD TOPPING

7 Layer the collard leaves on top of each other, roll them into a burrito, and cut them into very thin slices. To avoid long strips, cut the collard strips in half. Place the sliced collards into a large bowl, and add a few pinches of salt and 2 tbsp of balsamic vinegar. Mix well.

8 Mince the garlic and sun-dried tomatoes, and add to the collards.

9 Slice the mushrooms and place them in a small bowl. Mix the mushrooms with 2 tbsp of balsamic vinegar, and allow it to sit for 5 minutes. Add the mushrooms to the collards and mix well. Pour the olive oil onto the collards and mix well. Salt to taste.

To optimize your pizza experience, assemble it right before you are ready to serve. Take a slice of the crust, spread the white sauce on top, add several small spoonfuls of marinara, and top it with the juicy collards. Enjoy!

Nutrition Information Per Serving (based on 2,000 calorie daily intake): calories 504, protein 15g, total fat 32g, carbohydrate 48g, dietary fiber 18g, total sugars 17g, calcium 28%, iron 25%, sodium 28%, potassium 42%, zinc 17%, vitamin A 279%, vitamin E 38%, thiamin 211%, riboflavin 167%, niacin 98%, vitamin B6 150%, folate 56%, vitamin B12 33%, vitamin C 103%

Spring Pizza

CRUST

1 1/2 cups golden flaxseeds, whole	$1.50
5-7 collard greens	<$1.50
1 1/2 tsp sea salt	<$0.05
4 tsp apple cider vinegar	<$0.15
4 cloves garlic	$0.40
1 green bell pepper	$1.50
1/2 medium onions	$0.40
5 crimini mushrooms	$0.80
3 tbsp nutritional yeast	$0.75
1 tbsp extra virgin olive oil	$0.25

CHEESE

1 1/2 cup raw cashews, whole	$3.00
3 tbsp lemon juice	$0.35
1 pinch cayenne powder	<$0.05
7-12 tbsp water	$0.00
1 piece sun-dried tomatoes	$0.10
1 tsp Italian spices, dried	<$0.05
1 tsp balsamic vinegar	<$0.05
2 tbsp nutritional yeast	$0.50
sea salt to taste	<$0.05

TOMATO MARINARA

4 medium tomatoes	$2.00
6-9 pieces sun-dried tomatoes	<$0.90
1 tsp Italian herbs, dried	$0.50
1 clove garlic	$0.10
sea salt to taste	<$0.05

This is what pizza is supposed to be! This recipe is a beautiful combination of fresh ingredients, a crispy yet flaky crust, tangy arugula, creamy cheese, and a rich tomato marinara.

This recipe is simple, but it does have several components. Start the recipe the day before by soaking the seeds and cashews, and preparing the crust.

Preparation

Equipment needed: High-speed blender or food processor • Dehydrator

1 Soak the flaxseeds in 2 1/4 cups of water for 6+ hours or overnight.

2 Soak the cashews in water for 6+ hours or overnight.

CRUST

3 Put the soaked flaxseeds into a large bowl. Stir the flaxseeds to break up any clumps. Layer the collard greens on top of each other, rolling them into a burrito. Cut the collards into 1/4-inch thick slices. To avoid long strips, cut the collard strips in half. Add the collards, sea salt, and apple cider vinegar to the flaxseeds and stir.

4 Mince the garlic, dice the peppers and onions, and add to the collards. Slice the mushrooms and then slice them again into small strips. Add the mushrooms, nutritional yeast, and olive oil to the flaxseeds and mix very well. Mash out any flaxseed clumps.

5 Pour half of the mixture onto one Teflex sheet (or parchment paper) and spread it to 1/3-inch thickness. Repeat the process. Dehydrate the crust at 105-degrees for 12 hours (i.e. when the top of the crackers are dry). Then flip the crust, remove the Teflex sheet, score the crust into square slices with a sharp knife and return the crust back to the dehydrator for 12-24 hours. When the crust is done, break it into squares and store them in an airtight container or plastic bag.

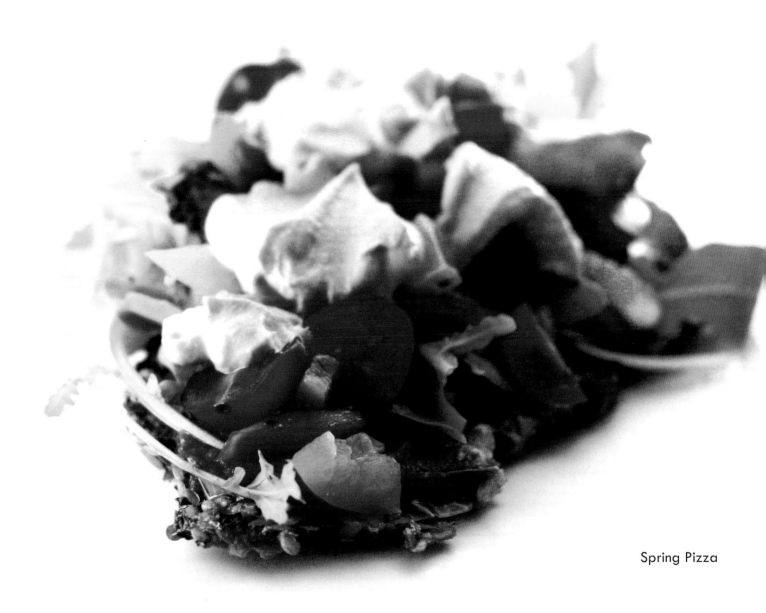

Spring Pizza

SAUTEED MUSHROOMS

8 crimini mushrooms	<$1.55
1 clove garlic	$0.10
1/4 medium onion	<$0.20
2 tsp balsamic vinegar	<$0.15
1 pinch sea salt	<$0.05
1/2 tsp dried Italian herbs	<$0.05
1 tsp extra virgin olive oil	$0.10

FRESH VEGETABLE TOPPING

1/2 pint cherry tomatoes	$1.00
1 medium red bell pepper	$3.00
2 1/2 cup arugula	$2.00
Total estimated cost	$23.20
Estimated cost per serving	$4.64

Tips to reduce the cost:

- Simplify the crust by leaving out the collard greens, mushrooms, and peppers!
- Replace the peppers in the vegetable topping with a less expensive crunchy vegetable like cucumbers, celery, or just use all tomatoes.
- Replace the collard greens with another hardy winter green like kale, mustard greens, or bok choy.

CHEESE

6 Blend the soaked cashews in a strong blender or food processor, adding water one tablespoon at a time to help the cashews blend. Be careful not to add too much water. Blend until very smooth.

7 Add the remaining ingredients and blend until smooth and creamy. You may need to add 1-3 tablespoons of water to help it blend. If you accidently add too much water, add a sun-dried tomato to thicken the cheese.

TOMATO MARINARA

8 Blend all of the ingredients in a food processor or blender until smooth. If you are using a food processor, soak the sun-dried tomatoes for 4 hours before using.

SAUTEED MUSHROOMS

9 Thinly slice the mushrooms and place them into a small bowl. Mince the garlic and slice the onions into thin strips. Add to the mushrooms and stir. Add the remaining ingredients and stir well. Allow the mushrooms to marinate for 20-60 minutes.

FRESH VEGETABLE TOPPING:

10 Dice the cherry tomatoes and bell pepper. Set aside.

To assemble the pizza, spread the marinara on top of a slice of crust. Add a small handful of arugula and a spoonful of sauteed mushrooms and vegetable topping. Lastly, top the pizza with a spoonful or two of cashew cheese.

The crust will last 2-3 weeks in an airtight plastic bag or container, and the toppings will last 5-6 days in the refrigerator.

Nutrition Information Per Serving (based on 2,000 calorie daily intake): calories 634, protein 24g, total fat 45g, carbohydrate 45g, dietary fiber 21g, total sugars 10g, calcium 24%, iron 40%, sodium 34%, potassium 42%, zinc 34%, vitamin A 57%, vitamin E 15%, thiamin 453%, riboflavin 356%, niacin 189%, vitamin B6 319%, folate 38%, vitamin B12 78%, vitamin C 82%

Chowmein Noodles

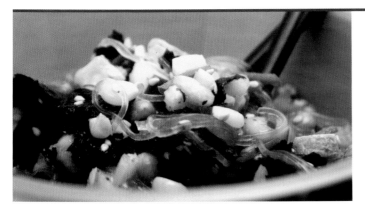

1/2 medium zucchini	<$0.15
1 ear fresh corn (about 1/2 cup)	$0.50
1/2 cup fresh peas	$1.00
2 stalks celery	<$0.25
1 medium carrot	$0.10
3 large florets of cauliflower	<$1.00
4 tsp white rice vinegar	<$0.35
1/4 tsp sea salt	<$0.05
1 cup kelp noodles	$1.25
2-3 sheets dried nori seaweed	<$0.90
extra virgin olive oil to taste	<$0.25
Total estimated cost	$5.80
Estimated cost per serving	$2.40

Tips to reduce the cost:

- Keep the recipe costs low by buying kelp noodles locally through a health food store or Asian market. Note that they can be difficult to find in some areas.

I was inspired to make this recipe by a good friend who also makes a wonderful raw stir-fry. However, it was only after I sun-baked a bowl of vegetables that I finally decided to make my own recipe. The key to this recipe is to allow the vegetables to marinate under the sun for 6 or more hours. They surprisingly come out tasting like chowmein!

Preparation

Equipment needed: Glass casserole dish or bowl with a glass lid for sun-baking

1 Dice the zucchini, celery, and cauliflower, and add to the glass casserole dish or bowl. Remove the corn from the ear using a knife and add. Cut the carrot into thin slices and add. Lastly, add the peas, vinegar, and salt, and mix well.

2 You will sun-bake the vegetables for 6-8 hours. To do this, cover the glass bowl or casserole dish with a glass lid and place it outside in a sunny location.

3 Once the vegetables have sun-baked, wash the kelp noodles by soaking them in a bowl of water with 1 tsp of vinegar for 5 minutes.

4 Take the kelp noodles out of the water and remove any excess moisture. Place the noodles into a large bowl and add the sun-baked vegetables. Mix very well until the noodles are well distributed. It may help to cut the noodles a little bit. Tear and sprinkle the nori sheets on top of the noodles, and mix well.

5 Finally, add olive oil to taste. You don't need a lot of olive oil for this recipe.

Nutrition Information Per Serving (based on 2,000 calorie daily intake): calories 202, protein 7g, total fat 8g, carbohydrate 28g, dietary fiber 8g, total sugars 7g, calcium 13%, iron 14%, sodium 20%, potassium 25%, zinc 8%, vitamin A 132%, vitamin E 13%, thiamin 18%, riboflavin 23%, niacin 12%, vitamin B6 16%, folate 42%, vitamin B12 0%, vitamin C 85%

Sun-Baked Gazpacho

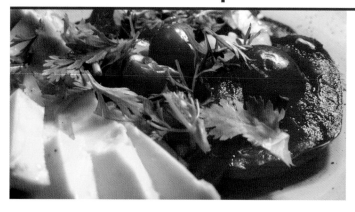

This is not your traditional gazpacho! Gazpacho is a cold Spanish soup that is typically made with tomatoes and other sweet summer vegetables. In this recipe, the tomatoes are sun-baked and when you bite into them, they melt into your mouth like a sweet summer soup. However, feel free to blend the tomatoes to make a more traditional-like soup.

Preparation

Equipment needed: Glass casserole dish or bowl with a glass lid for sun-baking

1 Using a large knife, slice the tomatoes into 1/4-inch slices and place them into a casserole dish or large bowl.

2 Mince the garlic and dice the white spring onion. Then add the garlic, salt, vinegar, and onion to the tomatoes and mix softly.

3 Cover the glass casserole dish or bowl with a glass lid and set outside to sun-bake for 6-8 hours.

4 Once the tomatoes have sun-baked, chop the cilantro and slice the avocado. Top the tomatoes with cilantro and olive oil, and serve with a few slices of avocado.

2 medium red tomatoes	$1.00
1/2 clove garlic	<$0.05
1/4 white spring onion	<$0.20
2 pinches sea salt	<$0.05
1 tsp apple cider vinegar	<$0.05
1 handful fresh cilantro	$0.25
1/2 medium avocado	$0.65
sprinkle extra virgin olive oil	<$0.15
Total estimated cost	$2.40
Estimated cost per serving	$2.40

Nutrition Information Per Serving (based on 2,000 calorie daily intake): calories 346, protein 5g, total fat 28g, carbohydrate 25g, dietary fiber 13g, total sugars 8g, calcium 5%, iron 9%, sodium 7%, potassium 38%, zinc 10%, vitamin A 50%, vitamin E 34%, thiamin 14%, riboflavin 15%, niacin 21%, vitamin B6 32%, folate 41%, vitamin B12 0%, vitamin C 78%

Tips to reduce the cost:

- Get the main ingredients from local farms, farmers markets, CSA programs, or grow them yourself!

'It Can Take It' Kale Salad

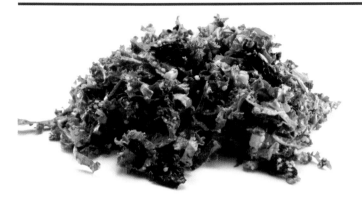

This salad is a nice combination of savory, crunchy, sour, cheesy, and nutty. And what I truly love about this salad is that I can add any vegetable to it and it will still taste good. In the past, I have added tomatoes, peas, peppers, celery, and carrots. Plus, the longer you let the recipe sit in the refrigerator, the better it will taste! And just look at the nutrition profile for this recipe! You can't lose!

Preparation
Equipment needed: Just a knife and cutting board!

1 Layer the kale leaves on top of each other, roll them into a burrito, and cut them into thin 1/4-inch slices. Place the sliced kale into a large bowl.

2 Add the salt and vinegar to the kale and mix well. Allow the greens to marinate while you prepare the rest of the recipe.

3 Mince the sun-dried tomatoes and add to the kale.

4 Tear and sprinkle the nori sheets on top of the kale, and mix well.

5 Add hemp seeds, sunflower seeds, and nutritional yeast to the kale and mix.

6 Add the olive oil and mix well. Enjoy!

5 leaves of green kale	$0.75
3-4 pinches sea salt	<$0.05
1 1/2 tbsp white rice vinegar	<$0.10
4-5 pieces sun-dried tomatoes	<$0.50
2 sheets nori seaweed	$0.60
2 tbsp hemp seeds	$0.60
1/4 cup raw sunflower seeds	$0.30
nutritional yeast to taste	$0.50
1 tsp extra virgin olive oil	<$0.10
Total estimated cost	$3.70
Estimated cost per serving	$3.00

Nutrition Information Per Serving (based on 2,000 calorie daily intake): calories 580, protein 31g, total fat 39g, carbohydrate 38g, dietary fiber 15g, total sugars 5g, calcium 51%, iron 78%, sodium 28%, potassium 62%, zinc 32%, vitamin A 147%, vitamin E 105%, thiamin 408%, riboflavin 325%, niacin 166%, vitamin B6 278%, folate 36%, vitamin B12 65%, vitamin C 468%

Tips to reduce the cost:

- If you make a lot of recipes with seaweed, buy the seaweed in 50-sheet packs at www.pangaia.cc.
- Buy your sea salt, sunflower seeds, and nutritional yeast from bulk bins at your local store.
- Avoid hemp seeds that are sold in bulk bins because they are often rancid. Instead, buy them in air-tight, sealed bags or containers.

Lemon Green Yum Kale Salad

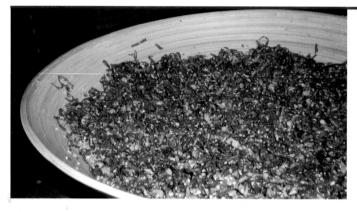

1 bunch lacinto kale	$1.50
sea salt to taste	<$0.05
2 tbsp apple cider vinegar	<$0.20
2 tsp garlic powder	<$0.10
1 tsp coriander, ground	<$0.10
1 tsp cumin, ground	<$0.10
3 tbsp nutritional yeast	$0.75
5 tbsp hemp seeds	$1.50
2 tbsp extra virgin olive oil	$0.25
Total estimated cost	$4.55
Estimated cost per serving	$1.14

This recipe is incredible! I have never made a vegetable recipe that has had such an impact! It made a 60-year old vegan a kale lover and my friend's children even did the dishes to persuade me to make the recipe again!

The recipe was affectionately named Lemon Green Yum Kale Salad by my friend's son who said it tasted like it had lemon in it.

Preparation
Equipment needed: Just a knife and cutting board!

1 Layer the kale leaves on top of each other, roll them into a burrito, and cut them into thin, 1/4-inch slices.

2 Place the sliced kale into a salad bowl, and massage the salt and vinegar into the kale.

3 Add the remaining ingredients on to the kale except for the oil and mix well.

4 Add the oil to the kale and mix well. Enjoy!

Nutrition Information Per Serving (based on 2,000 calorie daily intake): calories 214, protein 11g, total fat 14g, carbohydrate 16g, dietary fiber 5g, total sugars 0g, calcium 30%, iron 36%, sodium 16%, potassium 25%, zinc 10%, vitamin A 83%, vitamin E 14%, thiamin 255%, riboflavin 222%, niacin 114%, vitamin B6 197%, folate 9%, vitamin B12 49%, vitamin C 291%

Tips to reduce the cost:

- If you are purchasing kale at a grocery store, buy it on the day that it arrives so that it's fresh, crunchy, and will stay fresh longer.
- Buy spices from spice or bulk bins, so that you can buy the amounts you need.

Bok Choy Salad

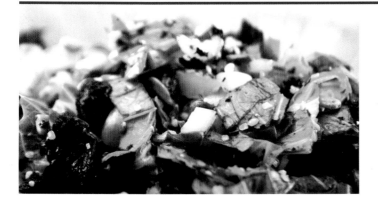

This recipe is probably the reason why I love bok choy so much. The dish is flavorful and savory, and super easy to make. You can also make the recipe creamier by adding an avocado.

This recipe uses a large variety of bok choy like china choy, which is different than baby bok choy. There benefits to using larger varieties of bok choy: they are more flavorful, less expensive, and frequently given in CSA programs.

1 large head or 3 medium heads of bok choy	$2.00
1/2 tbsp brown or white rice vinegar	<$0.15
sea salt to taste	<$0.05
3 sheets dried nori seaweed	$0.90
3 tbsp hemp seeds	$0.90
1/3 cup raw sunflower seeds	$0.40
1 tsp extra virgin olive oil	$0.25
1 clove garlic	$0.10
Total estimated cost	$4.75
Estimated cost per serving	$2.38

Tips to reduce the cost:

- The best way to get giant bok choy is from a farm, CSA program, farmers market, or Asian market.

Preparation
Equipment needed: Just a knife and cutting board!

1. Layer the bok choy leaves on top of each other, roll them into a burrito, and cut them into 1/3-inch slices. Chop the stalks of the bok choy into small pieces. Place the bok choy into a large bowl, and add the vinegar and a few pinches of salt. Mix well.

2. Mince the garlic and add to the bok choy. Mix.

3. Tear up the nori seaweed and sprinkle it on top of the bok choy.

4. Add the hemp seeds and sunflower seeds, and mix well.

5. Add the olive oil and mix well. Enjoy!

Nutrition Information Per Serving (based on 2,000 calorie daily intake): calories 370, protein 14g, total fat 32g, carbohydrate 11g, dietary fiber 7g, total sugars 2g, calcium 20%, iron 27%, sodium 10%, potassium 23%, zinc 17%, vitamin A 140%, vitamin E 77%, thiamin 50%, riboflavin 27%, niacin 9%, vitamin B6 23%, folate 37%, vitamin B12 0%, vitamin C 125%

Good Ole' Collards and Sweet Peppers

Makes 2 Servings

4 medium collard green leaves	<$0.75
1/4 tsp sea salt	<$0.05
1 tsp apple cider vinegar	<$0.05
juice from 1/4 lemon	<$0.10
1 medium sweet bell pepper	$3.00
14 brazil nuts	$1.40
1/4 tsp raw honey (optional)	<$0.10
Total estimated cost	$5.45
Estimated cost per serving	$2.75

Tips to reduce the cost:

- Purchase locally grown sweet peppers from farmer's markets or directly from a farm. Peppers are very affordable when they are in season.

This is a wonderful, light side salad for people who love the brilliant, sharp taste of collard greens. The brazil nuts add a creaminess that is tough to resist, and the peppers are fresh, crisp, and sweet.

Make this recipe in the fall when peppers are in season and inexpensive, and collards are coming into season. Choose collard greens that have medium-sized leaves (no larger than 10-inches, excluding the stalk) and no discolorations.

Preparation

Equipment needed: Coffee grinder, food processor, or high-speed blender

1 Layer the collard leaves on top of each other, roll them into a burrito, and cut them into thin 1/4-inch slices.

2 Place the sliced collards into a large bowl, and add the salt, vinegar, and lemon juice and mix well.

3 Dice the sweet bell peppers and add them to the greens.

4 Grind 10 brazil nuts into a flour using a coffee grinder, food processor, or high-speed blender.

5 Pour the nut flour onto the greens and mix until the greens are well coated.

6 Add on the honey and mix well.

7 Grind the remaining brazil nuts into a flour. Before serving, sprinkle the nut flour on top of the greens! Enjoy!

Nutrition Information Per Serving (based on 2,000 calorie daily intake): calories 283, protein 8g, total fat 24g, carbohydrate 16g, dietary fiber 7g, total sugars 7g, calcium 16%, iron 8%, sodium 13%, potassium 17%, zinc 12%, vitamin A 159%, vitamin E 35%, thiamin 21%, riboflavin 12%, niacin 9%, vitamin B6 24%, folate 42%, vitamin B12 0%, vitamin C 293%

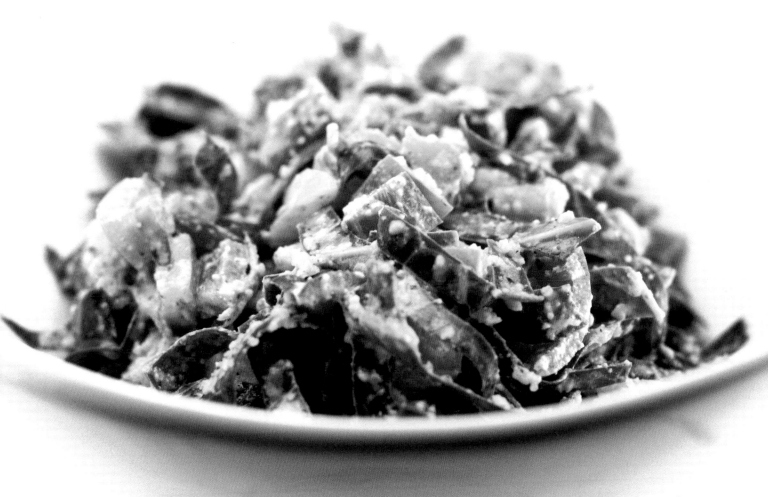

Good Ole' Collards and Sweet Peppers

Chinese Stir-Fry

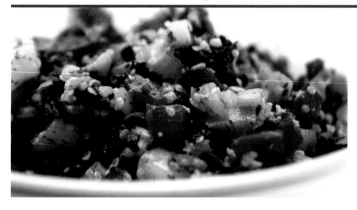

3 stalks celery	$0.25
1/3 large cucumber	$0.25
1/2 medium red bell pepper	$0.70
1 tsp brown or white rice vinegar	<$0.10
6 sprigs of cilantro	<$0.25
3 sheets dried nori seaweed	$0.90
1/8-1/4 tsp Chinese five spice powder	<$0.05
3 tbsp hemp seeds	$0.30
1/4 cup raw sunflower seeds	$0.30
1 tsp extra virgin olive oil	<$0.10
Total estimated cost	**$3.20**
Estimated cost per serving	**$3.20**

Tips to reduce the cost:
- Buy nori seaweed in bulk (e.g. 50 sheet packages)
- Buy Chinese five spice from the spice or bulk bin section at your local health food store.

This stir-fry was a wonderful, refreshing surprise! I was in the kitchen trying to figure out what to make for dinner, and this recipe came out of nowhere.

The recipe is lightly seasoned with Chinese five spice, which gives it a nice sweet and savory taste, and contains a good helping of fresh celery, cucumbers, and peppers. Plus, the sunflower and hemp seeds add a wonderful nutty flavor that is hard to resist.

Preparation
Equipment needed: Just a knife and cutting board!

1 Dice the celery stalks, cucumber, and red bell pepper, and place them into a large bowl.

2 Pour the vinegar onto the chopped vegetables and mix well.

3 Mince the cilantro and tear the sheets of nori seaweed into small pieces, and sprinkle on top of the chopped vegetables.

4 Add the Chinese five spice, hemp seeds, and sunflower seeds, and mix well.

5 Lastly, add the olive oil and mix until it's well distributed. If you like, add additional Chinese five spice. Enjoy!

Nutrition Information Per Serving (based on 2,000 calorie daily intake): calories 516, protein 23g, total fat 37g, carbohydrate 27g, dietary fiber 14g, total sugars 9g, calcium 18%, iron 42%, sodium 8%, potassium 47%, zinc 30%, vitamin A 90%, vitamin E 115%, thiamin 82%, riboflavin 52%, niacin 15%, vitamin B6 32%, folate 47%, vitamin B12 0%, vitamin C 181%

B12* Kale Salad

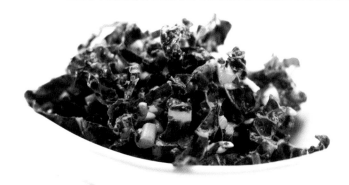

1 handful dried laver nori seaweed	<$1.00
5 leaves kale	$0.75
3-4 pinches sea salt	$0.50
1 tsp brown or white rice vinegar	<$0.10
1 clove garlic	$0.10
1/4 cup raw sunflower seeds	$0.30
2 tbsp nutritional yeast	$0.50
1 tsp extra virgin olive oil	<$0.10
Total estimated cost	**$3.35**
Estimated cost per serving	**$3.35**

Tips to reduce the cost:
- Buy laver nori seaweed in bulk (e.g. 1 pound bag) from online stores like Maine Sea Vegetables (www.seaveg.com).
- Buy the sea salt, sunflower seeds, and nutritional yeast from the spice or bulk bin section at your local health food store.

This is a great simple, tasty, filling salad that provides an estimated 7.8 grams of B12*! That's 130% of your recommended intake for the day! What more can you ask for?

I use dinosaur (or lacinto) kale to make this recipe, however, you can really use any type of kale or collards. You can also add other vegetables and nuts to the salad including peppers, hemp seeds, tomatoes, celery, etc.

Preparation
Equipment needed: Just a knife and cutting board!

1 Tear the laver seaweed into very small pieces. This can be done with a pair of scissors, high-speed blender, or coffee grinder. If you use a coffee grinder, break the laver up first. Set aside.

2 Layer the kale leaves on top of each other, roll them into a burrito, and cut them into thin 1/4-inch slices. Place the sliced kale into a large bowl, and add the salt and vinegar and mix well.

3 Mince the garlic and add to the kale. Mix.

4 Add the sunflower seeds, nutritional yeast, and seaweed to the kale and mix well.

5 Lastly, add the olive oil and mix well. Enjoy!

Nutrition Information Per Serving (based on 2,000 calorie daily intake): calories 394, protein 24g, total fat 25g, carbohydrate 31g, dietary fiber 11g, total sugars 1g, calcium 48%, iron 55%, sodium 26%, potassium 46%, zinc 20%, vitamin A 167%, vitamin E 90%, thiamin 707%, riboflavin 583%, niacin 304%, vitamin B6 520%, folate 49%, vitamin B12 130%, vitamin C 462%

*Based on current scientific evidence, it cannot yet be determined whether the vitamin B12 that is found in laver nori seaweed can be absorbed or utilized by the human body.

I made your Fig Freezer Cookies yesterday. Everyone I shared them with loved them!
-Narda

I want some!!!
-Nancy

I'm trying REALLY hard NOT to make the raw donut holes...***I'm Addicted***LOL!!! They are so DELISH - THEY WILL MAKE YOU DROP DOWN ON THE FLOOR - ROLL AROUND - JUMP UP AND SMACK THE FIRST PERSON YOU SEE!!! LOLOLOLOL
-Jaie

I had no idea raw foods looked so good!
-Maggie

I made the plum pie!!!
It was great!
-Shasta

I love the tip about saving the almond pulp for the carrot cake recipe. I go through a lot of almond milk... I may be making a LOT of carrot cake :)
-Judy

The apple pie is so delicious!!! Thank You!!!
-Jaie

Drooling. Not at all becoming.
-Kris

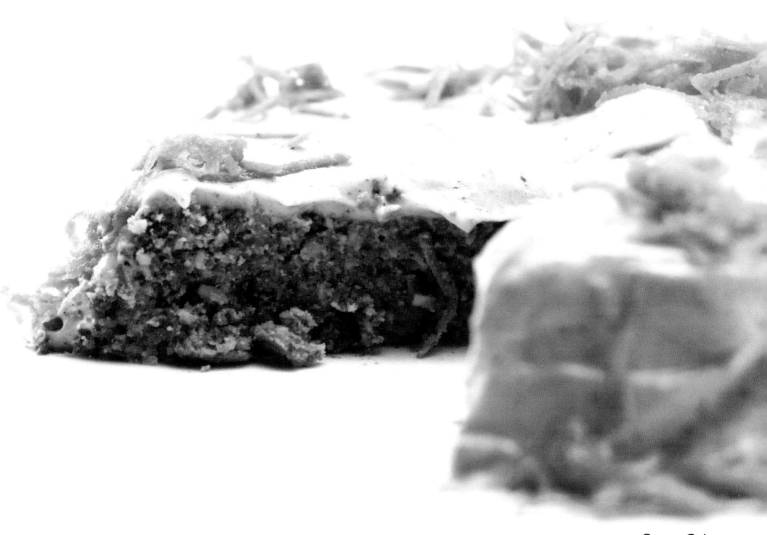

Carrot Cake
Page 232

Pies and Cakes

HOW TO SUN-BAKE

Sun-baking is a lot of fun! And it's super easy. All you need is a bowl, nutbag or cheesecloth, rubber band, and a sunny day! First, fill a medium-sized glass bowl or casserole dish with whatever you would like to sun-bake. Then cover the bowl with cheesecloth or a plastic nut bag (as shown in the picture below). Use a large rubber band to keep the cover in place. Make sure that there is no space underneath the rubber band. Now sun-bake!

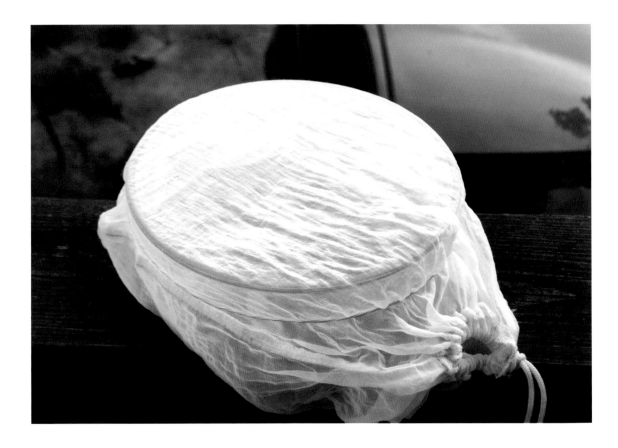

Quick Apple Pie

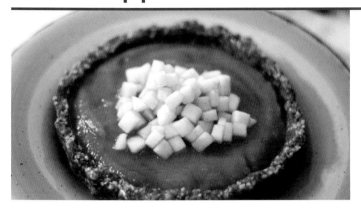

CRUST

1/2 cup raw shredded coconut	$0.25
1/2 cup raw sunflower seeds	$0.60
1/2 cup raw walnuts, whole	$1.00
1 tsp vanilla	<$0.25
1/2 tsp cinnamon	<$0.05
1 pinch sea salt	<$0.05
1 cup raisins	$1.00
1-2 tsp raw agave	<$0.20

FILLING

4 medium apples (baking)	$2.00
1/3 cup raisins	<$0.35
Total estimated cost	$5.75
Estimated cost per serving	$0.96

This pie is so moist and flavorful, yet it's so easy to make. In fact, you can make it in under 10 minutes. But be careful with this pie, you may find yourself eating 2 or 3 slices at a time!

Preparation
Equipment needed: Food processor • High-speed blender (optional) • Pie or dinner plate

CRUST

1 Process the shredded coconut in the food processor until the oils begin to come out of the coconut (about 30 seconds).

2 Add the sunflower seeds, walnuts, vanilla, cinnamon, and salt and process until the nuts and seeds are well broken down. Then add the raisins and process until they are completely broken down into small pieces. Lastly, add the agave and process until the dough begins to clump.

3 Press the dough onto a dinner or pie plate, forming a crust. Place the crust in the freezer for 30 minutes or until it hardens.

FILLING

4 Peel the apples and remove the cores. Using a food processor or strong blender, process the apples and raisins until liquefied.

5 Pour the mixture onto the crust and top with chopped apples. Serve.

Nutrition Information Per Serving (based on 2,000 calorie daily intake): calories 318, protein 7g, total fat 16g, carbohydrate 43g, dietary fiber 6g, total sugars 30g, calcium 5%, iron 12%, sodium 0%, potassium 15%, zinc 8%, vitamin A 1%, vitamin E 30%, thiamin 22%, riboflavin 7%, niacin 5%, vitamin B6 13%, folate 9%, vitamin B12 0%, vitamin C 9%

Sweet Glory Nectarine Pie

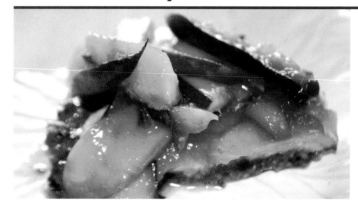

I made this pie for a potluck and it was amazing! The crust is succulent and moist, the coconut adds a nice creamy touch, and the luscious sun-baked nectarines are to die for.

You can make several substitutions when preparing this pie. Try using young coconut meat in place of coconut cream, or 1 cup of cashews (soaked 8 hours) and omit the coconut cream and meat. You can also replace 1/2 cup of the pecans with 1/2 cup of walnuts.

Preparation

Equipment needed: Food processor • High-speed blender (optional) • Dinner plate or pie plate • Large casserole dish or glass bowl • Cheesecloth or plastic nut bag

CRUST

1/2 cup raw sunflower seeds	$0.60
1 cup raw pecans, whole	$2.00
1/2 cup raisins	$0.50
1 tbsp agave	<$0.25
1 tsp cinnamon, ground	<$0.10
1 tsp vanilla	<$0.25
2 pinches nutmeg, ground	<$0.05
1 pinch sea salt	<$0.05

FILLING

1/4 cup raw coconut cream	$1.10
1/2 cup meat from 1 young coconut	$2.00
2 dates	$0.40
3-4 tbsp water	$0.00

1 Crack open the young coconut with a large knife and pour the water into a large glass. Scoop out the coconut meat with spoon. Remove any brown flakes from the meat and chop.

CRUST

2 Process the sunflower seeds in the food processor until a nutty flour forms. Add the pecans and process until they are well broken down. Add the remaining ingredients and process until a dough forms.

3 Press the crust onto the bottom of a pie plate or dinner plate. If you are using a pie plate, note that there will not be enough crust to press on the sides of the pie plate.

4 Place the crust in the freezer for 30 minutes or until it hardens.

FILLING

5 Blend the coconut cream, coconut meat, dates, and water using your high-speed blender or food processor. Be sure to only use enough water to blend the ingredients. Blend until the filling is smooth.

TOPPING

5 medium nectarines	$2.50
1/4 tsp vanilla	<$0.05
2 tsp raw agave	<$0.20
Total estimated cost	$10.05
Estimated cost per serving	$1.26

Tips to reduce the cost:

- Purchase nectarines from a local farm or farmers market.
- Try to buy all of the dry ingredients from bulk bins. This way you can buy the amounts you need.

6 Once the crust has hardened, spread the filling on top of the crust and place back in the freezer. Allow the filling to harden.

TOPPING

7 Slice the nectarines (leaving the skin on) into 1/3-inch thick slices and place into a medium bowl. Pour the vanilla and agave on the nectarines and softly stir.

8 Sun-bake the nectarines for 4+ hours. Refer to the sun-baking instructions on page 218.

When you are ready to serve the pie, scoop the sun-baked nectarines onto the frozen filling being careful not to take too much of the juice. Once the filling makes contact with the warm nectarines, it will soften, but the crust will remain firm until it melts in your mouth. Super, duper YUM!

Nutrition Information Per Serving (based on 2,000 calorie daily intake)**:** calories 301, protein 5g, total fat 21g, carbohydrate 27g, dietary fiber 5g, total sugars 18g, calcium 5%, iron 11%, sodium 0%, potassium 13%, zinc 10%, vitamin A 6%, vitamin E 27%, thiamin 23%, riboflavin 5%, niacin 9%, vitamin B6 9%, folate 8%, vitamin B12 0%, vitamin C 10%

Strawberry Cream Cobbler

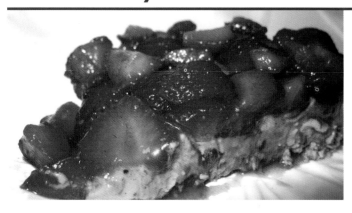

CRUST

1 1/2 cups raw shredded coconut	$0.75
1/2 cup raw pecans, whole	$1.00
1/2 tsp vanilla	<$0.15
1/2 tsp cinnamon, ground	<$0.05
6 dates	$1.20

FILLING

1 1/2 cups fresh strawberries	$1.50
1 cup meat from 2 young coconuts	$4.00
1 cup raw cashews, whole	$2.00
1/4 cup raw agave	<$1.00
2 tbsp water	$0.00

This is my best strawberry pie yet! It's the perfect combination of a creamy filling, buttery cookie crust, and strawberry freshness.

Prepare this recipe during the summer when strawberries are cheap and their most flavorful. This recipe calls for 5-7 cups of strawberries (about 2.5-3.5 pints), so the best way to keep your recipe costs low is to go fruit picking or grow your own strawberries.

Preparation

Equipment needed: High-speed blender • Food processor • Spring pan or pie plate

1 Soak 1 cup of cashews in water for 8+ hours or overnight.

2 Crack open the young coconuts with a large knife and pour the water into a large glass. Scoop out the coconut meat with spoon. Remove any brown flakes from the meat and chop.

CRUST

3 Process the shredded coconut in the food processor until the oils begin to come out of the coconut (about 30 sec). Add the pecans and process until they are well broken down. But be careful not to over process the pecans. Add the vanilla, cinnamon, and dates and process until the dates are well broken down.

4 Evenly press the crust mixture into a spring pan or pie plate. Place the crust in the freezer for 30 minutes or until it hardens.

FILLING

5 Blend the strawberries, coconut meat, soaked cashews, agave, and water until very smooth. If you would like a sweeter pie, add more agave.

TOPPING

4-5 cups fresh strawberries	$5.00
3 tbsp raw agave	$0.75
1/2 tsp cinnamon, ground	<$0.05
Total estimated cost	$17.45
Estimated cost per serving	$2.19

Tips to reduce the cost:

- Go fruit picking or grow your own strawberries. This recipe only cost me $11.75 because I grew the strawberries myself!

6

7 Pour the filling onto the hard crust. Put the pie in the refrigerator for 4-6 hours to allow the filling to set, and keep the pie in the refrigerator until it's time to serve.

TOPPING

8 Slice the strawberries into quarters or halves and place them into a mixing bowl.

9 Add the agave and cinnamon and mix well.

10 Refrigerate until you are ready to serve.

Before serving, remove the pie from the spring pan (if you are using one) and then pour the strawberry topping on top of the filling. Enjoy!

Nutrition Information Per Serving (based on 2,000 calorie daily intake): calories 342, protein 5g, total fat 22g, carbohydrate 34g, dietary fiber 8g, total sugars 20g, calcium 10%, iron 15%, sodium 0%, potassium 15%, zinc 12%, vitamin A 1%, vitamin E 5%, thiamin 9%, riboflavin 6%, niacin 6%, vitamin B6 10%, folate 12%, vitamin B12 0%, vitamin C 113%

Plum Pie

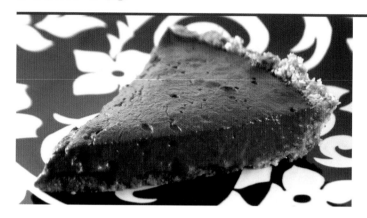

The objective was simple: make a plum pie. However, given that I have never made or eaten a plum pie, I didn't know what to expect. But, what I got was one of the coolest pies! The crust tastes like a cookie with a hint of fall spices, and the filling is creamy, plum goodness! You will not be disappointed with this pie! It even tastes better the next day...what more can you ask for?

Preparation
Equipment needed: High-speed blender • Food processor • Pie plate

CRUST

CRUST	
1 1/4 cups shredded coconut	<$0.65
1/4 cup raw pecans, whole	$0.50
1/4 cup raw sunflower seeds	$0.30
2 pinches clove, ground	<$0.05
1/4 tsp nutmeg, ground	<$0.05
1/2 tsp cinnamon, ground	<$0.05
1/2 tsp vanilla	<$0.15
1/8 cup raisins	<$0.15
1-2 tbsp raw agave	<$0.50

1 Process the shredded coconut in the food processor until the oils begin to come out of the coconut (about 30 seconds). Add the pecans and sunflower seeds and process until a nutty flour forms. Add the clove, nutmeg, cinnamon, vanilla, and raisins and process until the raisins are well broken down. Finally, add the agave and process until the mixture begins to clump together.

2 Evenly press the crust mixture into a pie plate. Place the crust in the freezer for 30 minutes or until it hardens.

FILLING

1 1/2 lbs red or purple plums	$3.75
1 tsp vanilla	<$0.25
1/2 cup raisins	$0.50
1 tbsp lemon juice	<$0.20
3-4 tbsp raw agave	<$1.00
1/4 tsp green stevia powder	<$0.05
3 tbsp arrowroot powder or 2 tbsp soy lecithin	<$0.50
1 tbsp raw coconut oil	$0.25
Total estimated cost	$8.75
Estimated cost per serving	$1.10

Tips to reduce the cost:

- Buy plums from a local farm or farmers market.
- Buy the spices and arrowroot from bulk bins. It's cheaper.
- If you don't have green stevia powder, use agave; but in the long-run, stevia is cheaper.

FILLING

3 Blend the plums, vanilla, raisins, lemon juice, agave, stevia, and arrowroot power until completely smooth (10-15 seconds). Check to make sure you don't see any plum skins floating around. Add the coconut oil (and soy lecithin) and blend for 15-20 seconds.

4 Pour the filling onto the hard crust. Put the pie in the refrigerator for 4-6 hours to allow the filling to set.

Refrigerate the pie until it's time to serve.

Nutrition Information Per Serving (based on 2,000 calorie daily intake): calories 222, protein 3g, total fat 14g, carbohydrate 25g, dietary fiber 5g, total sugars 15g, calcium 7%, iron 7%, sodium 0%, potassium 9%, zinc 5%, vitamin A 5%, vitamin E 12%, thiamin 11%, riboflavin 4%, niacin 11%, vitamin B6 6%, folate 4%, vitamin B12 0%, vitamin C 14%

Lemon Cream Pie

CRUST

1/2 cup raw shredded coconut	$0.50
zest from 1/2 lemon	<$0.20
1/3 cup raw almonds, whole	<$0.70
1/8 tsp green stevia powder	<$0.05
1/2 tsp vanilla	<$0.15
1 pinch sea salt	<$0.05
1 tbsp raw honey	<$0.25
2 dates	$0.40

FILLING

2/3 cup meat from 2 young coconuts	$3.00
1/4 cup raw almonds, whole	<$0.60
1 pinch green stevia powder	<$0.05
3 tsp lemon juice	<$0.20
1 date	$0.20
1/2 tsp vanilla	<$0.15
1 tbsp raw honey	<$0.25

Total estimated cost	$6.75
Estimated cost per serving	$1.35

Tips to reduce the cost:

- Buy lemons in bulk bags. Just be sure to use them all before they spoil! Or find a friend with a lemon tree!
- If you don't have green stevia, use agave instead.
- Use an inexpensive variety of dates like Deglet Noor dates.

If you love lemons, you will love this recipe! The crust is buttery and bursting with lemon flavor, and the filling is creamy and light. I made this pie for a few raw vegan friends and they all loved it!

Preparation

Equipment needed: Food processor • High-speed blender • Dinner plate

1 Crack open the young coconuts with a large knife and pour the water into a large glass. Scoop out the coconut meat with spoon. Remove any brown flakes from the meat and chop.

CRUST

2 Process the shredded coconut in the food processor until the oils begin to come out of the coconut (about 30 seconds).

3 Grate the rind from 1/2 lemon to create lemon zest, and add to the food processor.

4 Add the almonds, stevia, vanilla, and salt, and blend until the nuts are well broken down. Lastly, add the dates and honey, and process until they are completely broken down into small pieces.

5 Press the dough onto a dinner plate, forming a crust.

FILLING

6 Add the remaining ingredients to the blender, and blend until smooth. Add several tablespoons of water to help the ingredients blend.

7 Pour the mixture on top of the crust and serve.

Nutrition Information Per Serving (based on 2,000 calorie daily intake): calories 176, protein 2g, total fat 11g, carbohydrate 19g, dietary fiber 4g, total sugars 15g, calcium 3%, iron 5%, sodium 1%, potassium 6%, zinc 4%, vitamin A 0%, vitamin E 11%, thiamin 2%, riboflavin 4%, niacin 3%, vitamin B6 4%, folate 2%, vitamin B12 0%, vitamin C 1%

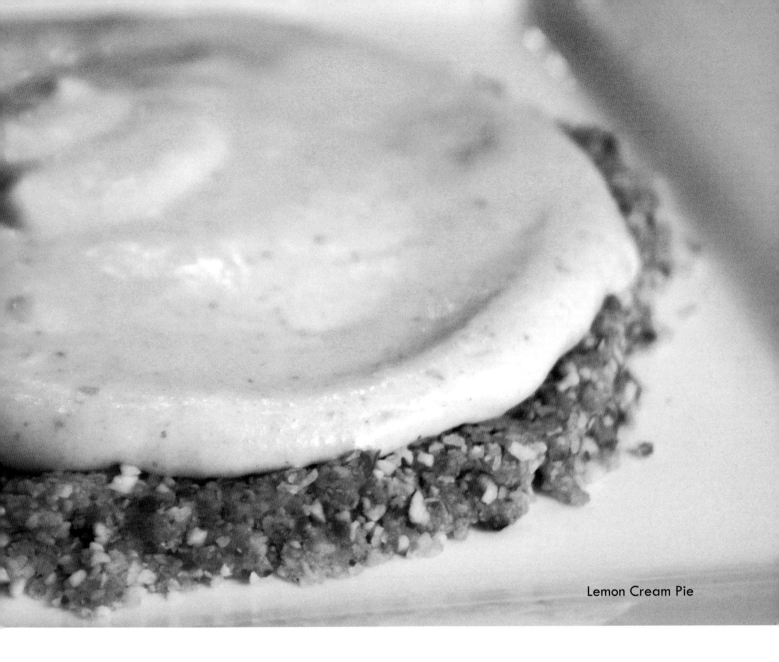

Lemon Cream Pie

Pumpkin Pie

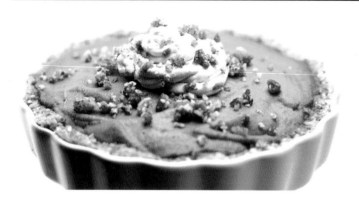

CRUST

1/2 cup raw shredded coconut	$0.25
5 raw brazil nuts	$0.50
1/4 cup raw pecans, whole	$0.50
1/4 cup raw walnuts, whole	$0.50
3 dates	$0.60
1/2 tsp vanilla	<$0.15

FILLING

1/4 cup raw cashews, whole	$0.50
2 medium apples	$1.00
1 1/2 cup sweet pumpkin (chopped)	$0.50
1/3 cup raisins	<$0.35
1/2 tsp cinnamon, ground	<$0.05
2 pinches nutmeg, ground	<$0.05
1 pinch clove, ground	<$0.05
1/2 tsp vanilla	<$0.15
2 tsp arrowroot	<$0.20

This pie celebrates the wonderful fall flavors of sweet pumpkins.

This recipes using a lot of ingredients, however, it's well worth it. And there are ways to simplify the recipe. Try reducing the number of nuts used in the crust to one type like brazil nuts, pecans, or walnuts. Omit the ground clove. Try using pumpkin pie spice in place of cinnamon and nutmeg. Substitute 1 tbsp of soy lecithin for arrowroot if that's what you have already in your kitchen.

Preparation
Equipment needed: High-speed blender • Food processor • Small 6-inch pie plate or dinner plate

1 Soak 1/4 and 1/2 cups of cashews in 2 separate cups of water for 6+ hours or overnight.

2 Crack open the young coconut with a large knife and pour the water into a large glass. Scoop out the coconut meat with spoon. Remove any brown flakes from the meat and chop. Set aside.

CRUST

3 Using a food processor, process the shredded coconut in the food processor until the oils begin to come out of the coconut (about 30 seconds).

4 Add all of the nuts and process until they are broken down. Lastly, add the vanilla and dates, and process until the dates are broken down into small pieces.

5 Press the dough onto a small pie or dinner plate, forming a crust.

WHIPPED TOPPING

1/2 cup raw cashews, whole	$0.50
1/4 cup meat from 1 young coconut	$1.00
2 dates	$0.40
1 tbsp raw agave	<$0.25
1/4 tsp vanilla	<$0.10
1 heavy pinch cinnamon, ground	<$0.05
1 small pinch nutmeg, ground	<$0.05
1 small pinch sea salt	<$0.05
1/4 cup water	$0.00

CRUNCHY TOPPING

1/4 cup raw pecans, whole	$0.50
2 dates	$0.40
1/4 tsp vanilla	<$0.10
1 pinch cinnamon, ground	<$0.05
1 small pinch nutmeg, ground	<$0.05

Total estimated cost	$8.40
Estimated cost per serving	$2.10

Tips to reduce the cost:

- Buy a small sweet pumpkin from a farm or local health food store.
- Purchase as many of the nuts, sweeteners, and spices that you can from bulk bins. This recipe uses a lot of ingredients, so try to buy what you need.
- Buy your young coconuts from an Asian market. They are cheaper and of the same quality you will find at larger health food and grocery stores.

FILLING

6 Peel and core the apples, and blend until liquefied. Remove the skin from the sweet pumpkin, chop the meat into 1-inch pieces, and add 1 1/2 cups to the blender. Add 1/4 cup of the soaked cashews, the raisins, cinnamon, nutmeg, clove, and vanilla, and blend until the pumpkin mixture is thick and smooth. Add the arrowroot and blend for 10 seconds.

7 Pour the filling into the crust and allow it to set in the refrigerator for 8 hours or overnight.

WHIPPED TOPPING

8 Remove the meat from the young coconuts and place it into the blender. Add the remaining ingredients (including the 1/2 cup of soaked cashews) and blend until smooth. You may need several extra tablespoons of water to help the ingredients blend.

CRUNCHY TOPPING

9 Process all of the ingredients in a dry food processor using the pulse button. Stop when all of the ingredients are broken down into small pieces.

When serving, place a generous dollop of whipped topping on each slice and sprinkle the crunchy topping on top.

Nutrition Information Per Serving (based on 2,000 calorie daily intake): calories 530, protein 9g, total fat 30g, carbohydrate 66g, dietary fiber 9g, total sugars 45g, calcium 10%, iron 17%, sodium 0%, potassium 25%, zinc 17%, vitamin A 66%, vitamin E 10%, thiamin 16%, riboflavin 10%, niacin 8%, vitamin B6 16%, folate 9%, vitamin B12 0%, vitamin C 13%

Butternut Cream Pie

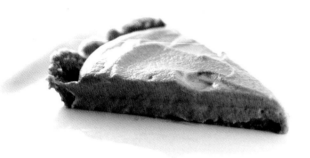

This is my best winter squash pie yet!!!! The filling is creamy and delicious, and the crust is a buttery celebration of fall and winter-warming spices.

For an extra treat, enjoy this pie warm by blending it extra long in the blender and pouring it into a cold crust. The contrast will delight your senses!

Preparation

Equipment needed: High-speed blender • Food processor • Pie plate • Plastic wrap

1 Soak 3/4 cup of cashews for 6+ hours or overnight.

CRUST

2 Using a food processor, process the shredded coconut until the oils begin to come out of the coconut (about 30 seconds).

3 Add the cashews, walnuts, and pecans and process until they are broken down. Add the clove, cinnamon, vanilla and dates, and process until the dates are broken down into small pieces. Finally, add the raw agave and process until it's well disbursed. The crust may begin to clump.

4 Now, you are ready to create the crust shell. Take a pie plate and line it with plastic wrap. Press the crust onto the lined plate. The crust will be thin and it may not rise very high on the sides of the pie plate.

5 Place the crust in the freezer for 30 minutes or until it hardens.

CRUST

1 cup raw shredded coconut	$0.50
1/4 cup raw cashews, whole	$0.50
1/4 cup raw walnuts, whole	$0.50
1/4 cup raw pecans, whole	$0.50
2 pinches clove, ground	<$0.05
1/2 tsp cinnamon, ground	<$0.05
1/2 tsp vanilla	<$0.25
4 dates	$0.80
1-2 tbsp raw agave	<$0.50

FILLING

1 medium apple	<$0.50
2 cups butternut squash	$2.00
3/4 cup cashews, whole	$1.50
1/2 tsp lemon juice	<$0.20
3/4 tsp vanilla	<$0.20
3 dates	$0.60
2 tbsp agave	$0.50
1/4 tsp green stevia powder	<$0.05
1/4 tsp cinnamon, ground	<$0.05
2 pinches of nutmeg, ground	<$0.05
1 tbsp arrowroot	<$0.10
Total estimated cost	$9.40
Estimated cost per serving	$1.18

Tips to reduce the cost:

- If you don't have ground clove, omit it!
- Use an inexpensive variety of dates such as Deglet Noor dates.
- Buy the butternut squash from a local farm. If you can find a giant squash (it usually costs a few dollars), then peel, cube, and store it in your freezer.

FILLING

6 Peel and core the apple, and blend until liquefied.

7 Remove the skin and seeds from the butternut squash, chop the meat into 1-inch pieces, and add it to the blender. Add all the remaining ingredients, except for the arrowroot, and blend until the mixture is thick and smooth. Add the arrowroot and blend until the mixture begins to warm up (25-35 seconds). Be careful not to cook it!

8 Remove the crust from the freezer and lift it out of the pie plate by carefully pulling up on the plastic wrap. Place the crust onto a plate and pour the butternut squash filling into the crust.

Serve the pie immediately if you would like to enjoy it warm. Otherwise, place it into the refrigerator until you are ready to serve.

Nutrition Information Per Serving (based on 2,000 calorie daily intake): calories 296, protein 5g, total fat 19g, carbohydrate 32g, dietary fiber 6g, total sugars 18g, calcium 8%, iron 12%, sodium 0%, potassium 14%, zinc 11%, vitamin A 75%, vitamin E 6%, thiamin 8%, riboflavin 5%, niacin 6%, vitamin B6 11%, folate 7%, vitamin B12 0%, vitamin C 15%

Carrot Cake

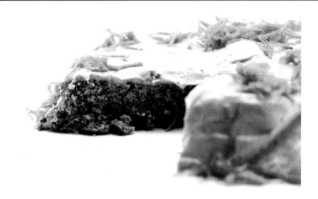

This is hands down one of the best (raw or cooked) carrot cakes I have ever tasted! The frosting is gooey and creamy, and is a perfect complement to the moist cake.

The key to this making cake is not to over process it in the food processor, which is pretty easy to do. You want the cake to be fluffy and moist, rather than thick and wet. So, keep an eye on the food processor and process the ingredients only as long as needed.

Preparation

Equipment needed: Food processor • High-speed blender (optional) • Medium-sized bowl or small casserole dish, • Plastic wrap or parchment paper

1 Soak 1 cup of cashews in water for 6+ hours or overnight.

CAKE

2 Using a food processor, process the shredded coconut until the oils begin to come out of the coconut (about 30 seconds). Add the shredded carrots and process until they well distributed.

3 Chop the dates and add to the coconut. Add the pumpkin pie spice, raisins, and vanilla, and process until the raisins are broken down into small chunks. Add almond pulp and process until it's well distributed. Add the orange juice and orange zest and process again. Scoop the cake into a large bowl.

4 Break the walnuts and pecans into small pieces by placing them into a bag and breaking them with your hands. Add and stir into the cake. Add the agave to taste.

5 Now you are ready to mold the cake. You can either do this by hand, or with a medium-sized bowl or small casserole dish. If you are taking the latter route, line the bowl or dish with parchment paper or plastic wrap. Softly, press the cake into the bowl and place the cake into the freezer for 20 minutes.

CAKE

1/2 cup raw shredded coconut	$0.25
3/4 cup shredded carrots	$0.20
4 dates	$0.80
3/4 tsp pumpkin pie spice	<$0.10
1/2 cup raisins	$0.50
1 tsp vanilla	<$0.25
1 cup almond pulp*	$0.00
2 tbsp oranges juice	<$0.20
1 pinch orange zest	<$0.25
1/4 cup raw walnuts, whole	$0.50
1/4 cup raw pecans, whole	$0.50
1-2 tbsp raw agave (or to taste)	<$0.50

FROSTING

1 cup raw cashews, whole	$2.00
1/2 cup almond milk	$0.35
1 tsp vanilla	<$0.25
1/4 tsp pumpkin pie spice	<$0.10
1 pinch orange zest	<$0.25
4 tbsp orange juice	<$0.25
3 dates	$0.60
1/4 cup raisins	$0.25
1/8 tsp green stevia powder	<$0.05
1-2 tbsp raw agave (or to taste)	<$0.50
Total estimated cost	$8.65
Estimated cost per serving	$1.08

Tips to reduce the cost:

- Make this recipe when you have left-over almond pulp from making almond milk. This way, the pulp is practically free. You will need to soak 1 1/2 cups of almonds to make 1 cup of almond pulp. To save your almond pulp, just place it in the freezer in an airtight container or plastic bag.
- Use an inexpensive variety of dates such as Deglet Noor dates.

*Almond pulp is the pulp that is leftover after preparing almond milk.

6 Remove the cake from the bowl by turning it upside onto a large plate. Place the cake into the refrigerator until the frosting is ready.

FROSTING

7 Blend all of the ingredients (including the soaked cashews) until very smooth using a blender or food processor. Sweeten to taste with agave.

8 Scoop the frosting into a small bowl, cover it, and allow it to get firm in the freezer for 20 minutes or so.

9 When the frosting is ready, spread it on the cake and decorate with shredded carrots.

Nutrition Information Per Serving (based on 2,000 calorie daily intake): calories 290, protein 5g, total fat 16g, carbohydrate 37g, dietary fiber 5g, total sugars 25g, calcium 6%, iron 11%, sodium 1%, potassium 14%, zinc 10%, vitamin A 42%, vitamin E 3%, thiamin 7%, riboflavin 5%, niacin 5%, vitamin B6 9%, folate 6%, vitamin B12 0%, vitamin C 12%

Aphroditie's Nectarine Cream Pie

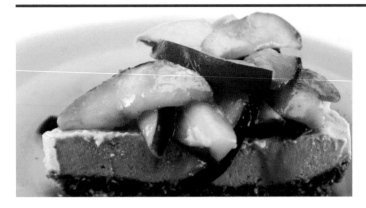

There is something sexy about this pie! I am not quite sure what it is, but this pie is quite an aphrodisiac. The filling is creamy and succulent and the sun-baked nectarines are sweet and beautiful.

Preparation

Equipment needed: Food processor • High-speed blender • Spring pan or pie plate • Glass casserole dish or large bowl for sun-baking • Cheesecloth or plastic nut bag

1 Soak 1 cup of cashews in water for 6+ hours or overnight.

2 Crack open the young coconuts with a large knife and pour the water into a large glass. Scoop out the coconut meat with spoon. Remove any brown flakes from the meat and chop. Set aside.

CRUST

3 In a food processor, process the sunflower seeds and shredded coconut until a nutty flour forms (about 30 seconds).

4 Add the pecans to the food processor, and process until they are well broken down. Add the remaining ingredients and process until a dough forms.

5 Press the crust onto the bottom of a spring pan or pie plate. Place the spring pan or pie plate in the freezer until the crust hardens.

FILLING

6 Remove the seeds from the nectarines and blend the meat until liquefied.

7 Add the remaining ingredients, except for the arrowroot or soy lecithin, to the nectarines and blend until smooth. Then add the arrowroot or soy lecithin and blend for 10-15 seconds.

CRUST

1/2 cup raw sunflower seeds	$0.60
1 cup raw shredded coconut	$0.50
1/2 cup raw pecans, whole	$1.00
1 tsp vanilla	<$0.25
2 dates	$0.20
1-2 tbsp raw agave	<$0.50

FILLING

4 medium nectarines	$2.00
1 cup raw cashews, whole	$2.00
1 cup meat from 2 young coconuts	$4.00
1/4 tsp green stevia powder	<$0.05
2 tbsp arrowroot or soy lecithin	<$0.20
4 dates	$0.80
1/4 tsp vanilla	<$0.10
1 pinch salt	<$0.05

TOPPING

5 medium nectarines	$2.50
1/4 tsp vanilla	<$0.10
2 tsp raw agave	<$0.50
Total estimated cost	$15.35
Estimated cost per serving	$1.92

Tips to reduce the cost:

- Make this recipe when nectarines are in season. Buy them from a local farm to obtain the best tasting, most inexpensive nectarines.
- Purchase Thai young coconuts from a local Asian market.
- Purchase arrowroot from the spice or bulk bin section at your local health food store.
- If you don't have green stevia powder, use agave; but in the long-run, stevia is cheaper.
- Soy lecithin can be expensive because it is often sold in large quantities. Consider borrowing some from a friend.

8 Once the crust has hardened, pour the filling on top of the crust. Place the pie in the refrigerator, allowing the filling to set for 6+ hours or overnight.

TOPPING

9 Slice the nectarines (leaving the skin on) into 1/3-inch thick slices and place them into a medium bowl. Add the vanilla and agave and softly stir. Sun-bake the nectarines for 4 or more hours. Refer to the sun-baking instructions on page 218.

When you are ready to serve the pie, scoop the sun-baked nectarines on top of the pie being careful not to take too much of the juice.

Nutrition Information Per Serving (based on 2,000 calorie daily intake): calories 397, protein 8g, total fat 25g, carbohydrate 42g, dietary fiber 8g, total sugars 27g, calcium 6%, iron 16%, sodium 0%, potassium 20%, zinc 15%, vitamin A 11%, vitamin E 31%, thiamin 24%, riboflavin 8%, niacin 14%, vitamin B6 12%, folate 12%, vitamin B12 0%, vitamin C 15%

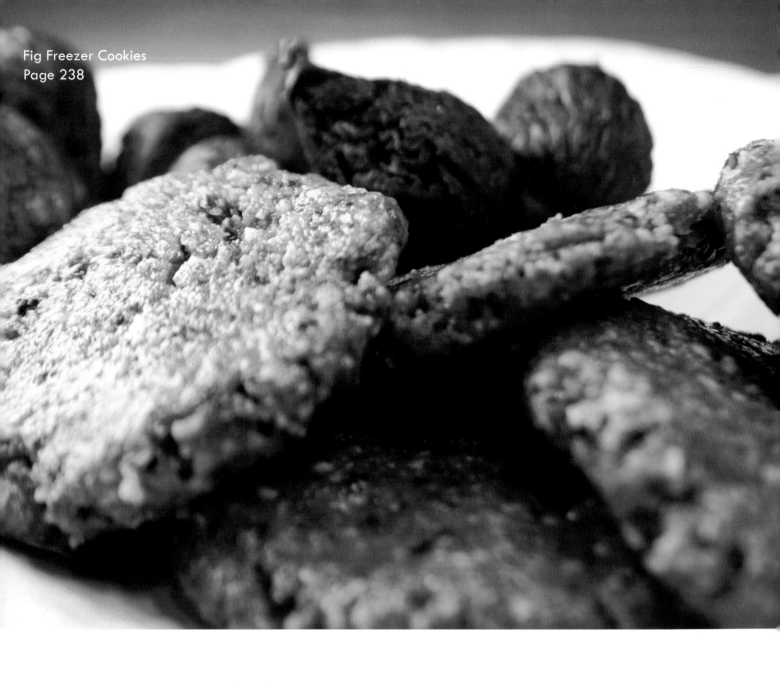

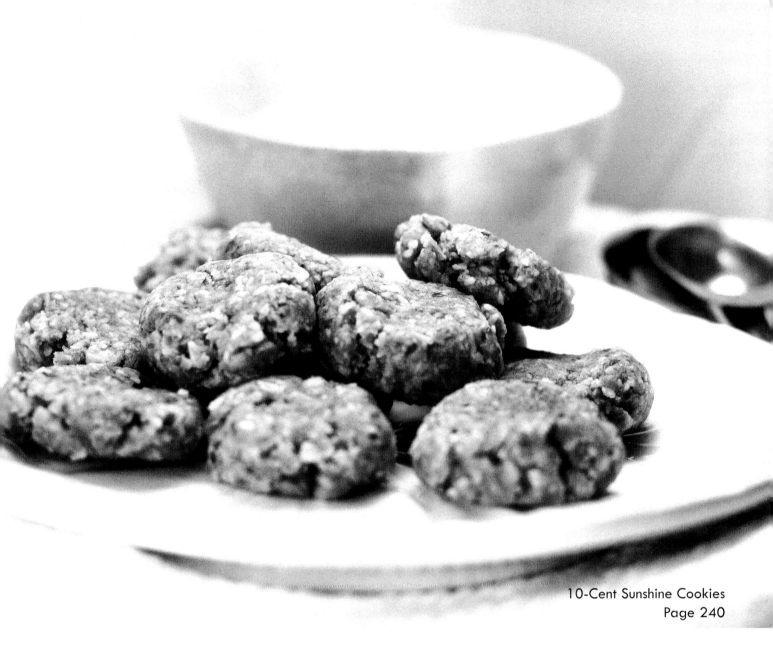

10-Cent Sunshine Cookies
Page 240

Cookies and Simple Pleasures

Fig Freezer Cookies

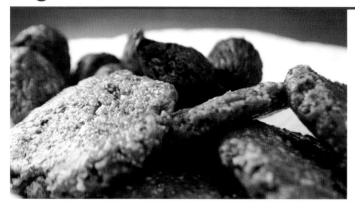

1/2 cup raw sunflower seeds	$0.60
1/4 cup raw walnuts, whole	$0.50
1/4 cup raisins	$0.25
6 pieces dried figs	$1.00
1/2 tsp vanilla	<$0.15
1 tbsp raw agave	<$0.25
Total estimated cost	$2.75
Estimated cost per cookie	$0.35

Tips to reduce the cost:

- Buy sunflower seeds, walnuts, figs, and raisins from the bulk bin section at your local health food store.

This recipe is awesome! Not only is it simple and cheap, the cookies are chewy and they taste like Fig Newtons! And you don't even need a dehydrator to make this recipe. All you need is a freezer!

Preparation

Equipment needed: Food processor

1 In a food processor, process the sunflower seeds and walnuts until a nutty flour forms.

2 Add the raisins, figs, and vanilla and process until a dough forms. Then add the agave (optional) and process until it's well combined.

3 Form the cookies by rolling them into a ball with your hands and pressing them flat with the palm of your hands.

4 Place the cookies on a plate and put them in the freezer for 30 minutes.

These cookies are best enjoyed right out of the freezer.

Nutrition Information Per Cookie (based on 2,000 calorie daily intake)**:** calories 107, protein 3g, total fat 7g, carbohydrate 10g, dietary fiber 2g, total sugars 6g, calcium 3%, iron 5%, sodium 0%, potassium 5%, zinc 4%, vitamin A 0%, vitamin E 21%, thiamin 15%, riboflavin 2%, niacin 3%, vitamin B6 5%, folate 6%, vitamin B12 0%, vitamin C 1%

Chocolate Cookies w/ Cashew Chunks

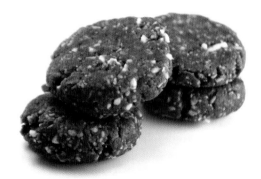

1/2 cup raw shredded coconut	$0.25
1/4 cup raw pumpkin seeds	$0.30
1/3 cup raw brazil nuts	$1.00
3/4 tsp vanilla	<$0.20
1/8 tsp green stevia powder	<$0.05
1/3 cup raw cacao powder	$0.75
2 dates	$0.40
1/4 cup raw cashews, whole	$0.50
2 tbsp raw agave	<$0.50
Total estimated cost	$3.95
Estimated cost per cookie	$0.33

Tips to reduce the cost:

• This is a great, inexpensive recipe to make when you have small quantities of a wide variety of nuts.

These cookies are super yummy. In addition to being choco-li-cious, the cookies are firm on the outside and soft in the middle. If you are anything like me, you will find yourself sneaking these cookies out of the dehydrator.

This is a very versatile recipe. You can substitute raw sunflower seeds for pumpkin seeds, raw agave for green stevia powder (be sure to add the agave last), macadamia nuts for brazil nuts, and raw carob powder for cacao powder.

Preparation
Equipment needed: Food processor • Dehydrator

1 Using a food processor, process the shredded coconut until the oils begin to come out of the coconut (about 30 seconds).

2 Add the pumpkin seeds, brazil nuts, vanilla, stevia, and cacao to the food processor, and process until the nuts are well broken down. Next, add the dates and process until they are completely broken down into small pieces. Add the cashews and process until they are broken into small chunks. Lastly, add the agave and process briefly until the dough begins to clump.

3 Form the dough into 12 1-inch cookies.

4 Dehydrate the cookies for 12-24 hours at 105-degrees or freeze for 2 hours to make freezer cookies.

Nutrition Information Per Cookie (based on 2,000 calorie daily intake)**:** calories 95, protein 2g, total fat 7g, carbohydrate 7g, dietary fiber 2g, total sugars 3g, calcium 3%, iron 7%, sodium 0%, potassium 4%, zinc 5%, vitamin A 0%, vitamin E 2%, thiamin 3%, riboflavin 2%, niacin 1%, vitamin B6 2%, folate 2%, vitamin B12 0%, vitamin C 0%

10-Cent Sunshine Cookies

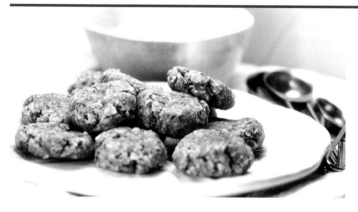

This recipe makes me feel like a kid again! The cookies are tasty and buttery, and they are super cheap, hence the name! Just remember that one cookie equals a serving, so don't go crazy!

You can also sun-bake the cookies instead of dehydrating them. Just sun-bake them for as long as possible or until the desired texture is achieved. Enjoy!

Preparation
Equipment needed: Food processor • Dehydrator

2 1/2 medium bananas	$0.50
1 cup pineapple (optional)	$1.00
1 cup raw shredded coconut	$0.50
1/3 cup raw walnuts, whole	<$0.70
1 tbsp raw agave	$0.25
1 tsp vanilla	<$0.25
1 pinch sea salt	<$0.05
3 dates	$0.60
Total estimated cost	$3.85
Estimated cost per cookie	$0.32

1 Slice the bananas and pineapple into ¼ inch slices.

2 Line the sliced fruit onto two dehydrator trays and dry for 10-12 hours at 105-degrees.

3 Once the bananas and pineapple have dried, remove them from the tray and set aside.

4 Using a food processor, process the shredded coconut until the oils begin to come out of the coconut (about 30 seconds).

5 Add the walnuts to the food processor, and process until they are well broken down. Then add the vanilla and salt, and process until distributed. While the blade is spinning, add the dried bananas and pineapple, and dates a few pieces at a time. Lastly, add the agave and blend until a dough forms.

6 Form the dough into 12 1-inch cookies.

7 Dehydrate the cookies for 10-12 hours at 105-degrees or sun-bake (see sun-baking tip on page 218).

Tips to reduce the cost:
- If you don't have walnuts at home, save yourself a trip to the grocery store by substituting them with another soft nut like cashews, brazil nuts, or pecans.
- Try to buy all of the dry ingredients from bulk bins. This way you can buy the amounts you need.

Nutrition Information Per Cookie (based on 2,000 calorie daily intake): calories 107, protein 2g, total fat 6g, carbohydrate 14g, dietary fiber 3g, total sugars 9g, calcium 2%, iron 3%, sodium 1%, potassium 6%, zinc 2%, vitamin A 1%, vitamin E 1%, thiamin 2%, riboflavin 2%, niacin 2%, vitamin B6 8%, folate 2%, vitamin B12 0%, vitamin C 12%

Pecan Delight Cookies

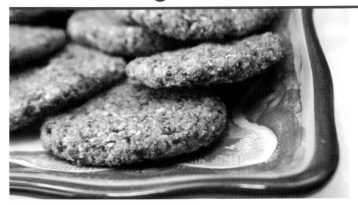

These are the perfect tea cookies. They are moist, yet firm to the touch, and have a rich, fall season pecan flavor. Enjoy these cookies with a cup of tea or a tea latte (recipe on page 164).

Preparation
Equipment needed: Food processor • Dehydrator

1 Using a food processor, process the pecans and sunflower seeds until they form a nutty flour. Be careful not to over process the pecans.

2 Add the almond pulp, nutmeg, cinnamon, and vanilla to the food processor, and process until they are well distributed. Then add the raisins and process until they are completely broken down into small pieces. Lastly, add the agave and process until the dough begins to clump.

3 Form the dough into 12 1-inch cookies.

4 Dehydrate the cookies for 12-24 hours at 105-degrees or freeze for 2 hours to make freezer cookies.

1/2 cup raw pecans, whole	$1.00
1/4 cup raw sunflower seeds	$0.30
1/4 cup almond pulp*	$0.00
1 pinch nutmeg, ground	<$0.05
1 tsp cinnamon, ground	<$0.10
1 tsp vanilla	<$0.25
1/2 cup raisins	$0.50
1 tbsp raw agave	$0.25
Total estimated cost	$2.45
Estimated cost per cookie	$0.21

Nutrition Information Per Cookie (based on 2,000 calorie daily intake): calories 69, protein 1g, total fat 5g, carbohydrate 6g, dietary fiber 1g, total sugars 4g, calcium 2%, iron 3%, sodium 0%, potassium 3%, zinc 3%, vitamin A 0%, vitamin E 7%, thiamin 7%, riboflavin 1%, niacin 1%, vitamin B6 2%, folate 2%, vitamin B12 0%, vitamin C 1%

Tips to reduce the cost:

• Prepare this recipe when you are making almond milk, so you can use the fresh almond pulp to make these cookies. Or, simply save the almond pulp in the freezer. It will stay fresh for up to 6 months.

*Almond pulp is the pulp that is left-over after preparing almond milk.

Donut Holes

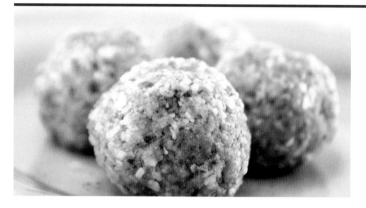

1 cup raw shredded coconut	$0.50
1/3 cup raw walnuts, whole	$0.70
1/2 tsp vanilla	<$0.15
1/4 tsp cinnamon, ground	<$0.05
1 pinch sea salt	<$0.05
4 dates	$0.80
2 tbsp raw agave	<$0.50
Total estimated cost	$2.75
Estimated cost per donut hole	$0.46

Tips to reduce the cost:

- Try to buy all of the dry ingredients from bulk bins. This way you can buy the amounts you need.

This recipe tastes just like glazed donut holes! It's so simple and delicious. And because they are so tasty, it's best to make this recipe when other people are coming over; otherwise, you just may eat them all yourself!

Preparation
Equipment needed: Food processor • Dehydrator (optional)

1 Using a food processor, process the shredded coconut until the oils begin to come out of the coconut (about 30 seconds).

2 Add the walnuts, vanilla, cinnamon, and salt to the food processor, and process until the walnuts are well broken down. Then add the dates and process until they are completely broken down into small pieces. Lastly, add the agave and process until the dough starts to clump.

3 Form the dough into 6 small balls.

4 To warm the donut holes, dehydrate at 105 degrees or set outside under the sun (see sun-baking tip on page 218). Warm for 3-4 hours.

These donut holes taste best when served warm.

Nutrition Information Per Donut Hole (based on 2,000 calorie daily intake)**:** calories 170, protein 3g, total fat 12g, carbohydrate 16g, dietary fiber 4g, total sugars 12g, calcium 4%, iron 5%, sodium 1%, potassium 6%, zinc 4%, vitamin A 1%, vitamin E 1%, thiamin 1%, riboflavin 2%, niacin 2%, vitamin B6 6%, folate 1%, vitamin B12 0%, vitamin C 1%

Peaches in My Dreams

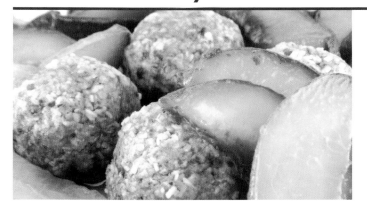

1 Donut Hole Recipe (page 242)	$2.75
3 medium peaches	$1.50
1/4 tsp vanilla	<$0.10
2 tbsp raw agave	<$0.50
Total estimated cost	$4.85
Estimated cost per serving	$0.81

Tips to reduce the cost:
- Buy the peaches from a local farm, farmers market, or CSA program.

This recipe appeared to me in my dreams! The donut holes are gooey, and the sun-baked peaches are sweet and silky. Make this dessert for several people or a party, otherwise you may eat it all yourself!

Preparation

Equipment needed: Glass casserole dish or large bowl for sun-baking • Cheesecloth or nutbag

1 Prepare the Donut Holes recipe. Keep the donut holes in the dehydrator at 105-degrees or under the sun until you are ready to serve this recipe.

2 Slice 3 peaches and place them in a casserole dish or large bowl. Add the vanilla and agave and stir gently.

3 Sun-bake the peaches for 4+ hours (see sun-baking tip on page 218).

4 When you are ready to serve the pie, scoop the sun-baked peaches (with their juice) on top of the donut holes. Enjoy!

Nutrition Information Per Serving (based on 2,000 calorie daily intake): calories 203, protein 4g, total fat 12g, carbohydrate 24g, dietary fiber 5g, total sugars 18g, calcium 6%, iron 6%, sodium 1%, potassium 11%, zinc 5%, vitamin A 6%, vitamin E 5%, thiamin 3%, riboflavin 3%, niacin 5%, vitamin B6 7%, folate 2%, vitamin B12 0%, vitamin C 9%

Cranberry Tea Squares

COOKIE

1/2 cup raw shredded coconut	$0.25
4 raw brazil nuts	$0.40
1/4 cup almond pulp*	$0.00
2 dates	$0.40
1 medium banana	$0.20
1/2 tsp vanilla	<$0.05
1 tbsp raw agave	$0.25
1 pinch nutmeg, ground	<$0.10
1/4 tsp cinnamon, ground	<$0.05
1/8 tsp green stevia powder	<$0.05
1 tbsp lemon juice	<$0.20

TOPPING

1/2 cup cranberries	$0.75
2 dates	$0.40
1 tbsp raw agave	$0.25
1 tbsp lemon juice	<$0.20

Total estimated cost	$3.55
Estimated cost per square	$0.18

Tips to reduce the cost:
- Make this recipe in the fall when cranberries are in season and their least expensive.
- Prepare this recipe when you making almond milk, so that you can use the pulp to make the cookies and milk to make a tea latte (recipe on page 164)!

These are fabulous little cranberry squares! They are the perfect sweet, tart snack that tastes wonderful alongside a warm tea latte (page 164).

This recipe uses a lot of ingredients; but, they are inexpensive and easy to find.

Preparation
Equipment needed: Food processor • Dehydrator

COOKIE

1 Using a food processor, process the shredded coconut until the oils begin to come out of the coconut (about 30 seconds).

2 Add the brazil nuts and almond pulp, and process until the nuts are well broken down. Then add the remaining ingredients and process until a thick batter forms.

3 Pour the entire mixture onto one Teflex sheet and spread to 1/4-inch thickness. Form the mixture into a 6 to 8-inch square. Set aside for now.

TOPPING

4 Using a food processor, process all the cranberries, dates, agave, and lemon juice. When the mixture rises on the sides of the processor, push it down with a spoon and continue to blend until you have a chunky mixture.

5 Pour the mixture on top of the cookie and softly spread it using a spoon.

6 Once the topping is evenly distributed, dehydrate the cookies at 105-degrees for 12 hours. When the top of the cookies are dry (after 12 hours), turn the cookies over and remove the Teflex sheet. Dehydrate for another 12-24 hours (depending on your texture preference).

Nutrition Information Per Square (based on 2,000 calorie daily intake): calories 40, protein 0.5g, total fat 2g, carbohydrate 6g, dietary fiber 1g, total sugars 4g, calcium 1%, iron 1%, sodium 0%, potassium 2%, zinc 3%, vitamin A 0%, vitamin E 1%, thiamin 1%, riboflavin 1%, niacin 1%, vitamin B6 2%, folate 1%, vitamin B12 0%, vitamin C 3%

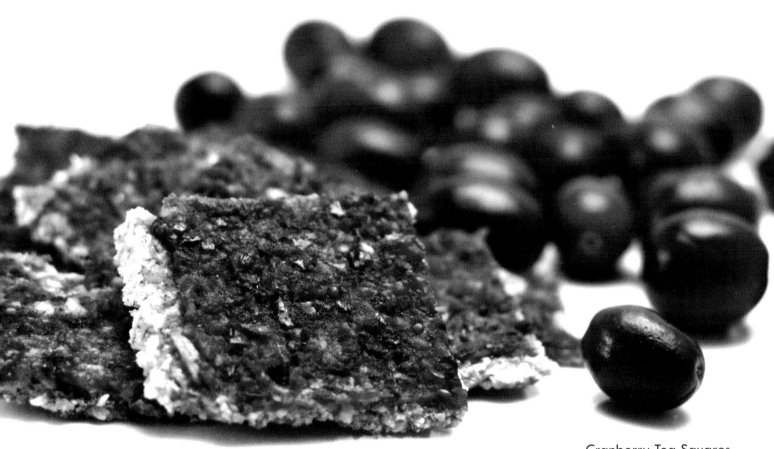

Cranberry Tea Squares

Sun-Kissed Fruit Cup

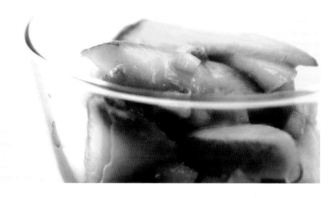

2 medium peaches	$1.00
1 medium nectarine	$0.50
4-inches of rhubarb (optional)	<$0.25
1-2 tbsp raw agave	<$0.50
1/4 tsp vanilla	<$0.10
Total estimated cost	$2.35
Estimated cost per serving	$1.18

Tips to reduce the cost:

- Make this recipe when you have ripe fruit that needs to be used immediately before it spoils.
- Buy fruit when it's in season.

This recipe tastes like the fruit cups we used to eat as kids... well, actually, it tastes a million times better! You and your kids will love this recipe. Just make it in the morning and leave it to sun-bake while you're at work. The dish makes a beautiful afternoon snack or after-dinner dessert.

You can use a variety of fruits in this recipe. As shown in the picture, I made this recipe with nectarines, peaches, and rhubarb, but you can also add strawberries, pears, apples, or other fruits that you may already have in your kitchen!

Preparation

Equipment needed: Glass casserole dish or large bowl for sun-baking • Cheesecloth or nutbag

1 Cut the peaches and nectarines into 1/8-inch slices, and add to a casserole or glass bowl.

2 Mice the rhubarb and add to the bowl. Mix.

3 Add the agave and vanilla, and softly mix.

4 Sun-bake the fruit for 6+ hours (see sun-baking tip on page 218).

Nutrition Information Per Serving (based on 2,000 calorie daily intake): calories 99, protein 2g, total fat 1g, carbohydrate 24g, dietary fiber 4g, total sugars 19g, calcium 5%, iron 4%, sodium 0%, potassium 13%, zinc 3%, vitamin A 15%, vitamin E 11%, thiamin 4%, riboflavin 4%, niacin 10%, vitamin B6 3%, folate 3%, vitamin B12 0%, vitamin C 25%

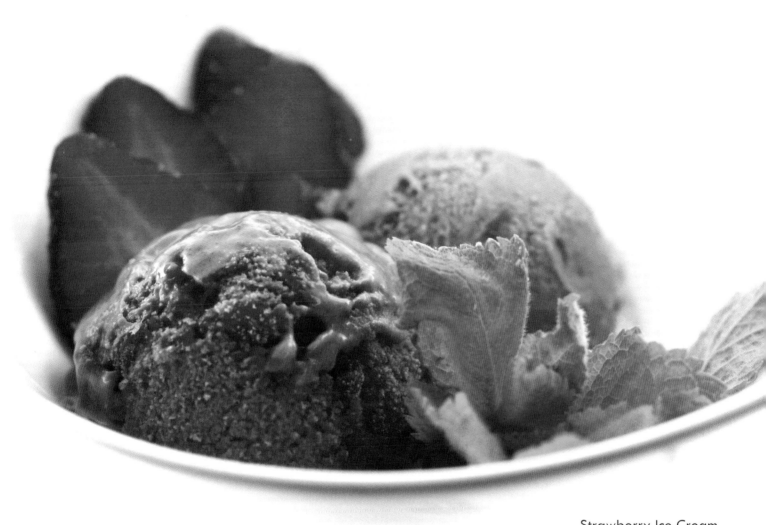

Strawberry Ice Cream
Page 248

Ice Creams and Sorbets

Strawberry Ice Cream

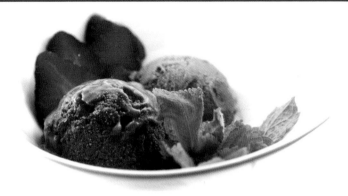

This ice cream is fluffy, flavorful, smooth, and filled with strawberry goodness. What I love about this recipe is that it actually tastes like fresh strawberries! Not many strawberry ice creams can make this claim.

Keep in mind that the flavor of this recipe will depend on the quality of strawberries you buy. So, if you buy amazing-tasting strawberries, you will make an amazing-tasting ice cream.

Preparation
Equipment needed: High-speed blender • Ice cream maker

1 Soak 1 cup of cashews in water for 6+ hours or overnight.

2 Crack open the young coconut with a large knife and pour the water into a large glass. Scoop out the coconut meat with spoon. Remove any brown flakes from the meat and chop. Set aside.

ICE CREAM

3 Blend all ingredients (including the soaked cashews) in a strong blender until very smooth. If you like, add additional agave to sweeten to taste.

4 Freeze the ice cream mixture for 1 hour or cool in the refrigerator overnight.

5 To make the ice cream, follow the manufacturer's instructions on your ice cream maker. Be sure to use the ice cream function if your ice cream maker has multiple functions. If your ice cream maker only holds 1 quart, you will need to make the recipe in 2 batches.

ICE CREAM

3 cups strawberries	$3.00
1 cup meat from 2 young coconuts	$4.00
1 cup raw cashews, whole	$2.00
1/2 cup water or coconut water	$0.00
4 dates	$0.80
1/3 cup raisins	$0.30
1/4 cup raw agave	<$1.00

TOPPING (OPTIONAL)

1/2 cup strawberries	$0.50
1 tbsp raw agave	$0.25
Total estimated cost	$11.85
Estimated cost per serving	$1.19

Tips to reduce the cost:

- Make this recipe during the height of strawberry season when strawberries are their most flavorful and least expensive.
- Buy your young coconuts from an Asian market. They are cheaper and the same quality you will find at larger health food and grocery stores.
- Omit the ice cream topping.

TOPPING (OPTIONAL)

6 Slice 1/2 cup of strawberries into thin strips and place them into them small bowl. Add the agave and mix.

7 Pour the glazed strawberries into the ice cream maker right before the ice cream is done. You may need to run the ice cream maker for an additional 5 minutes or so.

8 Pour the ice cream into a container with an air-tight lid. Store the container in the freezer to allow the ice cream to harden.

Allow the ice cream to soften before serving to maximize your ice cream experience! Enjoy!

Nutrition Information Per Serving (based on 2,000 calorie daily intake): calories 162, protein 3g, total fat 8g, carbohydrate 23g, dietary fiber 4g, total sugars 14g, calcium 6%, iron 9%, sodium 1%, potassium 9%, zinc 7%, vitamin A 0%, vitamin E 2%, thiamin 4%, riboflavin 4%, niacin 3%, vitamin B6 5%, folate 7%, vitamin B12 0%, vitamin C 61%

Strawberry-Cranberry Sorbet

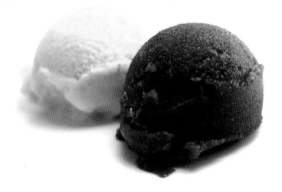

1/4 cup meat from 1 young coconuts	$1.00
1 medium apple	<$0.40
1/4 cup water	$0.00
2 cups cranberries	$2.00
2 cups strawberries, whole	$2.00
1/2 cup raisins	$0.50
1/8 tsp green stevia powder	<$0.05
3 tbsp raw agave	<$0.75
1 tsp vanilla	<$0.20
2 tbsp orange juice	<$0.75
Total estimated cost	$7.75
Estimated cost per serving	$0.98

Tips to reduce the cost:
- Make this recipe when cranberries are in season and least expensive.
- Omit the young coconut meat from the recipe.

OMG! This sorbet is amazing! The strawberries and cranberries create a beautiful balance that is tantalizing and truly spectacular! And the recipe is super simple.

Note that by the time cranberries come into season, strawberries are likely out of season. So if you are on the northern east coast like me, just use frozen strawberries. This is fine as long as you can get the best-tasting frozen strawberries available. I used the strawberries that I froze from my garden over the summer to make this fantastic recipe!

Preparation
Equipment needed: High-speed blender • Ice cream maker

1. Crack open the young coconut with a large knife and pour the water into a large glass. Scoop out the coconut meat with spoon. Remove any brown flakes from the meat and chop. Set aside.

2. Peel, core, and cube the apple and add to the blender. Add the water and blend until the apple and water are liquefied. Add the remaining ingredients and blend until completely smooth. Add additional agave to sweeten to taste.

3. Freeze the sorbet for 1 hour or let cool in the refrigerator overnight.

4. To make the sorbet, follow the manufacturer's instructions on your ice cream maker. Be sure to use the frozen yogurt function if your ice cream maker has multiple functions.

5. Pour the sorbet into a container with an air-tight lid. Store the container in the freezer to allow the sorbet to harden.

Allow the sorbet to soften for 20 minutes before serving.

Nutrition Information Per Serving (based on 2,000 calorie daily intake): calories 72, protein 1g, total fat 1g, carbohydrate 17g, dietary fiber 3g, total sugars 11g, calcium 4%, iron 3%, sodium 0%, potassium 5%, zinc 1%, vitamin A 1%, vitamin E 3%, thiamin 2%, riboflavin 2%, niacin 1%, vitamin B6 3%, folate 3%, vitamin B12 0%, vitamin C 49%

Peach Ice Cream

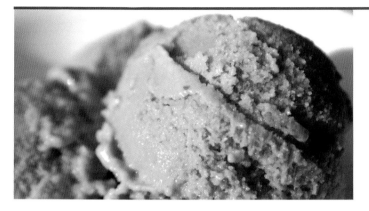

8 medium peaches	$4.00
1 cup raw cashews, whole	$2.00
1/2 tsp green stevia powder	<$0.05
1/4-1/2 cup raw agave	<$2.00
1/2 tsp vanilla	<$0.15
Total estimated cost	$8.20
Estimated cost per serving	$0.68

Tips to reduce the cost:

- Buy your peaches from local farms, farm stands, or a farmers market. This way, you can get the freshest peaches at the best price.

This is one of the best ice cream recipes I have ever made. This ice cream is so smooth and its flavor is incredible. I still can't believe this recipe turned out so well. And it makes a lot of ice cream!

Preparation

Equipment needed: High-speed blender • Ice cream maker

1 Soak the cashews for 6+ or overnight, in advance.

2 Blend all ingredients in a strong blender until very smooth. Sweeten to taste with agave.

3 Freeze the ice cream mixture for 1 hour or let cool in the refrigerator overnight.

4 To make the ice cream, follow the manufacturer's instructions on your ice cream maker. Be sure to use the ice cream function if your ice cream maker has multiple functions. If your ice cream maker only holds 1 quart, you will need to make this recipe in 2 batches.

5 Pour the ice cream into a container with an air-tight lid. Store the container in the freezer to allow the ice cream to harden.

Allow the ice cream to soften for 20 minutes before serving.

Nutrition Information Per Serving (based on 2,000 calorie daily intake): calories 110, protein 3g, total fat 6g, carbohydrate 14g, dietary fiber 2g, total sugars 9g, calcium 4%, iron 6%, sodium 0%, potassium 8%, zinc 5%, vitamin A 7%, vitamin E 6%, thiamin 3%, riboflavin 3%, niacin 5%, vitamin B6 3%, folate 3%, vitamin B12 0%, vitamin C 11%

Sweet Plum Sorbet

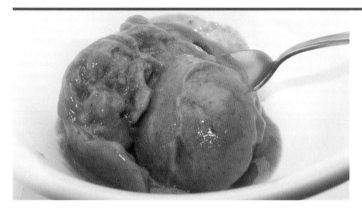

4 cups/1 quart of yellow sweet plums	$1.50
6 dates	$1.20
1/2 cup water or almond milk	$1.00
1/2 cup raisins	$0.50
1/2 tsp vanilla	<$0.10
1 tsp arrowroot powder	<$0.10
1/2 tsp tarragon leaves (optional)	<$0.25
Total estimated cost	**$4.65**
Estimated cost per serving	**$0.78**

Tips to reduce the cost:
- Buy sweet plums from a local farm or farmers market.
- Try to buy all of the dry ingredients from bulk bins. This way you can buy the amounts you need.

This is one of my favorite sorbets. The sorbet is sweet, slightly tart, creamy, and the fresh tarragon leaves add an amazing touch. However, if you don't have access to tarragon (I grow it in my yard), you can just leave it out of the recipe.

Preparation
Equipment needed: High-speed blender • Ice cream maker

1 Remove the seeds from the plums.

2 Blend the plums, dates, almond milk, raisins, vanilla, and arrowroot until very smooth.

3 Freeze the sorbet mixture for 1 hour or let cool in the refrigerator overnight.

4 To make the sorbet, follow the manufacturer's instructions on your ice cream maker. Be sure to use the frozen yogurt function if your ice cream maker has multiple functions.

5 Pour the sorbet into a container with an air-tight lid. Store the container in the freezer to allow the sorbet to harden.

Allow the sorbet to soften for 20 minutes before serving.

Nutrition Information Per Serving (based on 2,000 calorie daily intake): calories 156, protein 2g, total fat 0g, carbohydrate 41g, dietary fiber 4g, total sugars 34g, calcium 3%, iron 4%, sodium 0%, potassium 12%, zinc 2%, vitamin A 8%, vitamin E 2%, thiamin 4%, riboflavin 3%, niacin 5%, vitamin B6 6%, folate 2%, vitamin B12 0%, vitamin C 18%

Creamy Plum Sorbet

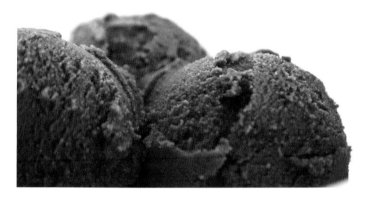

1/2 cup raw cashews, whole	$1.00
1 1/2 lbs red or purple plums	$3.75
1/2 tsp vanilla	<$0.10
1/4 cup raisins	$0.25
1/4 tsp green stevia powder	<$0.05
2 tsp raw agave	<$0.20
Total estimated cost	**$5.35**
Estimated cost per serving	**$0.90**

Tips to reduce the cost:

- Buy the plums from a local farm, farmers market, or CSA program.
- Because you need very few cashews and raisins for this recipe, buy them from bulk bins.
- If you don't have green stevia powder, use more agave instead. But, green stevia powder will save you more money in the long-run.

This sorbet is flavorful, creamy, sweet, slightly tart, and super simple to make. If you love plums, you will love this sorbet. And interestingly, if you love raspberries, you will love it too! For some reason, it tastes a little like raspberries!

Preparation

Equipment needed: High-speed blender • Ice cream maker

1 Soak the cashews in water for 6+ or overnight, in advance.

2 After the cashews have soaked, blend all the ingredients in a strong blender for 10-15 seconds until very smooth. You don't want to see any plum skins floating around.

3 Place the mixture in a container and freeze for 1 hour or let cool in the refrigerator overnight.

4 To make the sorbet, follow the manufacturer's instructions on your ice cream maker. Be sure to use the ice cream function, which makes a fluffier sorbet, if your ice cream maker has multiple functions.

5 Pour the sorbet into a container with an air-tight lid. Store the container in the freezer to allow the sorbet to harden.

Allow the sorbet to soften for 20 minutes before serving.

Nutrition Information Per Serving (based on 2,000 calorie daily intake): calories 134, protein 3g, total fat 6g, carbohydrate 21g, dietary fiber 2g, total sugars 14g, calcium 3%, iron 6%, sodium 0%, potassium 8%, zinc 5%, vitamin A 7%, vitamin E 3%, thiamin 4%, riboflavin 3%, niacin 3%, vitamin B6 4%, folate 3%, vitamin B12 0%, vitamin C 16%

Mint Gelato

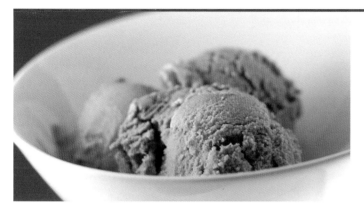

1 cup raw cashews, whole	$2.00
1 cup meat from 2 young coconuts	$4.00
1 1/2 cups water	$0.00
1/4 fresh mint leaves (or to taste)	$1.00
3/4 tsp green stevia powder	<$0.05
2 tbsp raw agave	<$0.50
2 dates	$0.40
1 1/2 tsp vanilla	<$0.40
1 tsp arrowroot powder	<$0.10
Total estimated cost	$8.45
Estimated cost per serving	$1.69

Tips to reduce the cost:

- Purchase inexpensive mint from a farmers market, local farm, friend, or grow it yourself.
- Buy young coconuts from an Asian market. They are cheaper and the same quality you find at larger health food and grocery stores.

This gelato is thick and minty! It's perfection!

This recipe tastes best with homegrown mint, but any mint will do. Add additional mint for a more minty flavor; however, too much mint may make the gelato slightly grainy.

Add cacao nibs to make a mint chocolate gelato or simply enjoy the gelato with a cookie.

Preparation
Equipment needed: High-speed blender • Ice cream maker

1 Soak the cashews in water for 6+ or overnight, in advance.

2 Crack open the young coconuts with a large knife and pour the water into a large glass. Scoop out the coconut meat with spoon. Remove any brown flakes from the meat and chop. Set aside.

3 Blend all the ingredients in a strong blender for 10-15 seconds until very smooth.

4 Pour the mixture into a container and freeze for 1 hour or cool in the refrigerator overnight.

5 To make the gelato, follow the manufacturer's instructions on your ice cream maker. Be sure to use the ice cream function if your ice cream maker has multiple functions.

6 Pour the gelato into a container with an air-tight lid. Store the container in the freezer to allow the gelato to harden.

It's important to allow the gelato to soften for 20 minutes before serving. Otherwise it will be too hard.

Nutrition Information Per Serving (based on 2,000 calorie daily intake): calories 279, protein 6g, total fat 19g, carbohydrate 24g, dietary fiber 3g, total sugars 11g, calcium 6%, iron 15%, sodium 1%, potassium 10%, zinc 14%, vitamin A 2%, vitamin E 2%, thiamin 6%, riboflavin 5%, niacin 4%, vitamin B6 6%, folate 8%, vitamin B12 0%, vitamin C 2%

Tamarind Banana Ice Cream

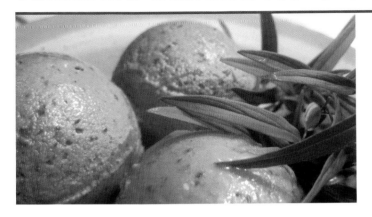

This is a wonderful creamy ice cream! The tamarind paste gives the ice cream a slight tart flavor and the banana and dates work together to even out the sweetness.

If you have never had tamarind, it can be found at most Asian and international markets. It has an amazing tangy, fruity flavor and is usually sold as a paste or in pods. Be sure to remove the seeds before using.

Preparation
Equipment needed: High-speed blender • Ice cream maker • Wire sieve

2-inch cube tamarind paste	$1.00
1 1/2 cups water or nut milk	$0.00
1 cup raw cashews, whole	$2.00
1 medium banana	$0.20
1 tsp vanilla	<$0.25
3 dates	$0.60
2 tbsp raw agave	<$0.50
1/4 tsp green stevia powder	<$0.05
Total estimated cost	$4.60
Estimated cost per serving	$1.15

Tips to reduce the cost:
- Inexpensive tamarind paste can be found at an Asian or international market.

1 Soak tamarind paste for 4+ hours in 1 cup of water, in advance. Soak the cashews in water for 6+ hours.

2 Once the paste has soaked, removed the seeds, and add it to the blender. Add the remaining ingredients and blend for 10-15 seconds until very smooth.

3 Strain the blended mixture through a wire sieve to remove the tamarind pulp.

4 Place the mixture in a container and freeze for 1 hour or let cool in the refrigerator overnight.

5 To make the ice cream, follow the manufacturer's instructions on your ice cream maker. Be sure to use the ice cream function if your ice cream maker has multiple functions.

6 Pour the ice cream into a container with an air-tight lid. Store the container in the freezer to allow the ice cream to harden.

Allow the ice cream to soften for 20 minutes before serving.

Nutrition Information Per Serving (based on 2,000 calorie daily intake): calories 300, protein 6g, total fat 16g, carbohydrate 38g, dietary fiber 4g, total sugars 22g, calcium 6%, iron 15%, sodium 0%, potassium 14%, zinc 14%, vitamin A 1%, vitamin E 2%, thiamin 8%, riboflavin 7%, niacin 6%, vitamin B6 13%, folate 8%, vitamin B12 0%, vitamin C 5%

Pecan Praline Ice Cream

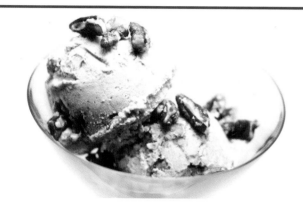

This recipe celebrates the rich, creamy flavor of pecans and is the perfect after dinner treat!

The key to making this an awesome ice cream experience, is to allow it to soften (can take 20-30 minutes) before serving! And feel free to add some lucuma to the ice cream for a nice caramel flavor.

Preparation

Equipment needed: High-speed blender • Ice cream maker • Dehydrator (optional)

1 Soak the cashews and pecans (separately) in water for 6+ hours or overnight.

2 Crack open the young coconut with a large knife and pour the water into a large glass. Scoop out the coconut meat with spoon. Remove any brown flakes from the meat and chop. Set aside.

ICE CREAM

3 Blend all the ingredients in a strong blender until very smooth.

4 Freeze the ice cream mixture for 1 hour or cool in the refrigerator overnight.

5 To make the ice cream, follow the manufacturer's instructions on your ice cream maker. Be sure to use the ice cream function if your ice cream maker has multiple functions.

ICE CREAM

1 cup raw cashews, whole	$2.00
1/3 cup raw pecans, whole	<$0.70
1 cup meat from 2 young coconuts	$4.00
1 1/2 cups water	$0.00
1/4 cup raisins	$0.25
1/3 tsp green stevia powder	<$0.05
5-6 dates	<$1.20
2 tsp vanilla	<$0.50
1 pinch sea salt	<$0.05

GLAZED PECAN TOPPING

1/3 cup raw pecans, whole	<$0.70
1 pinch cinnamon, ground	<$0.05
1 pinch nutmeg, ground	<$0.05
1/2 tbsp lucuma	<$0.25
2 tbsp raw agave	$0.50
1/4 tsp vanilla	<$0.10
Total estimated cost	$10.40
Estimated cost per serving	$1.30

Tips to reduce the cost:

- Buy your young coconuts from an Asian market. They are cheaper and the same quality you will find at larger health food and grocery stores.

GLAZED PECAN TOPPING

6 Break the pecans (unsoaked) into small pieces by placing them into a bag and crushing them. Place the broken pecans into a small bowl and add the remaining ingredients. Mix well.

7 For more of a crunch, try dehydrating the glazed pecans for 12 hours at 105-degrees before pouring them into the ice cream maker.

8 Pour the pecans into the ice cream maker right before the ice cream is done. Run the ice cream maker for an additional 5 minutes.

Allow the ice cream to soften for 10-20 minutes before serving.

Nutrition Information Per Serving (based on 2,000 calorie daily intake): calories 248, protein 4g, total fat 16g, carbohydrate 26g, dietary fiber 3g, total sugars 16g, calcium 4%, iron 9%, sodium 0%, potassium 9%, zinc 10%, vitamin A 1%, vitamin E 2%, thiamin 8%, riboflavin 4%, niacin 4%, vitamin B6 6%, folate 5%, vitamin B12 0%, vitamin C 1%

Ice Cream Candy Squares

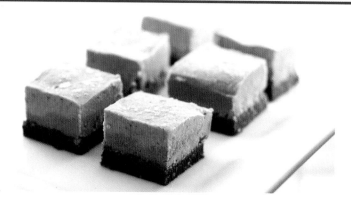

These squares look beautiful and fancy, yet they are simple to make. Plus, they are the perfect decadent, creamy treat. The gooey, chocolate crust complements the tamarind and mint layers.

If you are running short on ingredients, feel free to cut out a layer. Or try using a handful of tangy berries (e.g., raspberries) instead of the tamarind.

If you have never had tamarind, it can be found at most Asian and international markets. It has an amazing tangy, fruity flavor and is usually sold as a paste or in pods. Be sure to remove the seeds before using.

Preparation

Equipment needed: High-speed blender • Large dinner plate or platter

1 Soak the cashews in water for 6+ or overnight, in advance.

2 Crack open the young coconuts with a large knife and pour the water into a large glass. Scoop out the coconut meat with spoon. Remove any brown flakes from the meat and chop. Set aside.

CRUST

3 Process the shredded coconut in the food processor until the oils begin to come out of the coconut (about 30 seconds). Add the sunflower seeds, walnuts, cacao, vanilla, green stevia, and salt, and process until the nuts are well broken down. Then add the raisins and process until they are completely broken down into small pieces. Lastly, add the agave and process until the dough starts to clump.

4 Press the dough onto a dinner plate or platter, forming a square crust. Place the crust in the freezer while you prepare the remaining ingredients.

CRUST

1/2 cup raw shredded coconut	$0.25
1/3 cup raw sunflower seeds	$0.40
1/2 cup raw walnuts, whole	$1.00
1/3 cup raw cacao powder	$0.75
2 tsp vanilla	<$0.50
1/4 tsp green stevia powder	<$0.05
1 pinch sea salt	<$0.05
1/2 cup raisins	$0.50
raw agave to taste	<$0.25

TOPPING

Ingredient	Cost
2/3 cup raw cashews, whole	<$0.70
1 cup meat from 2 young coconuts	$4.00
1/8-1/4 cup tamarind meat	$1.00
1/8-1/4 cup fresh mint	$1.00
1/2 tsp vanilla	<$0.15
2 tbsp raw agave	$0.50
1/2 tsp green stevia powder	<$0.05
1/8 tsp sea salt	<$0.05
4 tbsp raisins	$0.25
3/4 cup water or coconut water	$0.00
Total estimated cost	**$11.45**
Estimated cost per serving	**$1.91**

Tips to reduce the cost:

- Purchase tamarind pods or paste and young coconuts from your local Asian or international markets. If possible, buy the tamarind pods (5-6 pods) instead of the paste. This way you can get the amount you need.
- Grow your own mint or get some from a friend! Mint is a very prolific plant and it's easy to grow!

TOPPING

5 To prepare the tamarind topping, blend 1/2 of the soaked cashews, 1/2 cup coconut meat, 1/4 tsp vanilla, 1 tbsp agave, 1/4 tsp green stevia powder, 1 pinch salt, 2 tbsp raisins, 6 tbsp of water, and the tamarind in a strong blender until creamy. Add additional tamarind if you want a more tangier flavor. Pour the tamarind topping into a small bowl and freeze for 1 hour.

6 To prepare the mint topping, take the remaining ingredients and 1/4 cup of the mint, and blend in a strong blender. Add additional mint if you want a mintier flavor. Pour the mint topping into a small bowl and freeze for 1 hour.

7 Remove the crust from the freezer and spread the tamarind topping on first and the mint topping on second.

8 Freeze the pie for 2+ hours or until the layers have completely hardened.

9 Cut the pie into 1-inch squares with sharp knife. Cover the squares with plastic wrap and keep them in the freezer until you are ready to eat them.

Before serving, allow the ice cream squares to partially thaw for 5-10 minutes. These squares can stay frozen in your freezer for up to 1 month.

Nutrition Information Per Square (based on 2,000 calorie daily intake): calories 85, protein 2g, total fat 6g, carbohydrate 7g, dietary fiber 1g, total sugars 4g, calcium 2%, iron 4%, sodium 0%, potassium 3%, zinc 3%, vitamin A 0%, vitamin E 5%, thiamin 5%, riboflavin 2%, niacin 1%, vitamin B6 3%, folate 2%, vitamin B12 0%, vitamin C 1%

Quick Mint Ice Cream

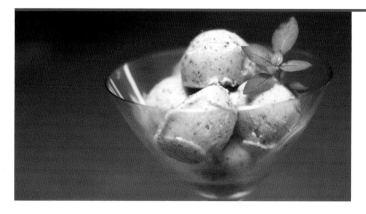

2 medium bananas	$0.40
leaves from 5-6 sprigs of mint	<$0.25
1 tbsp maple syrup	<$0.25
1/8 tsp of vanilla (optional)	<$0.05
Total estimated cost	$0.95
Estimated cost per serving	$0.48

Tips to reduce the cost:

- Grow your own mint or get some from a friend! Mint is a very prolific plant and it's easy to grow!

This is a delicious ice cream! I am not a big banana fan, but somehow this ice cream works!

This recipe does use maple syrup, which is not raw. You can substitute it with agave, dates, or honey.

Preparation
Equipment needed: Food processor or high-speed blender

1 Peel and freeze the bananas overnight.

2 Chop the bananas.

3 Place all the ingredients in your food processor or high speed blender, and blend until creamy.

Enjoy immediately or store in an air-tight container in the freezer.

Nutrition Information Per Serving (based on 2,000 calorie daily intake): calories 133, protein 1g, total fat 0g, carbohydrate 34g, dietary fiber 3g, total sugars 20g, calcium 2%, iron 3%, sodium 0%, potassium 13%, zinc 4%, vitamin A 3%, vitamin E 1%, thiamin 3%, riboflavin 5%, niacin 4%, vitamin B6 22%, folate 6%, vitamin B12 0%, vitamin C 18%

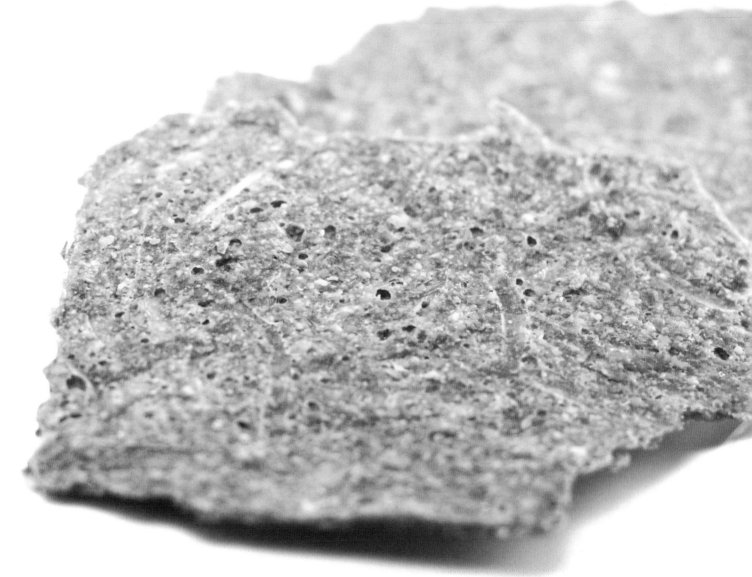

South of the Border Flatbread
Page 263

Breads and Crackers

Italian Flax Crackers

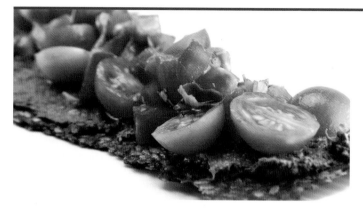

These are one of my favorite summer crackers! I make them in the summer, when basil and tomatoes taste their best! These crackers are super easy and incredibly flavorful.

Preparation
Equipment needed: Food processor or blender • Dehydrator • 2-3 teflex sheets (or parchment paper)

1 Soak the flaxseeds in 3 cups of water for at least 6 hours. A mixture of brown and golden flaxseeds works well. After the flaxseeds have soaked, pour them into a large bowl.

2 To make the flavoring for the flax crackers, place the remaining ingredients into the blender or food processor, except for the olive oil and 1/2 cup of the basil. Blend the ingredients until completely liquefied.

3 Pour the blended mixture onto the soaked flaxseeds and mix until well incorporated. Chop the remaining basil and stir into the mixture. Next, pour the olive oil onto the mixture and mix well. Taste the mixture and add additional salt if desired. You will want the mixture to taste slightly saltier than you would prefer.

4 Pour a portion of the flaxseed mixture onto one Teflex sheet (or parchment paper) and spread it to 1/8-inch thickness. Repeat the process until all of the mixture has been used.

5 Dehydrate the flax crackers at 105-degrees for 48 hours. When the top of the crackers are dry (about 12 hours), turn over and remove the Teflex sheets.

When the crackers are dry, break them into 4x4-inch pieces. Store them in an air-tight container or bag.

2 cups flaxseeds, whole	$2.00
3 medium red tomatoes	$1.50
1 cup fresh basil	$1.00
1 tsp fresh oregano	<$0.10
1/2 tsp fresh thyme	<$0.10
1/4 medium white onion	<$0.20
2 cloves garlic	$0.20
3 tbsp nutritional yeast	$0.75
1 tbsp balsamic vinegar	$0.15
1/3 cup extra virgin olive oil	<$1.80
1/2 tsp sea salt	<$0.05
Total estimated cost	$7.85
Estimated cost per cracker	$ 0.33

Tips to reduce the cost:
- Make this recipe in the summer when the ingredients are least expensive. Grow the herbs yourself or get them from a friend who has an herb garden.

Nutrition Information Per Cracker (based on 2,000 calorie daily intake): calories 109, protein 3g, total fat 9g, carbohydrate 5g, dietary fiber 4g, total sugars 1g, calcium 4%, iron 6%, sodium 2%, potassium 5%, zinc 4%, vitamin A 4%, vitamin E 4%, thiamin 56%, riboflavin 37%, niacin 20%, vitamin B6 34%, folate 4%, vitamin B12 8%, vitamin C 4%

South of the Border Flatbread

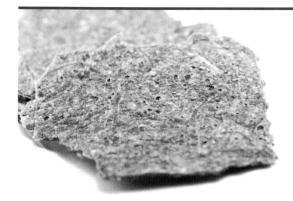

3 medium white onions	$2.25
3/4 cup raw sunflower seeds	$0.90
3/4 cup flaxseeds, whole	$0.75
3 medium red tomatoes	$1.50
1 cup sweet peppers	$2.25
1 3/4 tsp sea salt	<$0.05
1/4 tsp cumin, ground	<$0.05
1/4 tsp chipotle powder	<$0.05
1 tsp chili powder	<$0.05
2 whole green onions	<$0.20
1/2 bunch fresh cilantro	$0.50
1/2 cup extra virgin olive oil	$2.20
Total estimated cost	$10.75
Estimated cost per slice	$0.40

Tips to reduce the cost:
- Make this recipe in the summer when the ingredients are their least expensive.
- Buy the spices from the spice or bulk bin section at your local health food store.

This is such a splendid recipe. These crackers are a beautiful balance of fresh ingredients and flavorful spices. Enjoy these crackers with Mango Salsa, Pear Salsa, or Pineapple Salsa.

Preparation
Equipment needed: Mandoline • Food processor • High-speed blender/coffee grinder • Dehydrator • 2-3 teflex sheets

1 Using a mandoline, slice the onions translucent thin. Place the onions into a large bowl and set aside.

2 Separately grind the sunflower seeds and flax seeds into a powder using a coffee grinder or high-speed blender. Do not over grind the flaxseeds as the fats in the seeds will oxidize. Add the seed flours to the onions and mix until the onions are evenly coated.

3 In a blender or food processor, blend the tomatoes, sweet peppers, salt, cumin, chipotle, and chili. Blend until smooth and add to the onions. Mix well and allow the mixture to sit for 5 minutes.

4 Slice the green onions and chop the cilantro. Add to the onion mixture. Finally, add the water and olive oil, and mix well. Allow the mixture to sit for 5-10 minutes.

5 Pour one third of the mixture onto one Teflex sheet (or parchment paper) and spread it to 1/8-inch thickness. Repeat the process until all of the mixture has been used.

6 Dehydrate the flax crackers at 105-degrees for 36 hours. When the top of the crackers are dry (about 12 hours), turn over and remove the Teflex sheets.

When the flatbread is dry, break it into 4x4-inch pieces. Store them in an air-tight container or bag.

Nutrition Information Per Slice (based on 2,000 calorie daily intake): calories 96, protein 2g, total fat 8g, carbohydrate 5g, dietary fiber 2g, total sugars 2g, calcium 2%, iron 4%, sodium 6%, potassium 4%, zinc 3%, vitamin A 7%, vitamin E 15%, thiamin 12%, riboflavin 2%, niacin 2%, vitamin B6 5%, folate 6%, vitamin B12 0%, vitamin C 18%

Cozy Winter Crackers

3 medium white onions	$2.25
1/4 cup raw sunflower seeds	$0.30
1/4 cup raw pumpkin seeds	$0.30
3/4 flaxseeds, whole	$0.75
1 cup kabocha squash	$1.50
5 medium red tomatoes	$2.50
4 leaves kale	$0.75
3/4 cup sun-dried tomatoes	$1.50
1 clove garlic	$0.10
1-inch piece of ginger	$0.20
1/3 cup extra virgin olive oil	$1.50
2/3 tsp sea salt	<$0.05
Total estimated cost	$11.70
Estimated cost per cracker	$0.65

Tips to reduce the cost:
- Buy the smallest kabocha squash you can find. These squash are typically sold at Asian markets and health food stores.

These crackers celebrate the vibrant flavor of winter squash. They are perfect next to any soup, salad, or as a quick snack.

This recipe uses a kabocha squash; however, you can use other winter squash varieties like acorn or butternut squash.

Preparation
Equipment needed: Mandoline • High-speed blender or food processor • Dehydrator • 2-3 teflex sheets (or parchment paper)

1 Using a mandoline, slice the onions translucent thin. Place the onions into a large bowl and set aside.

2 Separately grind the sunflower, pumpkin, and flax seeds into a powder using a coffee grinder or high-speed blender. Do not over grind the flaxseeds as the fats in the seeds will oxidize. Add the seed flours to the onions and mix until the onions are evenly coated.

3 Cut off a large chunk of the kabocha squash, and peel and chop it into 1-inch pieces. Set aside.

4 Using a high-speed blender or food processor, blend the tomatoes until liquefied. Add 1 cup of kabocha and blend until smooth. Next, add the remaining ingredients and blend until smooth. Pour the mixture onto the onions and mix well. Allow the mixture to sit for 5 minutes.

5 Pour half of the mixture onto one Teflex sheet (or parchment paper) and spread it to 1/8-inch thickness. Repeat the process until all of the mixture has been used.

6 Dehydrate the flax crackers at 105-degrees for 36 hours. When the top of the crackers are dry (about 12 hours), turn over and remove the Teflex sheets.

Nutrition Information Per Cracker (based on 2,000 calorie daily intake): calories 120, protein 3g, total fat 9g, carbohydrate 8g, dietary fiber 3g, total sugars 3g, calcium 5%, iron 8%, sodium 6%, potassium 9%, zinc 5%, vitamin A 13%, vitamin E 10%, thiamin 14%, riboflavin 3%, niacin 5%, vitamin B6 7%, folate 6%, vitamin B12 0%, vitamin C 29%

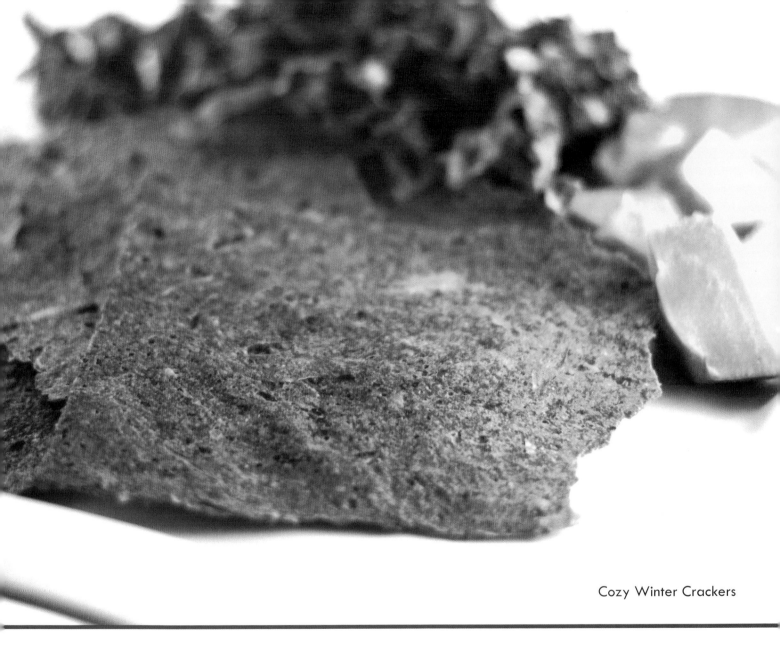
Cozy Winter Crackers

Seaweed Crackers

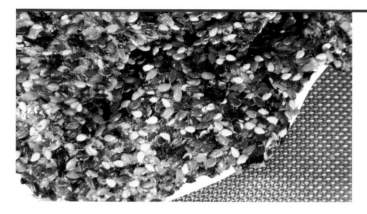

2 cups flaxseeds, whole	$2.00
3/4 cup sesame seeds, unhulled	$1.00
2 tbsp brown or white rice vinegar	<$0.50
1 tbsp raw nama shoyu	<$0.10
1 handful dried laver nori seaweed	$1.00
1 tbsp dried dulse seaweed	<$0.15
5 cloves garlic	<$0.50
1/3 cup raw sesame seed oil	<$0.85
sea salt to taste	<$0.05
Total estimated cost	$6.15
Estimated cost per cracker	$ 0.26

Tips to reduce the cost:

- Buy seaweed in bulk online. My 2 favorite seaweed websites are www.pangaia.cc and www.seaveg.com.
- If you cannot find sesame seed oil, use olive oil instead.

If you love seaweed, you will love these crackers. They are nutritious and a great snack.

Preparation

Equipment needed: Dehydrator • 2-3 teflex sheets (or parchment paper)

1 Soak the flaxseeds in 3 cups of water and sesame seeds in 2 cups of water for 6+ hours or overnight.

2 After the seeds have soaked, pour the flaxseeds and sesame seeds into one large bowl.

3 Pour the vinegars and nama shoyu onto the soaked seeds and mix. Break up the laver and dulse seaweeds into very small pieces (1/4-inch) using a knife or pair of scissors, and add to the soaked seeds. Mince the garlic and add, and mix very well. Lastly, add the sesame seed oil and mix.

4 Taste the mixture and salt to taste. You want the mixture to taste slightly saltier than you would normally prefer. Allow the mixture to sit for 5 minutes.

5 Pour a portion of the flaxseed mixture onto one Teflex sheet (or parchment paper) and spread it to 1/4-inch thickness. Repeat the process until all of the mixture has been used.

6 Dehydrate the flax crackers at 105-degrees for 48 hours. When the top of the crackers are dry (about 12 hours), turn over and remove the Teflex sheets.

When the crackers are dry, break them into 4x4-inch pieces. Store them in an air-tight container or bag.

Nutrition Information Per Cracker (based on 2,000 calorie daily intake): calories 127, protein 7g, total fat 11g, carbohydrate 6g, dietary fiber 5g, total sugars 0g, calcium 4%, iron 7%, sodium 5%, potassium 4%, zinc 7%, vitamin A 4%, vitamin E 1%, thiamin 19%, riboflavin 3%, niacin 4%, vitamin B6 5%, folate 5%, vitamin B12 0%, vitamin C 3%

Sweet Summer Salsa Crackers

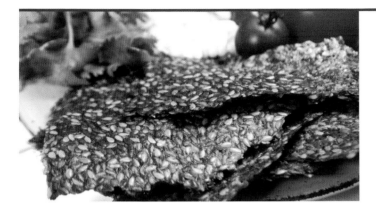

2 cups flaxseeds, whole	$2.00
1 ear corn	$0.50
2 medium red tomatoes	$1.00
1/2 medium red bell pepper	$1.50
1 whole jalapeno	$0.25
1/2 medium white onion	<$0.40
1 clove garlic	$0.10
1/4 cup extra virgin olive oil	$1.00
1/2 bunch fresh cilantro	$0.50
1/2 tsp sea salt	<$0.05
Total estimated cost	$7.30
Estimated cost per cracker	$ 0.30

Tips to reduce the cost:

- Buy most of the ingredients from local farms or grow them yourself!
- Make this recipe in the summer when the ingredients are their least expensive.
- Buy flaxseeds and sea salt from the spice or bulk bin section at your local health food store.

These crackers are one of my summer favorites. They taste wonderful with a simple salsa or by themselves.

Preparation

Equipment needed: High-speed blender or food processor • Dehydrator • 2-3 teflex sheets (or parchment paper)

1 Soak the flaxseeds in 3 cups of water for at least 6 hours. A mixture of brown and golden flaxseeds works well. After the flaxseeds have soaked, pour them into a large bowl.

2 Now you will make the flavoring for the flaxseeds. Remove the corn from the ear using a knife.

3 In a food processor or blender, blend the corn, tomatoes, red bell pepper, jalapeno, white onion, garlic, and olive oil until completely liquefied.

4 Pour the blended mixture onto the flaxseeds and mix until well incorporated. Chop the cilantro and stir into the mixture. Taste the mixture and salt to taste. You want the mixture to taste slightly saltier than you would prefer.

5 Pour a portion of the mixture onto one Teflex sheet (or parchment paper) and spread it to 1/4-inch thickness. Repeat the process until all of the mixture has been used.

6 Dehydrate the flax crackers at 105-degrees for 48 hours. When the top of the crackers are dry (about 12 hours), turn over and remove the Teflex sheets.

When the crackers are dry, break them into 4x4-inch pieces. Store them in an air-tight container or bag.

Nutrition Information Per Cracker (based on 2,000 calorie daily intake): calories 91, protein 3g, total fat 7g, carbohydrate 5g, dietary fiber 4g, total sugars 1g, calcium 3%, iron 4%, sodium 2%, potassium 4%, zinc 4%, vitamin A 4%, vitamin E 3%, thiamin 15%, riboflavin 2%, niacin 3%, vitamin B6 4%, folate 4%, vitamin B12 0%, vitamin C 8%

Fiesta Flax Crackers

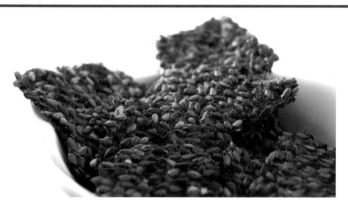

2 cups flaxseeds, whole	$2.00
2-3 cups of leftover juice pulp	$0.00
2 cloves garlic	$0.20
1 tbsp apple cider vinegar	$0.10
3-4 tbsp extra virgin olive oil	<$1.00
sea salt to taste	<$0.05
Total estimated cost	**$3.35**
Estimated cost per serving	**$0.14**

Tips to reduce the cost:
- I can't think of anything to reduce the costs of the recipe! This is the cheapest recipe in the whole book!

Do you have leftover pulp from juicing? Use it in this recipe! Try using a combination of vegetable and fruit pulp.

Enjoy these crackers with the BEST Pate Ever (on page 192) or by themselves.

Preparation
Equipment needed: Dehydrator • 2-3 teflex sheets (or parchment paper)

1 Soak the flaxseeds in 3 cups of water for at least 6 hours. A mixture of brown and golden flaxseeds works well. After the flaxseeds have soaked, pour them into a large bowl.

2 Sprinkle the leftover juice pulp onto the flaxseeds being careful to remove any hard peels and fibrous clumps. Stir very, very well.

3 Mince the garlic, and add the garlic and vinegar to the flaxseed mixture. Add the oil and mix well.

4 Lastly, taste the mixture and salt to taste. You want the mixture to taste slightly saltier than you would prefer. Allow the mixture to sit for 5 minutes.

5 Pour a portion of the mixture onto one Teflex sheet (or parchment paper) and spread it to 1/4-inch thickness. Repeat the process until all of the mixture has been used.

6 Dehydrate the flax crackers at 105-degrees for 36 hours. When the top of the crackers are dry (about 12 hours), turn over and remove the Teflex sheets.

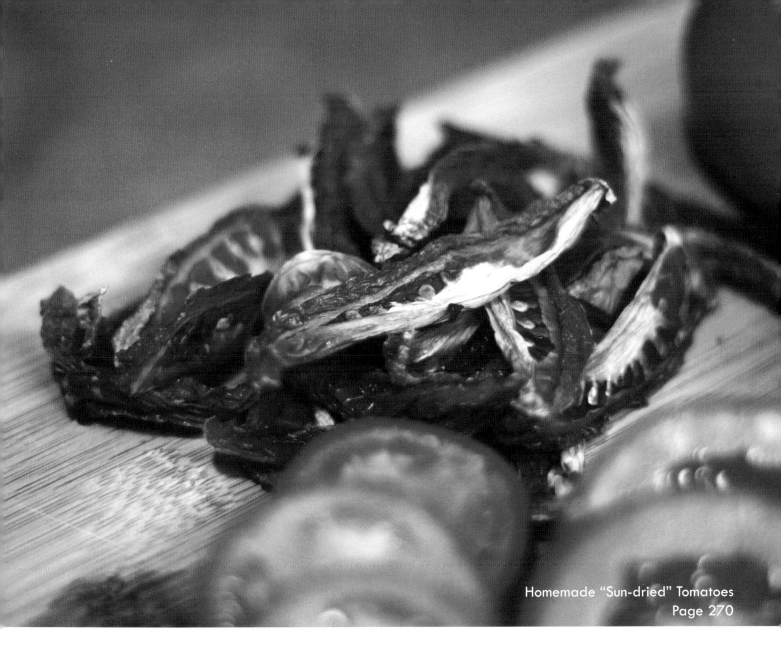

Homemade "Sun-dried" Tomatoes
Page 270

Dried and Frozen Foods

Homemade "Sun-dried" Tomatoes

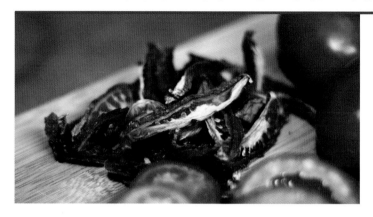

17 lbs Tomatoes (1/2 bushel)	$3.75
Total estimated cost	$3.75

Tips to reduce the cost:
- Buy tomatoes from local farms by the box or bushel (~48lbs) or grow them yourself!

Okay, so these are not really sun-dried tomatoes, but they taste so much better! They taste like candy and are super easy to make.

All you need are a lot of tomatoes and a dehydrator. Because you need so many tomatoes, try growing them yourself or buying them straight from a local farm by the box or bushel (48lbs). In the past, I have purchased bushels of tomatoes for $15 from a local farm via their CSA program. For more information on CSA programs, see page 63.

The taste of the dried tomatoes will depend on the type of tomatoes you use. Typical slicing or canning tomatoes taste like candy when you dry them, whereas roma tomatoes have a deeper tomato flavor. As a result, dried slicing tomatoes go well on salads, but dried roma tomatoes are great in sauces or recipes where you want a strong tomato flavor.

Preparation
Equipment needed: Dehydrator

1 Slice the tomatoes into 1/2 inch slices (see pictures on page 67). It helps to slice the tomatoes in half and then slice each half into 1/2 inch slices.

2 Line the sliced tomatoes on a dehydrator tray. Dehydrate the tomatoes at 145-degrees for 1 hour and then reduce the temperature to 105-degrees.

3 The tomatoes will take 2-2.5 days to dry completely. Store the tomatoes in mason jars or resealable plastic bags.

Depending on the type of dehydrator you have, you might find it useful to keep one tray empty. I have noticed that when I line all the trays in my 5-tray Excalibur dehydrator with tomatoes, the air circulation suffers and a few tomatoes begin to spoil as they dry. Usually this happens to the tomatoes on the bottom tray.

Freezing Fruits

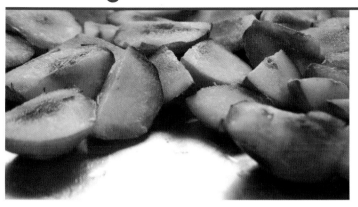

Freezing your own fruit during the summer is a great way to enjoy fruit all year round without breaking your budget. Just buy extra fruit like strawberries when they are in season and less expensive, and then freeze them. That's all.

Frozen fruit is great for making smoothies, ice creams, sorbets, and pies. You can use it in many of the recipes in this book like Peach Ice Cream (page 251) and Strawberry Ambrosia Green Smoothie (page 157).

Preparation
Equipment needed: Freezer-ready, resealable plastic bags • Baking sheet (optional)

BERRIES

1 When freezing berries (e.g. raspberries, blueberries), first wash the berries and allow them to dry completely. If the berries are left wet, they will stick together when frozen. One option is to not wash the berries at all.

2 Place the berries into resealable, plastic bags and freeze.

FRUITS CONTAINING SEEDS

3 When freezing stone fruit (e.g. peaches, nectarines) and fruits containing seeds (e.g. pears), first, wash the fruit and allow it to dry completely.

4 Slice the fruit into big chunks, removing the seeds or stones.

5 Place the cut fruit onto a baking sheet and freeze it for 3-4 hours (or until the fruit hardens on the outside).

6 Pour the fruit into plastic bags and freeze.

Tips to reduce the cost:

- To get high-quality fruit at the lowest price, buy fruit in bulk from local farms or through a CSA program.
- Buy fruit when it's in season. It's always cheaper.

Drying Herbs

Preparing your own dried herbs is inexpensive and easy. Plus, it's a great way to take advantage of the extra or leftover herbs you collect in the summer.

There are two ways to dry herbs: air dry or in a dehydrator. Herbs that air dry well tend to have low water content like oregano and thyme. Whereas, herbs that dry better in the dehydrator include basil and mint (i.e. herbs that contain more water). However, it's still possible to air dry these herbs as well.

Preparation
Equipment needed: Dehydrator (optional)

AIR DRYING

1 To air dry herbs that have low water content (e.g. oregano and thyme), take 6-8 stems and tie them together with a string or rubber band. Then tie a paper bag around the stem of the herbs so that the tops of the herbs are hanging upside down inside the bag. Write the date and name of the herbs on the bag and then hang in a dry location. The herbs will take 2-3 weeks to dry.

2 To dry high-moisture herbs like parsley and basil, line a baking sheet with paper towels. Lay the herbs on the tray and space them out so that they are not touching. You want to make sure that the herbs are exposed to as much air as possible. Cover the herbs with paper towels. The herbs will take 2-3 weeks to dry. An alternative is to allow the herbs to dry outside.

DEHYDRATING

3 Place your herbs on the dehydrator tray(s). Dehydrate at 105-degrees until dry.

Store all dry herbs in air-tight containers or plastic bags.

Freezing Greens and Herbs

Tips to reduce the cost:

- When you have leftover herbs, freeze them!
- Get low-cost herbs from local farms and CSA programs! Also, ask your gardener friends for extra herbs!
- Before leaving town, freeze your greens!

Freezing herbs and greens are a great way to preserve them! I freeze fresh herbs like basil in the summer and then use it to make amazing crackers in the winter. I also freeze greens before I leave town for vacation so that they won't spoil.

Use your frozen herbs and greens to make crackers, soups, green smoothies, and pates. Because greens and herbs lose their structure when they are frozen, it's best to use them in blended recipes.

Preparation
Equipment needed: Freezer-ready, resealable plastic bags

1 Wash and dry your herbs and greens.

2 Stuff them into freezer ready, resealable plastic bags.

3 Write the date and name of the green/herb on each bag. Store the greens in the freezer and that's it!

Dried Fruit Trail Mix

4 medium apples	$2.00
1 medium pear	$0.50
3 medium kiwi	$1.00
1 cup pineapple	$0.75
1 medium peach	$0.50
1 cup strawberries, whole	$1.00
1/2 cup raisins	$0.50
Total estimated cost	$6.25
Estimated cost per serving	$1.04

Tips to reduce the cost:
- Prepare this recipe when you have ripe fruit that needs to be used immediately.
- Buy local and in-season fruits.

I have been making my own dried fruit trail mix for years. It's the perfect treat for camping and backpacking trips, children's school lunches, and at work. Plus, you can use any type of fruit you want!

For dehydrating in your oven, read the tip on page 166.

Preparation
Equipment needed: Dehydrator

1 Peel and core the apples and pear, and cut them into 1/4-inch slices. Peel and slice the kiwi and pineapple into 1/4-inch slices. Lastly, slice the peaches and strawberries into 1/4-inch slices.

2 Dehydrate the fruit slices for 24 hours at 110-degrees.

3 After the fruit slices have dehydrated, place them into an air-tight container or bag, and add the raisins.

When stored in an airtight container or bag, the dried fruit will keep for 1 month.

Nutrition Information Per Serving (based on 2,000 calorie daily intake): calories 159, protein 2g, total fat 1g, carbohydrate 41g, dietary fiber 6g, total sugars 29g, calcium 4%, iron 4%, sodium 0%, potassium 14%, zinc 2%, vitamin A 4%, vitamin E 8%, thiamin 5%, riboflavin 5%, niacin 4%, vitamin B6 7%, folate 7%, vitamin B12 0%, vitamin C 123%

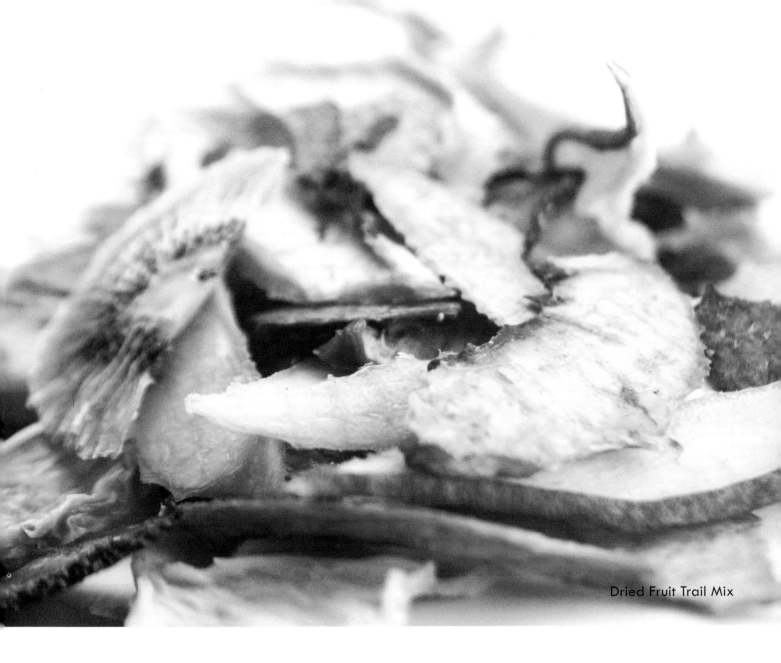

Dried Fruit Trail Mix

Easy Fruit Roll-Up

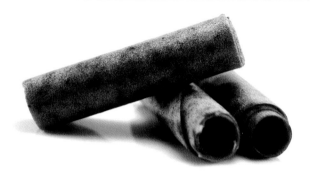

Fruit roll-ups are easy to make and fun to eat!

This recipe uses apples, bananas, and cranberries, but feel free to omit the cranberries and/or substitute them for other kid-friendly fruits like pineapples, raisins, strawberries, and so on.

Preparation
Equipment needed: Food processor or high-speed blender • Dehydrator

1 Peel, core, and cut the apples into 1-inch chunks.

2 Using a food processor, process all of the ingredients until completely smooth.

3 Pour the entire mixture onto one 14x14-inch Teflex sheet and spread to 1/4-inch thickness. Dehydrate the fruit mixture for 12-15 hours at 110 degrees Fahrenheit.

4 Cut the fruit roll-up into three large strips and roll up.

Store the fruit roll-up in an airtight container or bag. It will stay fresh for up to 1 month.

3 medium apples	<$1.15
1 medium banana	$0.20
1/2 cup cranberries	$0.75
1 date	$0.20
2 tbsp lemon juice	$0.35
1/4 tsp green stevia powder	<$0.05
1 tbsp raw agave	$0.25
Total estimated cost	$2.95
Estimated cost per serving	$0.99

Nutrition Information Per Serving (based on 2,000 calorie daily intake): calories 143, protein 1g, total fat 0g, carbohydrate 39g, dietary fiber 6g, total sugars 26g, calcium 4%, iron 3%, sodium 0%, potassium 11%, zinc 1%, vitamin A 3%, vitamin E 4%, thiamin 3%, riboflavin 4%, niacin 3%, vitamin B6 12%, folate 4%, vitamin B12 0%, vitamin C 28%

Tips to reduce the cost:

• Substitute the fruit in this recipe for whatever fruit is in season or that you already have in your kitchen.

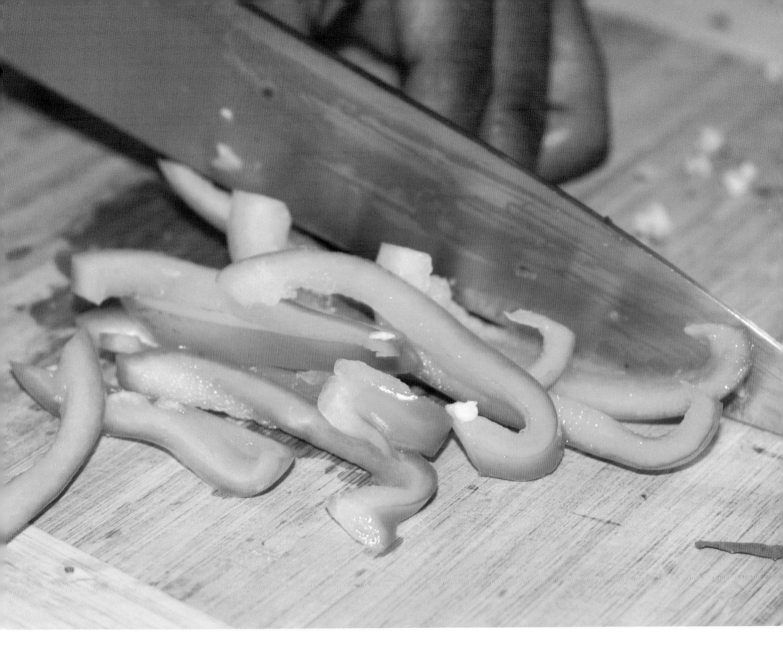

How this book came into being...

I'm not sure what made me start writing a new book immediately after I finished my last one. I was making the final edits to *Confessions of an East Coast Raw Vegan* and the idea for *Raw Foods on a Budget* popped up in my head. I immediately thought, "What a great topic for a book!" However, at the time, I didn't feel like I was in the perfect position to write such a book. I had just started to feel comfortable with my own budget and who was I to guide others in living a budget-conscious raw food lifestyle? So, I let the thought drift away, but the Universe had something else in mind.

One month later, I had a seven page outline detailing *Raw Foods on a Budget* and two committed editors by my side. I chose editors who knew me, could make a unique contribution to the writing style of the book, and would push me as a writer. I recruited Rufiena Jones, a close friend and true lover of language and words. I also recruited my close friend, GaBrilla Ballard of Urban Mama Song Productions. GaBrilla is a musician, poet, and mama advocate, and I knew that her ability to tell beautiful, powerful stories would add color to the tone of the book. Hence, my journey began with these two wise women at my side, and the Universe that connected us to everyone and everything.

As I expected, my editors pushed me. I thought my outline was already extensive, but they wanted more. These women were from my target audience and they told me what they needed. So, I listened...well, maybe I was a little stubborn at first, but the next thing I knew, I was writing a book for them and for people like them who needed real answers.

Then something miraculous happened. I found an online article about Beta Readers - i.e., readers that authors recruit to give them final feedback on their book before it's published. It was a great idea, but I thought it was strange that someone would wait so long to ask for feedback from their readers. So, I took the concept and made it my own. I recruited three Beta Readers from Facebook™ to give me continuous feedback as I wrote every chapter and recipe. The Universe sent me three amazing women: Nancy Cullinan, Tamar Wallace, and Cecelia Williams. They instantly became a part of the *Raw Foods on a Budget* team!

My beta readers pushed me just as hard as my editors. They were my readers and they told me what they wanted to see. So I gave them fruit and vegetable seasonal charts for each region of the United States, cost estimates for each recipe, and more activities and worksheets. Before I knew it, *Raw Foods on a Budget* had become a book that was being created for the readers by the readers. How cool!

From that moment on, I realized that my role was more than just writing the book--it was to help the book reach its full potential. So, I began releasing chapters of the book on my website to get more feedback from my target audience. And to my surprise, I received more comments like "you hit it right on the mark" and less of "The book needs..." or "The book is missing...". This was huge for me because I am a graduate student living in Central Pennsylvania with no children or a spouse, so it amazed me that people from all over the world were benefiting from my message. They liked it, and as the months went on I had the honor of watching it improve people's lives.

Then half way into writing the book, I decided to stop writing. I stopped because I felt like something was missing. I was receiving feedback from my readers, but it wasn't as frequent as I would have liked. I was committed to fulfilling a need, and I needed to know what people wanted. So, I opened myself up to the Universe for a solution and it sent me one: the Beta project, a free online program dedicated to teaching people how to live a budget-loving lifestyle. With *Raw Foods on a Budget* as the textbook for the program, I used the Beta Project as a platform to receive hands-on feedback about the book.

When I launched the Beta Project, the response was overwhelming. Everybody loves free stuff! But, I soon learned that not everybody is willing to do the work. The few people who participated in the program became my Angels. I welcomed them into my life for 2-3 months and they changed the way I thought about the book. Through our weekly conference calls I learned that *Raw Foods on a Budget* is more than just a list of strategies, it's a program that teaches people to how use their budget in ways that enhance their experience in the world.

After running the Beta Project twice, I was ready to start writing again. I had refocused my message and knew that what I had to say was helping people to live a more abundant life. And as I looked back, I saw how every aspect of this book had been co-created with the Universe. *Raw Foods on a Budget* was no accident; it was intentional and part of a bigger picture of excellence.

So, I wrote. I wrote when I wasn't working on my dissertation, when I took short breaks from school, and sometimes in my sleep! My readers kept me going. The positive changes they were making in their lives inspired me to keep on writing. They also inspired me to create a generous business model - one that meets people where they are by offering free video content, payment plans on books and programs, scholarships, and even multiple editions of *Raw Foods on a Budget* at varied prices.

Then, a few months before the release of the book, my *Raw Foods on a Budget* team was made complete. One of my closest friends, Alicia Ross-Beck, asked me if she could contribute her expertise to the book by serving as an editor and joining my book illustration team. I was a little hesitant because Alicia was already running a school-based clinic in Harlem, so I knew her time was limited. But through her sincere and generous commitment, persistence, and hard work, she showed me that she could take the book to the next level.

In the last week of completing the final edits for *Raw Foods on a Budget*, I learned an important lesson. It happened during a very scary moment when someone was attempting to break into my apartment at 3am. I just happened to up that night working on the book in my living room. In the moment of watching the knob of my front door turn, I got incredibly scared and braced myself. Once I realized that they couldn't get in because the door was locked (thank goodness!), my mind got very quiet. I wasn't freaked out, I just listened. I was consciously listening for the intruder, however, deep down I was really listening to Myself. My higher Self was telling me that it was not okay to work this way. It was not okay to work 15-hour days to finish this book and sacrifice so much of myself. At the time I wanted it done! I didn't want to write any more. I was tired. But in that quiet moment I realized that I did not want to finish the book this way. This book has been such a gift to me and I wanted to finish it in a way that would honor the book, my journey, and the lessons learned. So, I postponed the release of the book one week. And in that week, I found real balance.

It has been an honor to serve as a vehicle for this book. This book has taught me so much about Life, Truth, Abundance, and Generosity. And it taught me that these beautiful concepts could be interwoven into a household budget and my business. It has been a privileged to write this book.

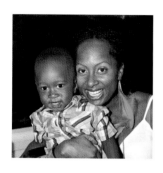

Rufiena Jones, Editor

I absolutely love food - good food. It excites me, energizes me and even inspires me. Tasting good food is such a blessing that enables us to explore and celebrate a sweet dimension of life on this beautiful planet. We are lucky.

At least once a week, I either visit an unfamiliar restaurant or try out a new recipe. These food escapades have proved fulfilling to my heart and imagination, but emptying to my wallet. So, thank God for this book! Since I began working on *Raw Foods on a Budget* with Brandi and this wonderful team of editors, my relationship with food has begun to… mature. Now I plan my meals better and eat most of what I buy which is helping me to save money, and finally those weekly culinary explorations are essentially guilt-free. As I integrate more and more raw food recipes and treats into my world, I'm exposing my loved ones and myself to a healthier way of being. I hope that you, too, will benefit in many ways from the strategies and overall point of view presented in this book. You may even influence and inspire those around you!

Rufiena enjoys exploring the world's cultures through their arts, languages and cuisines. She is an avid supporter of multicultural awareness and appreciation, and knows this can lead to a better human society.

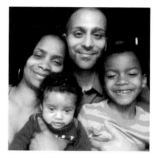

GaBrilla Ballard, Editor

I felt like I would imagine a midwife would feel when assisting a mother in bringing a child into the world. There have been times where I did not think I could continue as editor because of all the things going on in my life, but I knew this book was something special and I had to continue.

The process of editing *Raw Foods on a Budget* has allowed me to both learn and grow in my own process of being more mindful about how I "circulate" my money. It has stretched how I view the concept of abundance in a budget. I no longer see a budget as a means of depriving myself.

My contribution has been to support Brandi in keeping the spirit of celebration and abundance threaded throughout the book (something I am working on in my own work).

This book is such a massive contribution to the transformation of our consciousness around how we invest our money. I am deeply thankful to have been a part of its birth.

GaBrilla Ballard is a mama, writer, musician, creator of urban-mamasong.com, and is fiercely dedicated to her family, doing work she loves and supporting mamas to live amazing lives.

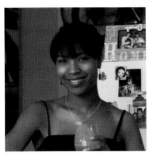

Alicia Ross-Beck, MSN, PNP, Editor

In my practice as a pediatric clinician I spend a great deal of time discussing the importance of healthy eating habits, and the most frequent response I'm given is that eating healthy is too expensive. So, when I joined Brandi's team to help edit *Raw Foods on a Budget* I was overjoyed by the opportunity to contribute to a book that not only has great recipes but also allows the reader to explore and improve their financial relationship with food.

At the beginning of this project I had no idea how much *Raw Foods on a Budget* would impact my consciousness regarding my own eating habits. I was born and raised a vegetarian, so maintaining a plant-based diet is innately natural for me. However, I now find myself at the grocery store rethinking my purchases and avoiding being an "Impulsive Ida." My entire approach to eating has improved from they way I store foods to the tools I use to prepare food. This book began as an informative collection of stories and tips and evolved into a self-improvement resource that will be life enhancing for any reader. I am so grateful to have been a part of this creative process. It has been a wonderful journey.

Alicia Ross-Beck is a Pediatric Nurse Practitioner whose work is passionately focused on chronic disease prevention and maintaining the overall health and well being of children.

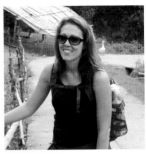

Tamar Wallace, Beta Reader

It was so great to be a part of this book as it developed. It was inspiring to see how many people were affected by Brandi's budgeting advice and wonderful recipes.

I've always thought of myself as someone who is careful with money, so I wasn't expecting to learn anything new from *Raw Foods on a Budget*, but the book really changed my perspective on how I buy food. I find I spend and waste a lot less now that I am more planful and feel less pressure to keep my fridge crammed full. I was not eating raw when I started working with Brandi so I was mainly interested in the recipes and how to buy seeds, nuts, and other raw ingredients I was less familiar with. As the book developed into a full program, I realized that Brandi was offering more than just tips on how to save money. She is helping people take control of their spending and change the way they think about prosperity. It was so great to be a part of this book as it grew, and inspiring to see how many people were affected by Brandi's budgeting advice and wonderful recipes.

Tamar Wallace is a photographer, writer, creator of crafty things, cook, dog owner, and blog writer of www.biggirllittlegirl.wordpress.com.

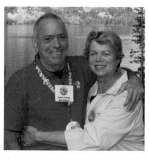

Nancy C. Cullinan, Beta Reader

I was a follower of Brandi on Facebook™ and looked forward to her tips about a raw food lifestyle. One day she had a request on Facebook™ for "beta readers" for her new book. On August 8, 2010, I emailed Brandi and applied to become a beta reader. I was new to raw foods and eager to learn more (so eager, in fact, that my e-mail was the first reply Brandi received!). Plus I thought that being a "beta reader" would be a fun thing to do.

After trying and abandoning webcam meetings, we three "beta readers" would meet with Brandi by phone to discuss the chapters and recipes which Brandi had emailed to us. As a result of reading the chapters and trying a lot of the recipes, my husband and I found ourselves adding and enjoying more raw foods.

It has been a fun year and exciting to be a small part of this developing project and to see how a book emerges from an idea. I have also enjoyed getting to know the other readers, Cecelia and Tamar. Thanks, Brandi!

Nancy Cullinan is a wife, mother, grandmother and retired CPA who is enjoying full-time meandering around North America with her husband in a 40 foot RV.

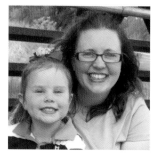

Cecelia Williams, Beta Reader

Working with Brandi on writing *Raw Foods on a Budget* was enlightening and I found that many of the methods that Brandi discussed are helpful in so many other areas of my life. I think assessing your cabinets and refrigerators before shopping is key to not spending a lot of money. One of the key things that makes such a difference is to eat before you shop so that you are not tempted to buy foods that are not within your budget *and* that would cause you to get off track with eating raw.

Cecelia Williams is an avid reader, friend, mama of three precious dogs, and student of life who enjoys engaging with others as we make this journey together.

Visit us at

www.rawfoodsonabudget.com

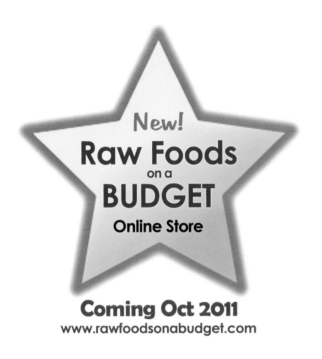

New!
Raw Foods
on a
BUDGET
Online Store

Coming Oct 2011
www.rawfoodsonabudget.com

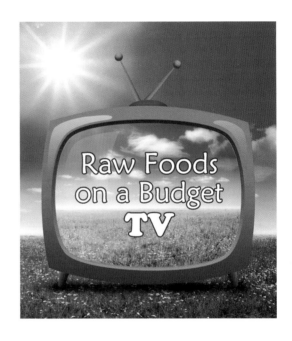

Raw Foods
on a Budget
TV

Raw Foods on a Budget
Newsletter

www.rawfoodsonabudget.com

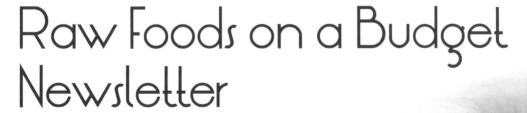

References

CHAPTER 3: IT'S NOT ABOUT THE PRICE

Blair, D., & Sobal, J. (2006). Lexus consumption: Wasting food resources through overeating. *Agriculture and Human Values, 23,* 63-74.

Sonesson, U., Anteson, F., Davis, J., & Sjoden, P. (2005). Home transport and wastage: Environmentally relevant household activities in the life cycle of food. *AMBIO, 34,* 371-375.

Parfitt, J., Barthel, M., & MacNaughton. (2010). Food waste within food supply chains: Quantification and potential for change to 2050. *Phil. Trans. R. Soc., 365,* 3065-3081.

Baker, D., Fear, J., & Denniss, R. (2009). What a waste: An analysis of household expenditure on food. (Policy Brief No. 9, ISSN 1836-9014). https://www.tai.org.au/index.php?q=node%2F19&act=display&pubid=696.

CHAPTER 7: IMPROVE HOW YOU BUY FOOD

Mela, D., Aaron, J., & Gatenby, S. (1996). Relationships of consumer characteristics and food deprivation to food purchasing behavior. *Physiology & Behavior, 60,* 1331-1335.

Nisbett, R., & Kanouse, D. (1969). Obesity, food deprivation, and supermarket shopping behavior. *Journal of Personality and Social Psychology, 12,* 289-294.

Read, D., & van Leeuwen, B. (1998). Predicting hunger: The effects of appetite and delay on choice. *Organizational Behavior and Human Decision Processes, 76,* 189-205.

Underhill, P. (2008). *Why we buy: The science of shopping--updated and revised for the Internet, the global consumer, and beyond.* New York, NY: Simon and Schuster.

CHAPTER 8: IMPROVE WHERE YOU BUY FOOD

United States Department of Agriculture-Agricultural Marketing Services Division. (2010). *Number of Operating Farmers Market.* Retrieved from http://www.ams.usda.gov/AMSv1.0/ams.fetchTemplateData.do?template=TemplateS&navID=WholesaleandFarmersMarkets&leftNav=WholesaleandFarmersMarkets&page=WFMFarmersMarketGrowth&description=Farmers%20Market%20Growth&acct=frmrdirmkt.

CHAPTER 10: IMPROVE HOW YOU STORE FOOD

U.S. Department of Health and Human Services, Center for the Evaluation of Risks to Human Reproduction. (2008). NTP-CERHR Monograph on the Potential Human Reproductive and Developmental Effects of Bisphenol A (Publication No. 08-5994). Retrieved at http://www.ncbi.nlm.nih.gov/pubmed/19407859.

U.S. Department of Health and Human Services. Bisphenol A (BPA) Information for Parents. Retrieved at http://www.hhs.gov/safety/bpa/index.html.

CHAPTER 11: IMPROVE HOW YOU PREPARE FOOD

University of Nebraska-Lincoln Extension. NebGuide: Stevia. Retrieved at http://elkhorn.unl.edu/epublic/live/g1634/build/g1634.pdf.

Index

Symbols

10-Cent Sunshine Cookies 246

A

Agave 145
Almond and Cashew Nut Butters 138
Almond Milk 167
Almonds 137
Aphroditie's Nectarine Cream Pie 240
Apple and Banana Granola 173
Apple Cider Vinegar 146
Apple-Collard Green Smoothie 160
Apple Sauce 198
Arrowroot Powder 148
Asian and International markets 71, 76
Ayurvedic medicine 117

B

Balsamic Vinegar 147
Beet Greens Smoothie 162
Berkeley Bowl 71
Better than Apple Sauce 198
Bisphenol A (BPA) 101
Blenders 150
Bok Choy Salad 215
Breads
    South of the Border Flatbread 271
Buckwheat Groats 138
Budget Books and Resources 37
Budgeting System, Creating a 36
Budgeting within a family 35
Butternut Cream Pie 236

Buy 3-4 days worth of food 49, 53
Buying Clubs 71
Buying food online 74
Buying from bulk bins 72
Buying in bulk 69–70, 76
Buy what's in season 49–50
Buy what you need 46–47, 52

C

Cakes
    Carrot Cake 238
Carrot Cake 238
Carrots Rejoice! 164
Cashew Nut Butters 138
Cashews 138
Casserole Bowl with Lid 150
Casseroles
    Green Beans in Italian Marinara 204
    Italian Spaghetti Squash Bowl 202
Celery Rejuvenation 164
Chili powder 143
Chinese Five Spice 143
Chinese Stir-Fry 218
Chipotle 143
Chocolate Cookies w/ Cashew
    Chunks 245
Chowmein Noodles 211
Cinnamon 144
Clark's Nutrition and Natural Food
    Market 71
Clove 144
Coconut Butter 136
Coconut Meat, Young or Thai 137
Coconut Oil 136
Coconut, Shredded 136
Coconut Water 137

Coffee Grinders 151
Compost 88–90
Conscious eating 114–115
    Books 122
    Unconscious eating 115
    Websites 122
Container gardening 89
Convenience produce 73
Cookies
    10-Cent Sunshine Cookies 246
    Chocolate Cookies w/ Cashew
        Chunks 245
    Cranberry Tea Squares 250
    Donut Holes 249
        Fig Freezer Cookies 244
    Ice Cream Candy Squares 266
    Pecan Delight Cookies 247
Coolers
    Lemon-Lime Cooler 163
    White Peach - Raspberry Cooler 163
Cooperative grocery stores 76
Coriander 143
Corn Salad 178
Cozy Winter Crackers 272
Crackers
    Cozy Winter Crackers 272
    Fiesta Flax Crackers 276
    Italian Flax Crackers 270
    Seaweed Crackers 274
    Sweet Summer Salsa Crackers 275
Cranberry Tea Squares 250
Creamy Apple Pie Breakfast Bars 172
Creamy Carrot-Beet Soup 186
Creamy Miso Soup 188
Creamy Plum Sorbet 259
Credit Cards 37

CSA programs 49, 50, 65, 66, 70, 75
Cumin 143
Curriculum 10–11
Cutting Board 151

D

Dates 109, 145
Dehydrator 151
Digestive cycle 117–118
Discount department stores 74, 76
Donut Holes 249
Dried Fruit Trail Mix 284
Drying herbs 280
Dulse 141

E

Eat all you have 46
Eating at home 121
Eating energy-dense foods 121
Eating goals 121
Eating when hungry 116, 123
Envelope Method 36
Envision your success 26
Equipment Start-Up Costs 149

F

Farmers markets 67–68, 75
Fiesta Flax Crackers 276
Fiesta Fruit & Nut Bars 171
Fig Freezer Cookies 244
Flaxseeds 139
Flu-Be-Gone Remedy Cocktail 166
Food diary 117, 123
Food Expense Log 33, 38
Food Monitoring System 103, 104
Food prices 16–17

Food Processor 152
Food spending goal 35
Food Start-Up Costs 135
Food wastage 16
Foraging 51, 53
Freecycle Network 92
Freezing Fruits 279
Freezing Greens and Herbs 281
Freezing produce 103
Fresh-Rite 71
Frother 152
Frozen Drinks
    Lemon-Lime Cooler 163
    White Peach - Raspberry Cooler 163
Fruit and Nut Bars
    Creamy Apple Pie Breakfast Bars 172
    Fiesta Fruit & Nut Bars 171
Fruit Cups
    Sun-Kissed Fruit Cup 252
Fruit flies 100
Fruit picking 67
Fruit Roll-Up 282
Fullness 117, 126

G

Gardening 80–98
    Acceptance 87
    Being practical 85
    Cash crops 85–86
    Finding the perfect fit 85
    Growing in containers 89
    Life cycles in your garden 87
    Location, locating the perfect 84
    Materials and Equipment
        Borrowing tools 92
        Composting 88–90

Create a test garden 92
Finding land 90
Online sources 92–93
Saving seeds 91
Seed Exchange 91
Planning 83–85, 95–97
Simple plants to grow 83
Starting small 82
Garlicky Pesto 194, 200
Garlicky Pesto with Cucumber Noodles 200
Gelatos
    Mint Gelato 262
Giving 34
Glorious Green Smoothie 160
Good Ole' Collards and Sweet
    Peppers 216
Granolas
    Apple and Banana Granola 173
    Quick Succulent Granola 174
Green Beans in Italian Marinara 204
Green Smoothies
    Apple-Collard Green Smoothie 160
    Beet Greens Smoothie 162
    Glorious Green Smoothie 160
    Strawberry Ambrosia Green
        Smoothie 161
    Strawberry and Banana Green
        Smoothie 161
Green stevia powder 107, 146
Grocery Stores, shopping at 70–74

H

Half-empty fridge 22
Health Food Stores, shopping at 70–74
Herb Italian Salad 183

Homemade Spiced Apple Cider 165
Homemade "Sun-dried" Tomatoes 278
Honey 145

I

Ice Cream
  Ice Cream Candy Squares 266
  Peach Ice Cream 260
  Pecan Praline Ice Cream 264
  Quick Mint Ice Cream 268
  Strawberry Ice Cream 254
  Tamarind Banana Ice Cream 263
Ice Cream Candy Squares 266
Ice Cream Maker 152
Infrequent bills 34
Italian Flax Crackers 270
Italian Spaghetti Squash Bowl 202
Italian Spices 143
'It Can Take It' Kale Salad 213

J

Japanese Mandoline 153
Juicer 153
Juices
  Carrots Rejoice! 164
  Celery Rejuvenation 164
  Flu-Be-Gone Remedy Cocktail 166
  Homemade Spiced Apple Cider 165
  Luscious Pink Cocktail 166
  Watermelon Juice 165
Julienne Peeler 153

K

Keep your recipes simple 111
Kelp 142

Knives 154
Know When to Eat 116

L

Launch-Pad Budget 41
Laver Nori 142
Lemon Cream Pie 230
Lemon Green Yum Kale Salad 214
Lemon-Lime Cooler 163
Local farms 64–70, 75
Low-Cost Websites, ordering from 74
Luscious Pink Cocktail 166

M

Macadamia Nuts 139
Mango Salsa 193
Master Gardener's Program 84, 86, 92
Meal planning 47, 52
  Worksheet 59
Mexican or Hot Spices 143
Mint 36
Mint Gelato 262
Mint Ice Cream 268
Mono meals 120

N

Nama Shoyu 147
Nature's Food Patch 71
Nature's Pantry 71
Nori Sheets 142
Nutmeg 144
Nut Milk Bag 154
Nut Milks
  Almond Milk 167
  Sunflower Seed Milk 167

Nutritional Yeast 148

O

Oatmeal 176
Olive Oil 141
Overeating 119

P

Pasta and Noodle Recipes
  Chowmein Noodles 211
  Garlicky Pesto with Cucumber
    Noodles 200
  Sweet Italian Herb Spaghetti 201
Pate
  The BEST Pate Ever! 196
Peaches in My Dreams 248
Peach Ice Cream 260
Pear Tomato Salsa 190
Pecan Delight Cookies 247
Pecans 139
Pesto
  Garlicky Pesto 194
  Simple Walnut Pesto 195
Pie Plate 154
Pies
  Aphroditie's Nectarine Cream Pie 240
  Butternut Cream Pie 236
  Lemon Cream Pie 230
  Plum Pie 228
  Pumpkin Pie 234
  Quick Apple Pie 232
  Strawberry Cream Cobbler 226
  Sweet Glory Nectarine Pie 223
Pineapple Avocado Salsa 191
Pizza

Spring Pizza 208
Winter Pizza 206
Plum Pie 228
Plum Sorbet 258, 259
Portion control 119–120
Portion sizes 118, 119–120, 128–129
Price comparison 76
Produce containers and bags 101
Produce delivery days 73
Pumpkin Pie 234
Pumpkin pie spice 144
Pumpkin Seeds 140

Q
Quick Apple Pie 232
Quicken Financial Software 36
Quick Mint Ice Cream 268

R
Rainbow Grocery 71
Raisins 108–110, 146
Raw Food Definitions 30
Rice Vinegars 147

S
Salad Dressings
    Strawberry - Rhubarb - Citrus
        Dressing 184
    Sweet Mustard Dressing 179
Salads
    Dark Leafy Green Salads
        B12 Kale Salad 219
        Bok Choy Salad 215
        Good Ole' Collards and Sweet
            Peppers 216
        'It Can Take It' Kale Salad 213

Lemon Green Yum Kale Salad 214
Light Salads
    Chinese Stir-Fry 218
    Corn Salad 178
    Herb Italian Salad 183
    Simple Savory Salad 180
    Summer Parsley Salad 182
    Sun-Baked Gazpacho 212
    Winter Salad & Sweet Mustard
        Dressing 179
Salad Spinner 154
Sales, shopping during 72
Salsas
    Mango Salsa 193
    Pear Tomato Salsa 190
    Pineapple Avocado Salsa 191
    Sweet Tomato Melody 192
Saving seeds 91
Savor your food 120, 130–131
Sea Salt 144
Seasonal Harvest Charts
    Make Your Own Local Seasonal
        Chart 58
    Midwestern Region of U.S. 55
    Northeastern Region of U.S. 54
    Southern Region of the U.S. 56
    Western Region of U.S. 57
Seaweed Crackers 274
Seaweeds 141
Seconds, buying 69, 73
Seed Exchange programs 91
Sesame Seed Oil 141
Setting spending goals 35
Shopping List, creating a
    Using a shopping list 48
    Worksheet 61

Shopping when you are hungry 48
Shredded Coconut 136
Simple meals 112
Simple recipes 111
Simple Savory Salad 180
Simple Walnut Pesto 195
Smoothies 160, 161, 162
    Apple-Collard Green Smoothie 160
    Beet Greens Smoothie 162
    Glorious Green Smoothie 160
    Strawberry Ambrosia Green
        Smoothie 161
    Strawberry and Banana Green
        Smoothie 161
Sorbet
    Creamy Plum Sorbet 259
    Strawberry-Cranberry Sorbet 256
    Sweet Plum Sorbet 258
Soups
    Creamy Carrot-Beet Soup 186
    Creamy Miso Soup 188
    Sun-Baked Gazpacho 212
Spices
    cayenne 180
    garlic 188
Spiralizer 155
Spring Pan 155
Spring Pizza 208
Sprout Tray 155
Stanley's 71
Start-Up Costs
    Food Start-Up Costs 135–148
    Equipment Start-Up Costs 149–156
Storing Raw Foods
    Fruits and Vegetables 100–101
    Nuts and seeds 102

Oils 102
   Protecting food from fruit flies 100
Strawberry Ambrosia 161
Strawberry and Banana 161
Strawberry-Cranberry Sorbet 256
Strawberry Cream Cobbler 226
Strawberry Ice Cream 254
Strawberry - Rhubarb - Citrus Dressing
   184
Substitutions
   Nuts 110–111
      Almonds 110, 111
      Arrowroot 110
      Cashews 110, 111
      Lecithin 110
      Macadamia nuts 110, 111
      Pecans 111
      Pumpkin seeds 111
      Shredded coconut 110
      Sunflower seeds 110, 111
      Walnuts 110, 111
      Young coconut 110
   Sweeteners 107–111
      Agave 109
      Dates 109
      Dried fruits 108–109
      Green stevia powder 107–108
      Honey 109
      Raisins 108–109
Summer Parsley Salad 182
Sun-Baked Gazpacho 212
Sun-Baked Recipes
   Aphroditie's Nectarine Cream Pie 240

Donut Holes 249
Peaches in My Dreams 248
Sun-Baked Gazpacho 212
Sun-Kissed Fruit Cup 252
Sweet Glory Nectarine Pie 223
Sunflower Seed Milk 167
Sunflower Seeds 140
Sun-Kissed Fruit Cup 252
Sweet Glory Nectarine Pie 223
Sweet Italian Herb Spaghetti 201
Sweet Plum Sorbet 258
Sweet Spices 144
Sweet Summer Salsa Crackers 275
Sweet Tomato Melody 192

T
Tamarind Banana Ice Cream 263
Tea Latte 168
Texflex Sheets 151
The BEST Pate Ever! 196
Timeline 11
Trail Mix
   Dried Fruit Trail Mix 284
Triggers for impulsive buying 37

U
Ume Plum Vinegar 148
Un-cooking philosophy 158

V
Vanilla 144
Variety in your diet 50

W
Walnuts 140
Warm Drinks 168
   Homemade Spiced Apple Cider 165
   Tea Latte 168
Watermelon Juice 165
White Peach - Raspberry Cooler 163
Winter Pizza 206
Winter Salad & Sweet Mustard Dressing
   179
Wire Sieve 155
Worksheets
   Create Your Own Gardening Plan!
      95–97
   Create Your Shopping List! 61
   Do Your Own Price Comparison! 77
   Envision Your Success 26–27
   It's Time to Savor Your Food 130–131
   Keep a Food Diary 123–125
   Launch-Pad Budget 41–43
   Plan Your Menu For the Next 3-4 Days!
      59–60
   Serve Yourself Less to Get More From
      Life 128–129
   Weekly Food Expense Log! 38–40
   What Does a Budget Mean to
      You? 24–25

Y
Young Coconuts 137